I0066548

Nutrition and Metabolism

Nutrition and Metabolism

Edited by
Kaden Hunt

Larsen & Keller
www.larsen-keller.com

Nutrition and Metabolism
Edited by Kaden Hunt
ISBN: 978-1-63549-202-6 (Hardback)

© 2017 Larsen & Keller

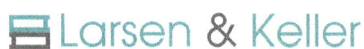

⊟ Larsen & Keller

Published by Larsen and Keller Education,
5 Penn Plaza,
19th Floor,
New York, NY 10001, USA

Cataloging-in-Publication Data

Nutrition and metabolism / edited by Kaden Hunt.
     p. cm.
Includes bibliographical references and index.
ISBN 978-1-63549-202-6
1. Nutrition. 2. Metabolism. 3. Health. I. Hunt, Kaden.
QP141 .N88 2017
613.2--dc23

This book contains information obtained from authentic and highly regarded sources. All chapters are published with permission under the Creative Commons Attribution Share Alike License or equivalent. A wide variety of references are listed. Permissions and sources are indicated; for detailed attributions, please refer to the permissions page. Reasonable efforts have been made to publish reliable data and information, but the authors, editors and publisher cannot assume any responsibility for the vaildity of all materials or the consequences of their use.

Trademark Notice: All trademarks used herein are the property of their respective owners. The use of any trademark in this text does not vest in the author or publisher any trademark ownership rights in such trademarks, nor does the use of such trademarks imply any affiliation with or endorsement of this book by such owners.

The publisher's policy is to use permanent paper from mills that operate a sustainable forestry policy. Furthermore, the publisher ensures that the text paper and cover boards used have met acceptable environmental accreditation standards.

Printed and bound in the United States of America.

For more information regarding Larsen and Keller Education and its products, please visit the publisher's website www.larsen-keller.com

Table of Contents

Preface   **VII**

Chapter 1 **Understanding Nutrition**   **1**
    a. Nutrition   1
    b. Human Nutrition   26
    c. Sports Nutrition   50
    d. Nutrition and Pregnancy   53

Chapter 2 **Introduction to Metabolism**   **58**
    a. Metabolism   58
    b. Digestion   74
    c. Microbial Metabolism   85
    d. Basal Metabolic Rate   96

Chapter 3 **Human Health and Nutrition**   **106**
    a. Diet (Nutrition)   106
    b. Healthy Diet   108
    c. Dietary Supplement   115
    d. Essential Amino Acid   121
    e. Obesity   125
    f. Malnutrition   145
    g. Eating Disorder   166

Chapter 4 **Processes Vital for Nutrition and Metabolism**   **185**
    a. Metabolic Pathway   185
    b. Ketogenesis   189
    c. Fatty Acid Metabolism   191
    d. Beta Oxidation   204
    e. Amino Acid Synthesis   210
    f. Fermentation   218
    g. Oxidative Phosphorylation   225

Chapter 5 **Nutritional Deficiencies**   **239**
    a. Mineral Deficiency   239
    b. Vitamin Deficiency   239
    c. Protein   240
    d. Kashin–Beck Disease   244
    e. Kwashiorkor   247
    f. Marasmus   249

Permissions

Index

Preface

This book provides comprehensive insights into the field of nutrition and metabolism. It provides deep insights about this field. Nutrition refers to interactions between food and nutrients and the use of food in catabolism, assimilation, excretion, absorption, biosynthesis, etc. Metabolism refers to the chemical transformations that take place within a cell when converting food to energy. Some of the diverse topics covered in this text address the varied branches that fall under this category. Such selected concepts that redefine this subject have been presented in it. This book aims to shed light on some of the unexplored aspects of this field. It is meant for students who are looking for an elaborate reference text on nutrition and metabolism.

To facilitate a deeper understanding of the contents of this book a short introduction of every chapter is written below:

Chapter 1- This chapter is an overview of the subject matter incorporating all the major aspects of nutrition. It informs its readers about the various fields of nutrition such as human nutrition, sports nutrition and nutrition. The following content provides with a deep understanding on the subject.

Chapter 2- Metabolism has three purposes which are the conversion of food to energy to run cellular processes, the conversion of fuel to building blocks for proteins and some carbohydrates and the elimination of nitrogenous wastes. This chapter discusses the process of metabolism and provides with key analysis to the subject matter by explaining digestion, microbial metabolism and the basal metabolic rate briefly.

Chapter 3- This chapter explains in detail the issues caused by the lack of nutrition and it elucidates the importance of nutrition and the issues caused by the lack of it. A detailed analysis of malnutrition, eating disorder, and obesity is dealt with. The aspects elucidated in this chapter are of vital importance, and provide a better understanding of nutrition and health.

Chapter 4- The following chapter elucidates the various processes that are related to nutrition and metabolism. The major categories that this chapter explains are processes like metabolic pathway, ketogenesis, fatty acid metabolism, fermentation and oxidative phosphorylation. The aspects elucidated are of vital importance, and provide a better understanding on the topic.

Chapter 5- This chapter serves as a source to understand nutritional deficiencies. Nutritional deficiencies are the result of your body not getting enough of the nutrients it needs. The major categories of nutritional deficiencies are discussed in this chapter; those include mineral deficiency, vitamin deficiency, protein-energy malnutrition, kwashiorkor and marasmus. Malnutrition has serious implications like marasmus and kwashiorkor; this chapter helps in the understanding of these deficiencies and is of great importance to broaden the existing knowledge of nutritional deficiencies.

Finally, I would like to thank the entire team involved in the inception of this book for their valuable time and contribution. This book would not have been possible without their efforts. I would also like to thank my friends and family for their constant support.

Editor

Understanding Nutrition

This chapter is an overview of the subject matter incorporating all the major aspects of nutrition. It informs its readers about the various fields of nutrition such as human nutrition, sports nutrition and nutrition. The following content provides with a deep understanding on the subject.

Nutrition

Sample Label for
Macaroni and Cheese

Start Here →

Nutrition Facts
Serving Size 1 cup (228g)
Servings Per Container 2

Amount Per Serving

Calories 250	Calories from Fat 110

	% Daily Value*
Total Fat 12g	18%
Saturated Fat 3g	15%
Trans Fat 1.5g	
Cholesterol 30mg	10%
Sodium 470mg	20%
Total Carbohydrate 31g	10%
Dietary Fiber 0g	0%
Sugars 5g	
Protein 5g	

Vitamin A	4%
Vitamin C	2%
Calcium	20%
Iron	4%

Limit these Nutrients

Get Enough of these Nutrients

Quick Guide to % DV

5% or less is low
20% or more is high

* Percent Daily Values are based on a 2,000 calorie diet. Your Daily Values may be higher or lower depending on your calorie needs:

	Calories:	2,000	2,500
Total Fat	Less than	65g	80g
Sat Fat	Less than	20g	25g
Cholesterol	Less than	300mg	300mg
Sodium	Less than	2,400mg	2,400mg
Total Carbohydrate		300g	375g
Dietary Fiber		25g	30g

Footnote

The "Nutrition Facts" table displayed on packaged food labels in the United States and Canada indicates the amounts of nutrients recommended by the US Food and Drug Administration to limit or consume according to the Daily Value

Nutrition is the science that interprets the interaction of nutrients and other substances in food (e.g. phytonutrients, anthocyanins, tannins, etc.) in relation to maintenance, growth, reproduction, health and disease of an organism. It includes food intake, absorption, assimilation, biosynthesis, catabolism and excretion.

The diet of an organism is what it eats, which is largely determined by the availability, the processing and palatability of foods. A healthy diet includes preparation of food and storage methods that preserve nutrients from oxidation, heat or leaching, and that reduce risk of food-born illnesses.

Registered dietitian nutritionists (RDs or RDNs) are health professionals qualified to provide safe, evidence-based dietary advice which includes a review of what is eaten, a thorough review of nutritional health, and a personalized nutritional treatment plan. They also provide preventive and therapeutic programs at work places, schools and similar institutions. Certified Clinical Nutritionists or CCNs, are trained health professionals who also offer dietary advice on the role of nutrition in chronic disease, including possible prevention or remediation by addressing nutritional deficiencies before resorting to drugs. Government regulation especially in terms of licensing, is currently less universal for the CCN than that of RD or RDN. Another advanced Nutrition Professional is a Certified Nutrition Specialist or CNS. These Board Certified Nutritionists typically specialize in obesity and chronic disease. In order to become board certified, potential CNS candidate must pass an examination, much like Registered Dieticians. This exam covers specific domains within the health sphere including; Clinical Intervention and Human Health.

A poor diet may cause health problems, causing deficiency diseases such as blindness, anemia, scurvy, preterm birth, stillbirth and cretinism; health-threatening conditions like obesity and metabolic syndrome; and such common chronic systemic diseases as cardiovascular disease, diabetes, and osteoporosis. A poor diet can cause the wasting of kwashiorkor in acute cases, and the stunting of marasmus in chronic cases of malnutrition.

History

Antiquity

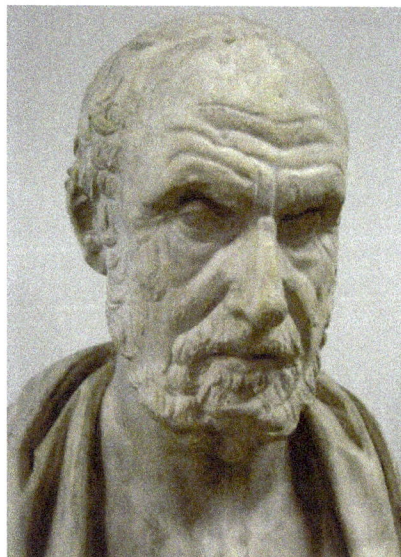

Hippocrates lived about 400 BC, and Galen and the understanding of nutrition followed him for centuries.

The first recorded dietary advice, carved into a Babylonian stone tablet in about 2500 BC, cautioned those with pain inside to avoid eating onions for three days. Scurvy, later found to be a vitamin C deficiency, was first described in 1500 BC in the Ebers Papyrus.

According to Walter Gratzer, the study of nutrition probably began during the 6th century BC. In China, the concept of *Qi* developed, a spirit or "wind" similar to what Western Europeans later called *pneuma*. Food was classified into "hot" (for example, meats, blood, ginger, and hot spices) and "cold" (green vegetables) in China, India, Malaya, and Persia. *Humours* developed perhaps first in China alongside *qi*. Ho the Physician concluded that diseases are caused by deficiencies of elements (Wu Xing: fire, water, earth, wood, and metal), and he classified diseases as well as prescribed diets. About the same time in Italy, Alcmaeon of Croton (a Greek) wrote of the importance of equilibrium between what goes in and what goes out, and warned that imbalance would result in disease marked by obesity or emaciation.

The first recorded nutritional experiment with human subjects is found in the Bible's Book of Daniel. Daniel and his friends were captured by the king of Babylon during an invasion of Israel. Selected as court servants, they were to share in the king's fine foods and wine. But they objected, preferring vegetables (pulses) and water in accordance with their Jewish dietary restrictions. The king's chief steward reluctantly agreed to a trial. Daniel and his friends received their diet for ten days and were then compared to the king's men. Appearing healthier, they were allowed to continue with their diet.

Around 475 BC, Anaxagoras stated that food is absorbed by the human body and, therefore, contains "homeomerics" (generative components), suggesting the existence of nutrients. Around 400 BC, Hippocrates, who recognized and was concerned with obesity, which may have been common in southern Europe at the time, said, "Let food be your medicine and medicine be your food." The works that are still attributed to him, *Corpus Hippocraticum*, called for moderation and emphasized exercise.

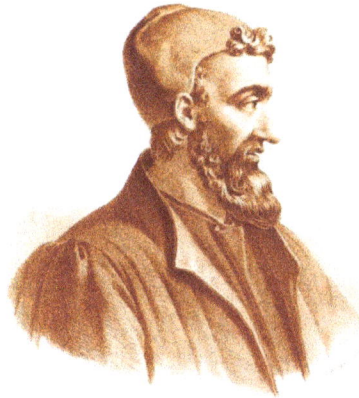

Followed for a millennium and a half, Galen (1st century) created the first coherent (although mistaken) theory of nutrition.

Salt, pepper and other spices were prescribed for various ailments in various preparations for example mixed with vinegar. In the 2nd century BC, Cato the Elder believed that cabbage (or the urine of cabbage-eaters) could cure digestive diseases, ulcers, warts, and intoxication. Living about the turn of the millennium, Aulus Celsus, an ancient Roman doctor, believed in "strong" and "weak" foods (bread for example was strong, as were older animals and vegetables).

Galen to Lind

One mustn't overlook the doctrines of Galen: In use from his life in the 1st century AD until the 17th century, it was heresy to disagree with him for 1500 years. Galen was physician to gladiators in Pergamon, and in Rome, physician to Marcus Aurelius and the three emperors who succeeded him. Most of Galen's teachings were gathered and enhanced in the late 11th century by Benedictine monks at the School of Salerno in *Regimen sanitatis Salernitanum*, which still had users in the 17th century. Galen believed in the bodily *humours* of Hippocrates, and he taught that *pneuma* is the source of life. Four elements (earth, air, fire and water) combine into "complexion", which combines into states (the four temperaments: sanguine, phlegmatic, choleric, and melancholic). The states are made up of pairs of attributes (hot and moist, cold and moist, hot and dry, and cold and dry), which are made of four humours: blood, phlegm, green (or yellow) bile, and black bile (the bodily form of the elements). Galen thought that for a person to have gout, kidney stones, or arthritis was scandalous, which Gratzer likens to Samuel Butler's *Erehwon* (1872) where sickness is a crime.

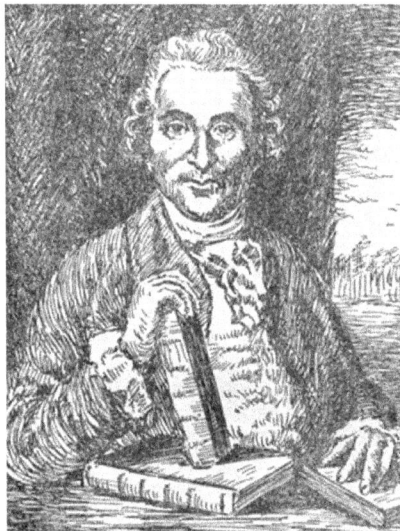

James Lind conducted in 1747 the first controlled clinical trial in modern times,
and in 1753 published *Treatise on Scurvy*.

In the 1500s, Paracelsus was probably the first to criticize Galen publicly. Also in the 16th century, scientist and artist Leonardo da Vinci compared metabolism to a burning candle. Leonardo did not publish his works on this subject, but he was not afraid of thinking for himself and he definitely disagreed with Galen. Ultimately, 16th century works of Andreas Vesalius, sometimes called the father of modern medicine, overturned Galen's ideas. He was followed by piercing thought amalgamated with the era's mysticism and religion sometimes fueled by the mechanics of Newton and Galileo. Jan Baptist van Helmont, who discovered several gases such as carbon dioxide, performed the first quantitative experiment. Robert Boyle advanced chemistry. Sanctorius measured body weight. Physician Herman Boerhaave modeled the digestive process. Physiologist Albrecht von Haller worked out the difference between nerves and muscles.

Sometimes overlooked during his life, James Lind, a physician in the British navy, performed the first scientific nutrition experiment in 1747. Lind discovered that lime juice saved sailors that had been at sea for years from scurvy, a deadly and painful bleeding disorder. Between 1500 and 1800, an estimated two million sailors had died of scurvy. The discovery was ignored for forty years, after which British sailors became known as "limeys." The essential vitamin C within citrus fruits would not be identified by scientists until 1932.

Lavoisier and Modern Science

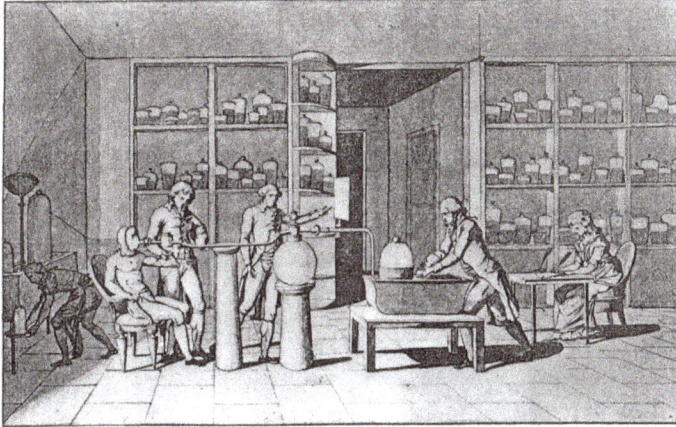

By containing his assistant, Armand Seguin, inside a rubber suit fitted with a tube sealed to his mouth with putty, Antoine Lavoisier first measured basal metabolic rate. Drawing by Madame Lavoisier (seated at right).

Around 1770, Antoine Lavoisier discovered the details of metabolism, demonstrating that the oxidation of food is the source of body heat. Called the most fundamental chemical discovery of the 18th century, Lavoisier discovered the principle of conservation of mass. His ideas made the phlogiston theory of combustion obsolete.

In 1790, George Fordyce recognized calcium as necessary for the survival of fowl. In the early 19th century, the elements carbon, nitrogen, hydrogen, and oxygen were recognized as the primary components of food, and methods to measure their proportions were developed.

In 1816, François Magendie discovered that dogs fed only carbohydrates (sugar), fat (olive oil), and water died evidently of starvation, but dogs also fed protein survived, identifying protein as an essential dietary component. William Prout in 1827 was the first person to divide foods into carbohydrates, fat, and protein. During the 19th century, Jean-Baptiste Dumas and Justus von Liebig quarreled over their shared belief that animals get their protein directly from plants (animal and plant protein are the same and that humans do not create organic compounds). With a reputation as the leading organic chemist of his day but with no credentials in animal physiology, Liebig grew rich making food extracts like beef bouillon and infant formula that were later found to be of questionable nutritious value. In the 1860s, Claude Bernard discovered that body fat can be synthesized from carbohydrate and protein, showing that the energy in blood glucose can be stored as fat or as glycogen.

In the early 1880s, Kanehiro Takaki observed that Japanese sailors (whose diets consisted almost entirely of white rice) developed beriberi (or endemic neuritis, a disease causing heart problems and paralysis), but British sailors and Japanese naval officers did not. Adding various types of vegetables and meats to the diets of Japanese sailors prevented the disease, (not because of the increased protein as Takaki supposed but because it introduced a few parts per million of thiamine to the diet, later understood as a cure).

In 1896, Eugen Baumann observed iodine in thyroid glands. In 1897, Christiaan Eijkman worked with natives of Java, who also suffered from beriberi. Eijkman observed that chickens fed the native diet of white rice developed the symptoms of beriberi but remained healthy when fed unprocessed brown rice with the outer bran intact. Eijkman cured the natives by feeding them brown rice, discovering that food can cure disease. Over two decades later, nutritionists learned that the outer rice bran contains vitamin B1, also known as thiamine.

From 1900 to the Present

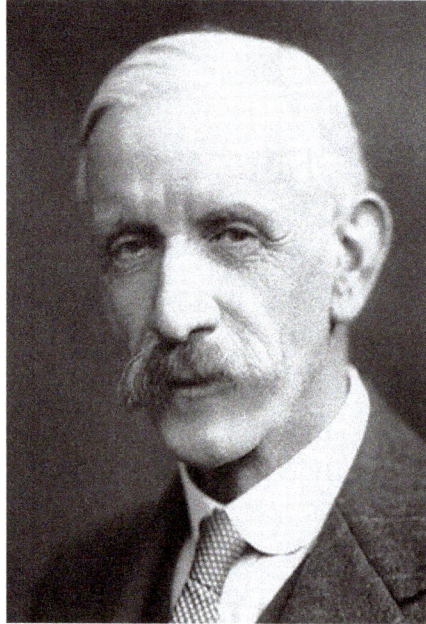

Frederick Hopkins discovered vitamins, for which he shared a Nobel prize with Eijkman.

In the early 20th century, Carl von Voit and Max Rubner independently measured caloric energy expenditure in different species of animals, applying principles of physics in nutrition. In 1906, Edith G. Willcock and Frederick Hopkins showed that the amino acid tryptophan aids the well-being of mice but it did not assure their growth. In the middle of twelve years of attempts to isolate them, Hopkins said in a 1906 lecture that "unsuspected dietetic factors," other than calories, protein, and minerals, are needed to prevent deficiency diseases. In 1907, Stephen M. Babcock and Edwin B. Hart conducted the single-grain experiment, which took nearly four years to complete.

Vitamin	Year Isolated
Thiamin	1926
Vitamin C	1926
Vitamin A	1939
Vitamin D	1931
Vitamin E	1936
Niacin	1937
Biotin	1939
Vitamin K	1939
Pantothenic acid	1939

Folate	1939
Riboflavin	1933
Vitamin B6	1936

Oxford University closed down its nutrition department after World War II because the subject seemed to have been completed between 1912 and 1944.

In 1912, Casimir Funk coined the term vitamin, a vital factor in the diet, from the words "vital" and "amine," because these unknown substances preventing scurvy, beriberi, and pellagra, were thought then to be derived from ammonia. The vitamins were studied in the first half of the 20th century.

In 1913, Elmer McCollum and Marguerite Davis discovered the first vitamin, fat-soluble vitamin A, then water-soluble vitamin B (in 1915; now known to be a complex of several water-soluble vitamins) and named vitamin C as the then-unknown substance preventing scurvy. Lafayette Mendel and Thomas Osborne also performed pioneering work on vitamins A and B. In 1919, Sir Edward Mellanby incorrectly identified rickets as a vitamin A deficiency because he could cure it in dogs with cod liver oil. In 1922, McCollum destroyed the vitamin A in cod liver oil, but found that it still cured rickets. Also in 1922, H.M. Evans and L.S. Bishop discover vitamin E as essential for rat pregnancy, originally calling it "food factor X" until 1925.

In 1925, Hart discovered that trace amounts of copper are necessary for iron absorption. In 1927, Adolf Otto Reinhold Windaus synthesized vitamin D, and was awarded the Nobel Prize in Chemistry in 1928. In 1928, Albert Szent-Györgyi isolated ascorbic acid, and in 1932 proved that it is vitamin C by preventing scurvy. In 1935, he synthesized it, and in 1937, he won a Nobel Prize for his efforts. Szent-Györgyi concurrently elucidated much of the citric acid cycle.

In the 1930s, William Cumming Rose identified essential amino acids, necessary protein components that the body cannot synthesize. In 1935, Underwood and Marston independently discovered the necessity of cobalt. In 1936, Eugene Floyd DuBois showed that work and school performance are related to caloric intake. In 1938, Erhard Fernholz discovered the chemical structure of vitamin E and then he tragically disappeared. It was synthesised the same year by Paul Karrer.

In 1940, rationing in the United Kingdom during and after World War II took place according to nutritional principles drawn up by Elsie Widdowson and others. In 1941, the first Recommended Dietary Allowances (RDAs) were established by the National Research Council.

In 1992, The U.S. Department of Agriculture introduced the Food Guide Pyramid. In 2002, a Natural Justice study showed a relation between nutrition and violent behavior. In 2005, one inconclusive study found that obesity could be caused by adenovirus in addition to bad nutrition.

World leaders are looking at alternatives like genetically modified foods to tackle the problem of world hunger and food shortages.

Nutrients

The list of nutrients that people are known to require is, in the words of Marion Nestle, "almost certainly incomplete". As of 2014, nutrients are thought to be of two types: macro-nutrients which are needed in relatively large amounts, and micronutrients which are needed in smaller quantities. A type of carbohydrate, dietary fiber, i.e. non-digestible material such as cellulose, is required, for both mechanical and biochemical reasons, although the exact reasons remain unclear. Other micronutrients include antioxidants and phytochemicals, which are said to influence (or protect) some body systems. Their necessity is not as well established as in the case of, for instance, vitamins.

Most foods contain a mix of some or all of the nutrient types, together with other substances, such as toxins of various sorts. Some nutrients can be stored internally (e.g., the fat-soluble vitamins), while others are required more or less continuously. Poor health can be caused by a lack of required nutrients or, in extreme cases, too much of a required nutrient. For example, both salt and water (both absolutely required) will cause illness or even death in excessive amounts.

Macronutrients

The macronutrients are carbohydrates, fiber, fats, protein, and water. The macronutrients (excluding fiber and water) provide structural material (amino acids from which proteins are built, and lipids from which cell membranes and some signaling molecules are built) and energy. Some of the structural material can be used to generate energy internally, and in either case it is measured in Joules or kilocalories (often called "Calories" and written with a capital C to distinguish them from little 'c' calories). Carbohydrates and proteins provide 17 kJ approximately (4 kcal) of energy per gram, while fats provide 37 kJ (9 kcal) per gram, though the net energy from either depends on such factors as absorption and digestive effort, which vary substantially from instance to instance. Vitamins, minerals, fiber, and water do not provide energy, but are required for other reasons.

Molecules of carbohydrates and fats consist of carbon, hydrogen, and oxygen atoms. Carbohydrates range from simple monosaccharides (glucose, fructose, galactose) to complex polysaccharides (starch). Fats are triglycerides, made of assorted fatty acid monomers bound to a glycerol backbone. Some fatty acids, but not all, are essential in the diet: they cannot be synthesized in the body. Protein molecules contain nitrogen atoms in addition to carbon, oxygen, and hydrogen. The fundamental components of protein are nitrogen-containing amino acids, some of which are essential in the sense that humans cannot make them internally. Some of the amino acids are convertible (with the expenditure of energy) to glucose and can be used for energy production, just as ordinary glucose, in a process known as gluconeogenesis. By breaking down existing protein, the carbon skeleton of the various amino acids can be metabolized to intermediates in cellular respiration; the remaining ammonia is discarded primarily as urea in urine. This occurs normally only during prolonged starvation.

Carbohydrates

Carbohydrates may be classified as monosaccharides, disaccharides, or polysaccharides depending on the number of monomer (sugar) units they contain. They constitute a large part of foods such as rice, noodles, bread, and other grain-based products. Monosaccharides, disaccharides, and polysaccharides contain one, two, and three or more sugar units, respectively. Polysaccharides are often referred to as *complex* carbohydrates because they are typically long, multiple branched chains of sugar units.

Traditionally, simple carbohydrates are believed to be absorbed quickly, and therefore to raise blood-glucose levels more rapidly than complex carbohydrates. This, however, is not accurate. Some simple carbohydrates (e.g., fructose) follow different metabolic pathways (e.g., fructolysis) that result in only a partial catabolism to glucose, while, in essence, many complex carbohydrates may be digested at the same rate as simple carbohydrates. Glucose stimulates the production of insulin through food entering the bloodstream, which is grasped by the beta cells in the pancreas.

Fiber

Dietary fiber is a carbohydrate that is incompletely absorbed in humans and in some animals. Like all carbohydrates, when it is metabolized it can produce four Calories (kilocalories) of energy per gram. However, in most circumstances it accounts for less than that because of its limited absorption and digestibility. Dietary fiber consists mainly of cellulose, a large carbohydrate polymer which is indigestible as humans do not have the required enzymes to disassemble it. There are two subcategories: soluble and insoluble fiber. Whole grains, fruits (especially plums, prunes, and figs), and vegetables are good sources of dietary fiber. There are many health benefits of a high-fiber diet. Dietary fiber helps reduce the chance of gastrointestinal problems such as constipation and diarrhea by increasing the weight and size of stool and softening it. Insoluble fiber, found in whole wheat flour, nuts and vegetables, especially stimulates peristalsis – the rhythmic muscular contractions of the intestines, which move digesta along the digestive tract. Soluble fiber, found in oats, peas, beans, and many fruits, dissolves in water in the intestinal tract to produce a gel that slows the movement of food through the intestines. This may help lower blood glucose levels because it can slow the absorption of sugar. Additionally, fiber, perhaps especially that from whole grains, is thought to possibly help lessen insulin spikes, and therefore reduce the risk of type 2 diabetes. The link between increased fiber consumption and a decreased risk of colorectal cancer is still uncertain.

Fat

A molecule of dietary fat typically consists of several fatty acids (containing long chains of carbon and hydrogen atoms), bonded to a glycerol. They are typically found as triglycerides (three fatty acids attached to one glycerol backbone). Fats may be classified as saturated or unsaturated depending on the detailed structure of the fatty acids involved. Saturated fats have all of the carbon atoms in their fatty acid chains bonded to hydrogen atoms, whereas unsaturated fats have some of these carbon atoms double-bonded, so their molecules have relatively fewer hydrogen atoms than a saturated fatty acid of the same length. Unsaturated fats may be further classified as monounsaturated (one double-bond) or polyunsaturated (many double-bonds). Furthermore, depending on the location of the double-bond in the fatty acid chain, unsaturated fatty acids are classified as omega-3 or omega-6 fatty acids. Trans fats are a type of unsaturated fat with *trans*-isomer bonds; these are rare in nature and in foods from natural sources; they are typically created in an industrial process called (partial) hydrogenation. There are nine kilocalories in each gram of fat. Fatty acids such as conjugated linoleic acid, catalpic acid, eleostearic acid and punicic acid, in addition to providing energy, represent potent immune modulatory molecules.

Saturated fats (typically from animal sources) have been a staple in many world cultures for millennia. Unsaturated fats (e. g., vegetable oil) are considered healthier, while trans fats are to be avoided. Saturated and some trans fats are typically solid at room temperature (such as butter or lard), while unsaturated fats are typically liquids (such as olive oil or flaxseed oil). Trans fats are very rare in nature, and have been shown to be highly detrimental to human health, but have properties useful in the food processing industry, such as rancidity resistance.

Essential Fatty Acids

Most fatty acids are non-essential, meaning the body can produce them as needed, generally from other fatty acids and always by expending energy to do so. However, in humans, at least two fatty acids are essential and must be included in the diet. An appropriate balance of essential fatty acids—omega-3 and omega-6 fatty acids—seems also important for health, although definitive experimental demonstration has been elusive. Both of these "omega" long-chain polyunsaturated fatty acids are substrates for a class of eicosanoids known as prostaglandins, which have roles throughout the human body. They are hormones, in some respects. The omega-3 eicosapentaenoic acid (EPA), which can be made in the human body from the omega-3 essential fatty acid alpha-linolenic acid (ALA), or taken in through marine food sources, serves as a building block for series 3 prostaglandins (e.g., weakly inflammatory PGE3). The omega-6 dihomo-gamma-linolenic acid (DGLA) serves as a building block for series 1 prostaglandins (e.g. anti-inflammatory PGE1), whereas arachidonic acid (AA) serves as a building block for series 2 prostaglandins (e.g. pro-inflammatory PGE 2). Both DGLA and AA can be made from the omega-6 linoleic acid (LA) in the human body, or can be taken in directly through food. An appropriately balanced intake of omega-3 and omega-6 partly determines the relative production of different prostaglandins, which is one reason why a balance between omega-3 and omega-6 is believed important for cardiovascular health. In industrialized societies, people typically consume large amounts of processed vegetable oils, which have reduced amounts of the essential fatty acids along with too much of omega-6 fatty acids relative to omega-3 fatty acids.

The conversion rate of omega-6 DGLA to AA largely determines the production of the prostaglandins PGE1 and PGE2. Omega-3 EPA prevents AA from being released from membranes, thereby skewing prostaglandin balance away from pro-inflammatory PGE2 (made from AA) toward anti-inflammatory PGE1 (made from DGLA). Moreover, the conversion (desaturation) of DGLA to AA is controlled by the enzyme delta-5-desaturase, which in turn is controlled by hormones such as insulin (up-regulation) and glucagon (down-regulation). The amount and type of carbohydrates consumed, along with some types of amino acid, can influence processes involving insulin, glucagon, and other hormones; therefore, the ratio of omega-3 versus omega-6 has wide effects on general health, and specific effects on immune function and inflammation, and mitosis (i.e., cell division).

Protein

Proteins are structural materials in much of the animal body (e.g. muscles, skin, and hair). They also form the enzymes that control chemical reactions throughout the body. Each protein molecule is composed of amino acids, which are characterized by inclusion of nitrogen and sometimes sulphur (these components are responsible for the distinctive smell of burning protein, such as the keratin in hair). The body requires amino acids to produce new proteins (protein retention) and to replace damaged proteins (maintenance). As there is no protein or amino acid storage provision, amino acids must be present in the diet. Excess amino acids are discarded, typically in the urine. For all animals, some amino acids are *essential* (an animal cannot produce them internally) and some are *non-essential* (the animal can produce them from other nitrogen-containing compounds). About twenty amino acids are found in the human body, and about ten of these are essential and, therefore, must be included in the diet. A diet that contains adequate amounts of amino acids (especially those that are essential) is particularly important in some situations: during early development and maturation, pregnancy, lactation, or injury (a burn, for instance). A *complete* protein source contains all the essential amino acids; an *incomplete* protein source lacks one or more of the essential amino acids.

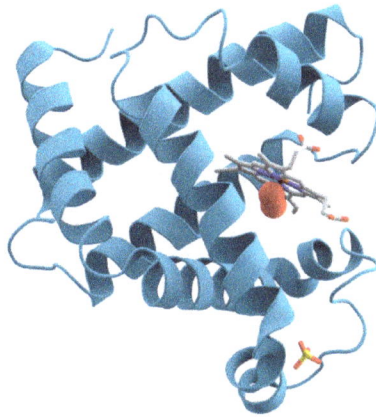

Proteins are chains of amino acids found in most nutritional foods.

It is possible with protein combinations of two incomplete protein sources (e.g., rice and beans) to make a complete protein source, and characteristic combinations are the basis of distinct cultural cooking traditions. However, complementary sources of protein do not need to be eaten at the same meal to be used together by the body. Excess amino acids from protein can be converted into glucose and used for fuel through a process called gluconeogenesis. The amino acids remaining after such conversion are discarded.

Water

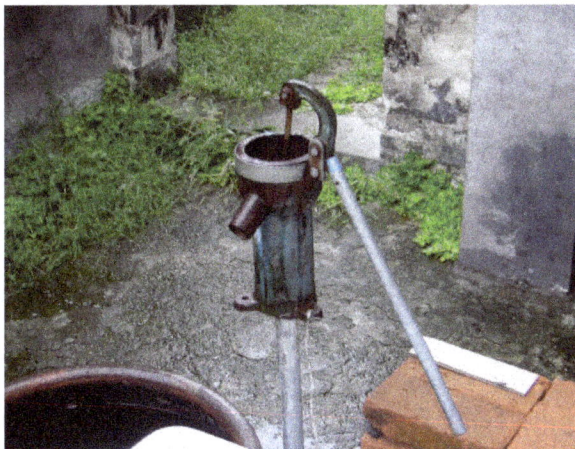

A manual water pump in China

Water is excreted from the body in multiple forms; including urine and feces, sweating, and by water vapour in the exhaled breath. Therefore, it is necessary to adequately rehydrate to replace lost fluids.

Early recommendations for the quantity of water required for maintenance of good health suggested that 6–8 glasses of water daily is the minimum to maintain proper hydration. However the notion that a person should consume eight glasses of water per day cannot be traced to a credible scientific source. The original water intake recommendation in 1945 by the Food and Nutrition Board of the National Research Council read: "An ordinary standard for diverse persons is 1 milliliter for each calorie of food. Most of this quantity is contained in prepared foods." More recent comparisons of well-known recommendations on fluid intake have revealed large discrepancies in the volumes of water we need to consume for good health. Therefore, to help standardize guidelines, recommendations for water consumption are included in two recent European Food Safety Authority (EFSA) documents (2010): (i) Food-based dietary guidelines and (ii) Dietary reference values for water or adequate daily intakes (ADI). These specifications were provided by calculating adequate intakes from measured intakes in populations of individuals with "desirable osmolarity values of urine and desirable water volumes per energy unit consumed." For healthful hydration, the current EFSA guidelines recommend total water intakes of 2.0 L/day for adult females and 2.5 L/day for adult males. These reference values include water from drinking water, other beverages, and from food. About 80% of our daily water requirement comes from the beverages we drink, with the remaining 20% coming from food. Water content varies depending on the type of food consumed, with fruit and vegetables containing more than cereals, for example. These values are estimated using country-specific food balance sheets published by the Food and Agriculture Organisation of the United Nations. Other guidelines for nutrition also have implications for the beverages we consume for healthy hydration- for example, the World Health Organization (WHO) recommend that added sugars should represent no more than 10% of total energy intake.

The EFSA panel also determined intakes for different populations. Recommended intake volumes in the elderly are the same as for adults as despite lower energy consumption, the water requirement of this group is increased due to a reduction in renal concentrating capacity. Pregnant and breastfeeding women require additional fluids to stay hydrated. The EFSA panel proposes that pregnant women should consume the same volume of water as non-pregnant women, plus an increase in proportion to the higher energy requirement, equal to 300 mL/day. To compensate for additional fluid output, breastfeeding women require an additional 700 mL/day above the recommended intake values for non-lactating women.

For those who have healthy kidneys, it is somewhat difficult to drink too much water, but (especially in warm humid weather and while exercising) it is dangerous to drink too little. While overhydration is much less common than dehydration, it is also possible to drink far more water than necessary, which can result in water intoxication, a serious and potentially fatal condition. In particular, large amounts of de-ionized water are dangerous.

Micronutrients

Minerals

Dietary minerals are inorganic chemical elements required by living organisms, other than the four elements carbon, hydrogen, nitrogen, and oxygen that are present in nearly all organic molecules.

The term "mineral" is archaic, since the intent is to describe simply the less common elements in the diet. Some are heavier than the four just mentioned, including several metals, which often occur as ions in the body. Some dietitians recommend that these be supplied from foods in which they occur naturally, or at least as complex compounds, or sometimes even from natural inorganic sources (such as calcium carbonate from ground oyster shells). Some minerals are absorbed much more readily in the ionic forms found in such sources. On the other hand, minerals are often artificially added to the diet as supplements; the most famous is likely iodine in iodized salt which prevents goiter.

Macrominerals

Many elements are essential in relative quantity; they are usually called "bulk minerals". Some are structural, but many play a role as electrolytes. Elements with recommended dietary allowance (RDA) greater than 150 mg/day are, in alphabetical order (with informal or folk-medicine perspectives in parentheses):

- Calcium, a common electrolyte, but also needed structurally (for muscle and digestive system health, bone strength, some forms neutralize acidity, may help clear toxins, provides signaling ions for nerve and membrane functions)

- Chlorine as chloride ions; very common electrolyte

- Magnesium, required for processing ATP and related reactions (builds bone, causes strong peristalsis, increases flexibility, increases alkalinity)

- Phosphorus, required component of bones; essential for energy processing

- Potassium, a very common electrolyte (heart and nerve health)

- Sodium, a very common electrolyte; in general not found in dietary supplements, despite being needed in large quantities, because the ion is very common in food: typically as sodium chloride, or common salt. Excessive sodium consumption can deplete calcium and magnesium, leading to high blood pressure and osteoporosis.

- Sulfur, for three essential amino acids and therefore many proteins (skin, hair, nails, liver, and pancreas). Sulfur is not consumed alone, but in the form of sulfur-containing amino acids

Trace minerals

Many elements are required in trace amounts, usually because they play a catalytic role in enzymes. Some trace mineral elements (RDA < 200 mg/day) are, in alphabetical order:

- Cobalt required for biosynthesis of vitamin B12 family of coenzymes. Animals cannot biosynthesize B12, and must obtain this cobalt-containing vitamin in their diet.

- Copper required component of many redox enzymes, including cytochrome c oxidase

- Chromium required for sugar metabolism

- Iodine required not only for the biosynthesis of thyroxine but also — it is presumed — for other important organs as breast, stomach, salivary glands, thymus, etc; for this reason iodine is needed in larger quantities than others in this list, and sometimes classified with the macrominerals

- Iron required for many enzymes, and for hemoglobin and some other proteins

- Manganese (processing of oxygen)

- Molybdenum required for xanthine oxidase and related oxidases

- Selenium required for peroxidase (antioxidant proteins)

- Zinc required for several enzymes such as carboxypeptidase, liver alcohol dehydrogenase, and carbonic anhydrase

Vitamins

As with the minerals discussed above, some vitamins are recognized as organic essential nutrients, necessary in the diet for good health. (Vitamin D is the exception: it can be synthesized in the skin, in the presence of UVB radiation.) Certain vitamin-like compounds that are recommended in the diet, such as carnitine, are thought useful for survival and health, but these are not "essential" dietary nutrients because the human body has some capacity to produce them from other compounds. Moreover, thousands of different phytochemicals have recently been discovered in food (particularly in fresh vegetables), which may have desirable properties including antioxidant activity; however, experimental demonstration has been suggestive but inconclusive. Other essential nutrients that are not classified as vitamins include essential amino acids, choline, essential fatty acids, and the minerals discussed in the preceding section.

Vitamin deficiencies may result in disease conditions, including goitre, scurvy, osteoporosis, impaired immune system, disorders of cell metabolism, certain forms of cancer, symptoms of premature aging, and poor psychological health (including eating disorders), among many others. Excess levels of some vitamins are also dangerous to health (notably vitamin A). Deficient or excess levels of minerals can also have serious health consequences.

Healthy Diets

Whole Plant Food Diet

Heart disease, cancer, obesity, and diabetes are commonly called "Western" diseases because these maladies were once rarely seen in developing countries. An international study in China found some regions had virtually no cancer or heart disease, while in other areas they reflected "up to a 100-fold increase" coincident with shifts from diets that were found to be entirely plant-based to heavily animal-based, respectively. In contrast, diseases of affluence like cancer and heart disease are common throughout the developed world, including the United States. Adjusted for age and exercise, large regional clusters of people in China rarely suffered from these "Western" diseases possibly because their diets are rich in vegetables, fruits, and whole grains, and have little dairy and meat products. Some studies show these to be, in high quantities, possible causes of some cancers. There are arguments for and against this controversial issue.

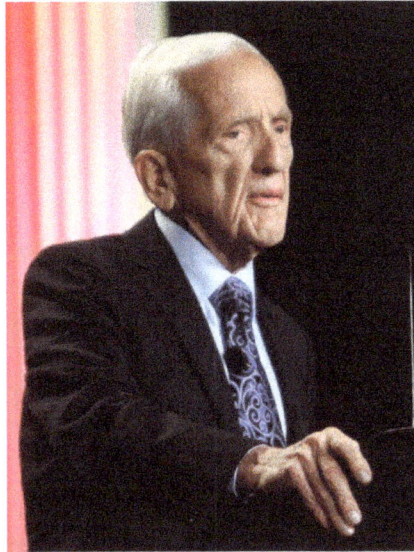

T. Colin Campbell is among the scientists who advocate a plant-based diet

The United Healthcare/Pacificare nutrition guideline recommends a whole plant food diet, and recommends using protein only as a condiment with meals. A *National Geographic* cover article from November 2005, entitled *The Secrets of Living Longer*, also recommends a whole plant food diet. The article is a lifestyle survey of three populations, Sardinians, Okinawans, and Adventists, who generally display longevity and "suffer a fraction of the diseases that commonly kill people in other parts of the developed world, and enjoy more healthy years of life." In common with all three groups is to "Eat fruits, vegetables, and whole grains."

The *National Geographic* article noted that an NIH funded study of 34,000 Seventh-day Adventists between 1976 and 1988 "...found that the Adventists' habit of consuming beans, soy milk, tomatoes, and other fruits lowered their risk of developing certain cancers. It also suggested that eating whole grain bread, drinking five glasses of water a day, and, most surprisingly, consuming four servings of nuts a week reduced their risk of heart disease."

The French "Paradox"

The French paradox is the observation that the French suffer a relatively low incidence of coronary heart disease, despite having a diet relatively rich in saturated fats. A number of explanations have been suggested:

- Saturated fat consumption does not cause heart disease

- Reduced consumption of processed carbohydrate and other junk foods.

- Regular consumption of red wine.

- Higher consumption of artificially produced trans-fats by Americans, which has been shown to have greater lipoprotein effects per gram than saturated fat.

However, statistics collected by the World Health Organization from 1990–2000 show that the incidence of heart disease in France may have been underestimated and, in fact, may be similar to that of neighboring countries.

Phytochemicals

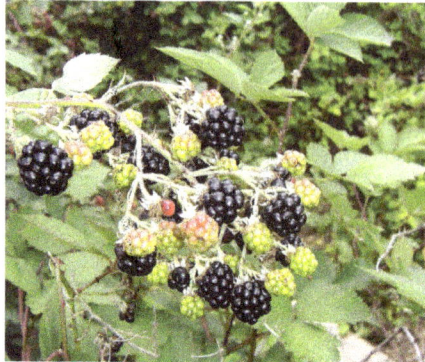

Blackberries are a source of polyphenols

Phytochemicals such as polyphenols are compounds produced naturally in plants. In general, the term is used to refer to those chemicals under research to assess whether they have biological significance. To date, there is no evidence in humans that polyphenols or other non-nutrient compounds from plants have health effects. Further, dietary supplements containing phytochemicals also have no proven health benefit.

While initial studies sought to reveal if antioxidant or phytochemical supplements might promote health, later large clinical trials did not detect any benefit and showed instead that excess supplementation could be harmful.

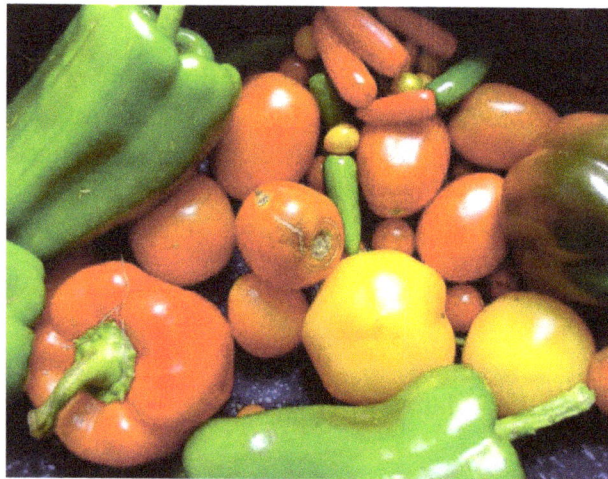

Colorful fruits and vegetables can be components of a healthy diet.

Intestinal Bacterial Flora

Animal intestines contain a large population of gut flora. In humans, the four dominant phyla are Firmicutes, Bacteroidetes, Actinobacteria, and Proteobacteria. They are essential to digestion and are also affected by food that is consumed. Bacteria in the gut perform many important functions for humans, including breaking down and aiding in the absorption of otherwise indigestible food; stimulating cell growth; repressing the growth of harmful bacteria, training the immune system to respond only to pathogens; producing vitamin B_{12}; and defending against some infectious diseases.

Animal Nutrition

Nutritional science investigates the metabolic and physiological responses of the body to diet. With advances in the fields of molecular biology, biochemistry, nutritional immunology, molecular medicine and genetics, the study of nutrition is increasingly concerned with metabolism and metabolic pathways: the sequences of biochemical steps through which substances in living things change from one form to another.

Carnivore and herbivore diets are contrasting, with basic nitrogen and carbon proportions vary for their particular foods. "The nitrogen content of plant tissues averages about 2%, while in fungi, animals, and bacteria it averages about 5% to 10%." Many herbivores rely on bacterial fermentation to create digestible nutrients from indigestible plant cellulose, while obligate carnivores must eat animal meats to obtain certain vitamins or nutrients their bodies cannot otherwise synthesize. All animals' diets must provide sufficient amounts of the basic building blocks they need, up to the point where their particular biology can synthesize the rest. Animal tissue contains chemical compounds, such as water, carbohydrates (sugar, starch, and fiber), amino acids (in proteins), fatty acids (in lipids), and nucleic acids (DNA and RNA). These compounds in turn consist of elements such as carbon, hydrogen, oxygen, nitrogen, phosphorus, calcium, iron, zinc, magnesium, manganese, and so on. All of these chemical compounds and elements occur in various forms and combinations (e.g. hormones, vitamins, phospholipids, hydroxyapatite).

Animal tissue consists of elements and compounds ingested, digested, absorbed, and circulated through the bloodstream to feed the cells of the body. Except in the unborn fetus, the digestive system is the first system involved. Digestive juices break chemical bonds in ingested molecules, and modify their conformations and energy states. Though some molecules are absorbed into the bloodstream unchanged, digestive processes release them from the matrix of foods. Unabsorbed matter, along with some waste products of metabolism, is eliminated from the body in the feces.

Studies of nutritional status must take into account the state of the body before and after experiments, as well as the chemical composition of the whole diet and of all material excreted and eliminated from the body (in urine and feces). Comparing the food to the waste can help determine the specific compounds and elements absorbed and metabolized in the body. The effects of nutrients may only be discernible over an extended period, during which all food and waste must be analyzed. The number of variables involved in such experiments is high, making nutritional studies time-consuming and expensive, which explains why the science of animal nutrition is still slowly evolving.

In particular, the consumption of whole-plant foods slows digestion and allows better absorption, and a more favorable balance of essential nutrients per Calorie, resulting in better management of cell growth, maintenance, and mitosis (cell division), as well as better regulation of appetite and blood sugar. Regularly scheduled meals (every few hours) have also proven more wholesome than infrequent or haphazard ones.

Plant Nutrition

Plant nutrition is the study of the chemical elements that are necessary for plant growth. There are several principles that apply to plant nutrition. Some elements are directly involved in plant metabolism. However, this principle does not account for the so-called beneficial elements, whose presence, while not required, has clear positive effects on plant growth.

A nutrient that is able to limit plant growth according to Liebig's law of the minimum is considered an essential plant nutrient if the plant cannot complete its full life cycle without it. There are 16 essential plant soil nutrients, besides the three major elemental nutrients carbon and oxygen that are obtained by photosynthetic plants from carbon dioxide in air, and hydrogen, which is obtained from water.

Plants uptake essential elements from the soil through their roots and from the air (consisting of mainly nitrogen and oxygen) through their leaves. Green plants obtain their carbohydrate supply from the carbon dioxide in the air by the process of photosynthesis. Carbon and oxygen are absorbed from the air, while other nutrients are absorbed from the soil. Nutrient uptake in the soil is achieved by cation exchange, wherein root hairs pump hydrogen ions (H^+) into the soil through proton pumps. These hydrogen ions displace cations attached to negatively charged soil particles so that the cations are available for uptake by the root. In the leaves, stomata open to take in carbon dioxide and expel oxygen. The carbon dioxide molecules are used as the carbon source in photosynthesis.

Although nitrogen is plentiful in the Earth's atmosphere, very few plants can use this directly. Most plants, therefore, require nitrogen compounds to be present in the soil in which they grow. This is made possible by the fact that largely inert atmospheric nitrogen is changed in a nitrogen fixation process to biologically usable forms in the soil by bacteria.

Plant nutrition is a difficult subject to understand completely, partially because of the variation between different plants and even between different species or individuals of a given clone. Elements present at low levels may cause deficiency symptoms, and toxicity is possible at levels that are too high. Furthermore, deficiency of one element may present as symptoms of toxicity from another element, and vice versa.

Environmental Nutrition

Research in the field of nutrition has greatly contributed in finding out the essential facts about how environmental depletion can lead to crucial nutrition-related health problems like contamination, spread of contagious diseases, malnutrition, etc. Moreover, environmental contamination due to discharge of agricultural as well as industrial chemicals like organocholrines, heavy metal, and radionucleotides may adversely affect the human and the ecosystem as a whole. As far as safety of the human health is concerned, then these environmental contaminants can reduce people's nutritional status and health. This could directly or indirectly cause drastic changes in their diet habits. Hence, food-based remedial as well as preventive strategies are essential to address global issues like hunger and malnutrition and to enable the susceptible people to adapt themselves to all these environmental as well as socio-economic alterations.

Advice and Guidance

U.S. Government Policies

In the US, dietitians are registered (RD) or licensed (LD) with the Commission for Dietetic Registration and the American Dietetic Association, and are only able to use the title "dietitian," as described by the business and professions codes of each respective state, when they have met specific educational and experiential prerequisites and passed a national registration or licensure examination, respectively. In California, registered dietitians must abide by the *"Business and Professions Code of Section 2585-2586.8"*. Anyone may call themselves a nutritionist, including unqualified dietitians, as this term is unregulated. Some states, such as the State of Florida, have begun to include the title "nutritionist" in state licensure requirements. Most governments provide guidance on nutrition, and some also impose mandatory disclosure/labeling requirements for processed food manufacturers and restaurants to assist consumers in complying with such guidance.

In the US, nutritional standards and recommendations are established jointly by the US Department of Agriculture and US Department of Health and Human Services. Dietary and physical activity guidelines from the USDA are presented in the concept of MyPlate, which superseded the food pyramid, which replaced the Four Food Groups. The Senate committee currently responsible for oversight of the USDA is the *Agriculture, Nutrition and Forestry Committee*. Committee hearings are often televised on C-SPAN.

The U.S. Department of Health and Human Services provides a sample week-long menu that fulfills the nutritional recommendations of the government. Canada's Food Guide is another governmental recommendation.

Government Programs

Federal and state governmental organizations have been working on nutrition literacy interventions in non-primary health care settings to address the nutrition information problem in the U.S. Some programs include:

The Family Nutrition Program (FNP) is a free nutrition education program serving low-income adults around the U.S. This program is funded by the Food Nutrition Service's (FNS) branch of the United States Department of Agriculture (USDA) usually through a local state academic institution that runs the program. The FNP has developed a series of tools to help families participating in the Food Stamp Program stretch their food dollar and form healthful eating habits including nutrition education.

Expanded Food and Nutrition Education Program (ENFEP) is a unique program that currently operates in all 50 states and in American Samoa, Guam, Micronesia, Northern Marianas, Puerto Rico, and the Virgin Islands. It is designed to assist limited-resource audiences in acquiring the knowledge, skills, attitudes, and changed behavior necessary for nutritionally sound diets, and to contribute to their personal development and the improvement of the total family diet and nutritional well-being.

An example of a state initiative to promote nutrition literacy is Smart Bodies, a public-private partnership between the state's largest university system and largest health insurer, Louisiana State Agricultural Center and Blue Cross and Blue Shield of Louisiana Foundation. Launched in 2005, this program promotes lifelong healthful eating patterns and physically active lifestyles for children and their families. It is an interactive educational program designed to help prevent childhood obesity through classroom activities that teach children healthful eating habits and physical exercise.

Education

Nutrition is taught in schools in many countries. In England and Wales, the Personal and Social Education and Food Technology curricula include nutrition, stressing the importance of a balanced diet and teaching how to read nutrition labels on packaging. In many schools, a Nutrition class will fall within the Family and Consumer Science or Health departments. In some American schools, students are required to take a certain number of FCS or Health related classes. Nutrition is offered at many schools, and, if it is not a class of its own, nutrition is included in other FCS or Health classes such as: Life Skills, Independent Living, Single Survival, Freshmen Connection, Health etc. In many Nutrition classes, students learn about the food groups, the food pyramid, Daily Recommended Allowances, calories, vitamins, minerals, malnutrition, physical activity, healthful food choices, portion sizes, and how to live a healthy life.

A 1985, US National Research Council report entitled *Nutrition Education in US Medical Schools* concluded that nutrition education in medical schools was inadequate. Only 20% of the schools surveyed taught nutrition as a separate, required course. A 2006 survey found that this number had risen to 30%.

Nutrition Literacy

At the time of this entry, we were not able to identify any specific nutrition literacy studies in the U.S. at a national level. However, the findings of the 2003 National Assessment of Adult Literacy (NAAL) provide a basis upon which to frame the nutrition literacy problem in the U.S. NAAL introduced the first ever measure of "the degree to which individuals have the capacity to obtain, process and understand basic health information and services needed to make appropriate health decisions" – an objective of Healthy People 2010 and of which nutrition literacy might be considered an important subset. On a scale of below basic, basic, intermediate and proficient, NAAL found 13 percent of adult Americans have proficient health literacy, 44% have intermediate literacy, 29 percent have basic literacy and 14 percent have below basic health literacy. The study found that health literacy increases with education and people living below the level of poverty have lower health literacy than those above it.

Another study examining the health and nutrition literacy status of residents of the lower Mississippi Delta found that 52 percent of participants had a high likelihood of limited literacy skills. While a precise comparison between the NAAL and Delta studies is difficult, primarily because of methodological differences, Zoellner et al. suggest that health literacy rates in the Mississippi Delta region are different from the U.S. general population and that they help establish the scope of the problem of health literacy among adults in the Delta region. For example, only 12 percent of study participants identified the My Pyramid graphic two years after it had been launched by the USDA. The study also found significant relationships between nutrition literacy and income level and nutrition literacy and educational attainment further delineating priorities for the region.

These statistics point to the complexities surrounding the lack of health/nutrition literacy and reveal the degree to which they are embedded in the social structure and interconnected with other problems. Among these problems are the lack of information about food choices, a lack of understanding of nutritional information and its application to individual circumstances, limited or difficult access to healthful foods, and a range of cultural influences and socioeconomic constraints such as low levels of education and high levels of poverty that decrease opportunities for healthful eating and living.

The links between low health literacy and poor health outcomes has been widely documented and there is evidence that some interventions to improve health literacy have produced successful results in the primary care setting. More must be done to further our understanding of nutrition literacy specific interventions in non-primary care settings in order to achieve better health outcomes.

Malnutrition

Malnutrition refers to insufficient, excessive, or imbalanced consumption of nutrients by an organism. In developed countries, the diseases of malnutrition are most often associated with nutritional imbalances or excessive consumption. In developing countries, malnutrition is more likely to be caused by poor access to a range of nutritious foods or inadequate knowledge. In Mali the International Crops Research Institute for the Semi-Arid Tropics (ICRISAT) and the Aga Khan Foundation, trained women's groups to make *equinut*, a healthy and nutritional version of the traditional recipe *di-dèguè* (comprising peanut paste, honey and millet or rice flour). The aim was to boost nutrition and livelihoods by producing a product that women could make and sell, and which would be accepted by the local community because of its local heritage.

Although there are more organisms in the world who are malnourished due to insufficient consumption, increasingly more organisms suffer from excessive over-nutrition; a problem caused by an over abundance of sustenance coupled with the instinctual desire (by animals in particular) to consume all that it can.

Nutritionism is the view that excessive reliance on food science and the study of nutrition can lead to poor nutrition and to ill health. It was originally credited to Gyorgy Scrinis, and was popularized by Michael Pollan. Since nutrients are invisible, policy makers rely on nutrition experts to advise on food choices. Because science has an incomplete understanding of how food affects the human body, Pollan argues, nutritionism can be blamed for many of the health problems relating to diet in the Western World today.

Insufficient

In general, *under-consumption* refers to the long-term consumption of insufficient sustenance in relation to the energy that an organism expends or expels, leading to poor health.

Excessive

In general, *over-consumption* refers to the long-term consumption of excess sustenance in relation to the energy that an organism expends or expels, leading to poor health and, in animals, obesity. It can cause excessive hair loss, brittle nails, and irregular premenstrual cycles for females.

Unbalanced

When too much of one or more nutrients is present in the diet to the exclusion of the proper amount of other nutrients, the diet is said to be unbalanced.

Illnesses Caused by Improper Nutrient Consumption

Nutrients	Deficiency	Excess
Macronutrients		
Calories	Starvation, marasmus	Obesity, diabetes mellitus, cardiovascular disease
Simple carbohydrates	Low energy levels.	Obesity, diabetes mellitus, cardiovascular disease
Complex carbohydrates	Micronutrient deficiency	Obesity, cardiovascular disease (high glycemic index foods)
Protein	Kwashiorkor	Rabbit starvation, ketoacidosis (in diabetics)
Saturated fat	Low testosterone levels, vitamin deficiencies.	Obesity, cardiovascular disease
Trans fat	None	Obesity, cardiovascular disease
Unsaturated fat	Fat-soluble vitamin deficiency	Obesity, cardiovascular disease
Micronutrients		
Vitamin A	Xerophthalmia and night blindness	Hypervitaminosis A (cirrhosis, hair loss)
Vitamin B_1	Beri-Beri	?
Vitamin B_2	Skin and corneal lesions	?
Niacin	Pellagra	Dyspepsia, cardiac arrhythmias, birth defects
Vitamin B_{12}	Pernicious anemia	?
Vitamin C	Scurvy	Diarrhea causing dehydration
Vitamin D	Rickets	Hypervitaminosis D (dehydration, vomiting, constipation)
Vitamin E	Neurological disease	Hypervitaminosis E (anticoagulant: excessive bleeding)
Vitamin K	Hemorrhage	Liver damage
Omega-3 fats	Cardiovascular Disease	Bleeding, Hemorrhages, Hemorrhagic stroke, reduced glycemic control among diabetics
Omega-6 fats	None	Cardiovascular Disease, Cancer
Cholesterol	None	Cardiovascular Disease
Macrominerals		
Calcium	Osteoporosis, tetany, carpopedal spasm, laryngospasm, cardiac arrhythmias	Fatigue, depression, confusion, nausea, vomiting, constipation, pancreatitis, increased urination, kidney stones
Magnesium	Hypertension	Weakness, nausea, vomiting, impaired breathing, and hypotension
Potassium	Hypokalemia, cardiac arrhythmias	Hyperkalemia, palpitations
Sodium	Hyponatremia	Hypernatremia, hypertension
Trace minerals		
Iron	Anemia	Cirrhosis, Hereditary hemochromatosis, heart disease
Iodine	Goiter, hypothyroidism	Iodine toxicity (goiter, hypothyroidism)

Mental Agility

Research indicates that improving the awareness of nutritious meal choices and establishing long-term habits of healthy eating have a positive effect on cognitive and spatial memory capacity, with potential to increase a student's ability to process and retain academic information.

Some organizations have begun working with teachers, policymakers, and managed foodservice contractors to mandate improved nutritional content and increased nutritional resources in school cafeterias from primary to university level institutions. Health and nutrition have been proven to have close links with overall educational success. Currently, less than 10% of American college students report that they eat the recommended five servings of fruit and vegetables daily. Better nutrition has been shown to affect both cognitive and spatial memory performance; a study showed those with higher blood sugar levels performed better on certain memory tests. In another study, those who consumed yogurt performed better on thinking tasks when compared to those that consumed caffeine-free diet soda or confections. Nutritional deficiencies have been shown to have a negative effect on learning behavior in mice as far back as 1951.

> "Better learning performance is associated with diet-induced effects on learning and memory ability".

> The "nutrition-learning nexus" demonstrates the correlation between diet and learning and has application in a higher education setting.

> "We find that better-nourished children perform significantly better in school, partly because they enter school earlier and thus have more time to learn but mostly because of greater learning productivity per year of schooling."

> 91% of college students feel that they are in good health, whereas only 7% eat their recommended daily allowance of fruits and vegetables.

> Nutritional education is an effective and workable model in a higher education setting.

> More "engaged" learning models that encompass nutrition is an idea that is picking up steam at all levels of the learning cycle.

There is limited research available that directly links a student's Grade Point Average (G.P.A.) to their overall nutritional health. Additional substantive data is needed to prove that overall intellectual health is closely linked to a person's diet, rather than just another correlation fallacy.

Mental Disorders

Nutritional supplement treatment may be appropriate for major depression, bipolar disorder, schizophrenia, and obsessive compulsive disorder, the four most common mental disorders in developed countries. Supplements that have been studied most for mood elevation and stabilization include eicosapentaenoic acid and docosahexaenoic acid (each of which an omega-3 fatty acid contained in fish oil but not in flaxseed oil), vitamin B12, folic acid, and inositol.

Cancer

Cancer is now common in developing countries. According to a study by the International Agency for Research on Cancer, "In the developing world, cancers of the liver, stomach and esophagus were more common, often linked to consumption of carcinogenic preserved foods, such as smoked or salted food, and parasitic infections that attack organs." Lung cancer rates are rising rapidly in poorer nations because of increased use of tobacco. Developed countries "tended to have cancers linked to affluence or a 'Western lifestyle' — cancers of the colon, rectum, breast and prostate — that can be caused by obesity, lack of exercise, diet and age."

Metabolic Syndrome

Several lines of evidence indicate lifestyle-induced hyperinsulinemia and reduced insulin function (i.e., insulin resistance) as a decisive factor in many disease states. For example, hyperinsulinemia and insulin resistance are strongly linked to chronic inflammation, which in turn is strongly linked to a variety of adverse developments such as arterial microinjuries and clot formation (i.e., heart disease) and exaggerated cell division (i.e., cancer). Hyperinsulinemia and insulin resistance (the so-called metabolic syndrome) are characterized by a combination of abdominal obesity, elevated blood sugar, elevated blood pressure, elevated blood triglycerides, and reduced HDL cholesterol. The negative effect of hyperinsulinemia on prostaglandin PGE1/PGE2 balance may be significant.

The state of obesity clearly contributes to insulin resistance, which in turn can cause type 2 diabetes. Virtually all obese and most type 2 diabetic individuals have marked insulin resistance. Although the association between overweight and insulin resistance is clear, the exact (likely multifarious) causes of insulin resistance remain less clear. It is important to note that it has been demonstrated that appropriate exercise, more regular food intake, and reducing glycemic load all can reverse insulin resistance in overweight individuals (and thereby lower blood sugar levels in those with type 2 diabetes).

Obesity can unfavourably alter hormonal and metabolic status via resistance to the hormone leptin, and a vicious cycle may occur in which insulin/leptin resistance and obesity aggravate one another. The vicious cycle is putatively fuelled by continuously high insulin/leptin stimulation and fat storage, as a result of high intake of strongly insulin/leptin stimulating foods and energy. Both insulin and leptin normally function as satiety signals to the hypothalamus in the brain; however, insulin/leptin resistance may reduce this signal and therefore allow continued overfeeding despite large body fat stores. In addition, reduced leptin signalling to the brain may reduce leptin's normal effect to maintain an appropriately high metabolic rate.

There is a debate about how and to what extent different dietary factors— such as intake of processed carbohydrates, total protein, fat, and carbohydrate intake, intake of saturated and trans fatty acids, and low intake of vitamins/minerals—contribute to the development of insulin and leptin resistance. In any case, analogous to the way modern man-made pollution may possess the potential to overwhelm the environment's ability to maintain homeostasis, the recent explosive introduction of high glycemic index and processed foods into the human diet may possess the potential to overwhelm the body's ability to maintain homeostasis and health (as evidenced by the metabolic syndrome epidemic).

Hyponatremia

Excess water intake, without replenishment of sodium and potassium salts, leads to hyponatremia, which can further lead to water intoxication at more dangerous levels. A well-publicized case occurred in 2007, when Jennifer Strange died while participating in a water-drinking contest. More usually, the condition occurs in long-distance endurance events (such as marathon or triathlon competition and training) and causes gradual mental dulling, headache, drowsiness, weakness, and confusion; extreme cases may result in coma, convulsions, and death. The primary damage comes from swelling of the brain, caused by increased osmosis as blood salinity decreases. Effective fluid replacement techniques include water aid stations during running/cycling races, trainers providing water during team games, such as soccer, and devices such as Camel Baks, which can provide water for a person without making it too hard to drink the water.

Antinutrient

Antinutrients are natural or synthetic compounds that interfere with the absorption of nutrients. Nutrition studies focus on antinutrients commonly found in food sources and beverages.

Sugar Consumption in the United States

The relatively recent increased consumption of sugar has been linked to the rise of some afflictions such as diabetes, obesity, and more recently heart disease. Increased consumption of sugar has been tied to these three, among others. Obesity levels have more than doubled in the last 30 years among adults, going from 15% to 35% in the United States. Obesity and diet also happen to be high risk factors for diabetes. In the same time span that obesity doubled, diabetes numbers quadrupled in America. Increased weight, especially in the form of belly fat, and high sugar intake are also high risk factors for heart disease. Both sugar intake and fatty tissue increase the probability of elevated LDL cholesterol in the bloodstream. Elevated amounts of Low-density lipoprotein (LDL) cholesterol, is the primary factor in heart disease. In order to avoid all the dangers of sugar, moderate consumption is paramount.

Processed Foods

Since the Industrial Revolution some two hundred years ago, the food processing industry has invented many technologies that both help keep foods fresh longer and alter the fresh state of food as they appear in nature. Cooling is the primary technology used to maintain freshness, whereas many more technologies have been invented to allow foods to last longer without becoming spoiled. These latter technologies include pasteurisation, autoclavation, drying, salting, and separation of various components, all of which appearing to alter the original nutritional contents of food. Pasteurisation and autoclavation (heating techniques) have no doubt improved the safety of many common foods, preventing epidemics of bacterial infection. But some of the (new) food processing technologies have downfalls as well.

Modern separation techniques such as milling, centrifugation, and pressing have enabled concentration of particular components of food, yielding flour, oils, juices, and so on, and even separate fatty acids, amino acids, vitamins, and minerals. Inevitably, such large-scale concentration changes the nutritional content of food, saving certain nutrients while removing others. Heating techniques may also reduce food's content of many heat-labile nutrients such as certain vitamins and phytochemicals, and possibly other yet-to-be-discovered substances. Because of reduced nutritional value, processed foods are often 'enriched' or 'fortified' with some of the most critical nutrients (usually certain vitamins) that were lost during processing. Nonetheless, processed foods tend to have an inferior nutritional profile compared to whole, fresh foods, regarding content of both sugar and high GI starches, potassium/sodium, vitamins, fiber, and of intact, unoxidized (essential) fatty acids. In addition, processed foods often contain potentially harmful substances such as oxidized fats and trans fatty acids.

A dramatic example of the effect of food processing on a population's health is the history of epidemics of beri-beri in people subsisting on polished rice. Removing the outer layer of rice by polishing it removes with it the essential vitamin thiamine, causing beri-beri. Another example is the development of scurvy among infants in the late 19th century in the United States. It turned out that the vast majority of sufferers were being fed milk that had been heat-treated (as suggested by Pasteur) to control bacterial disease. Pasteurisation was effective against bacteria, but it destroyed the vitamin C.

As mentioned, lifestyle- and obesity-related diseases are becoming increasingly prevalent all around the world. There is little doubt that the increasingly widespread application of some modern food processing technologies has contributed to this development. The food processing industry is a major part of modern economy, and as such it is influential in political decisions (e.g., nutritional recommendations, agricultural subsidising). In any known profit-driven economy, health considerations are hardly a priority; effective production of cheap foods with a long shelf-life is more the trend. In general, whole, fresh foods have a relatively short shelf-life and are less profitable to produce and sell than are more processed foods. Thus, the consumer is left with the choice between more expensive, but nutritionally superior, whole, fresh foods, and cheap, usually nutritionally inferior, processed foods. Because processed foods are often cheaper, more convenient (in both purchasing, storage, and preparation), and more available, the consumption of nutritionally inferior foods has been increasing throughout the world along with many nutrition-related health complications.

Human Nutrition

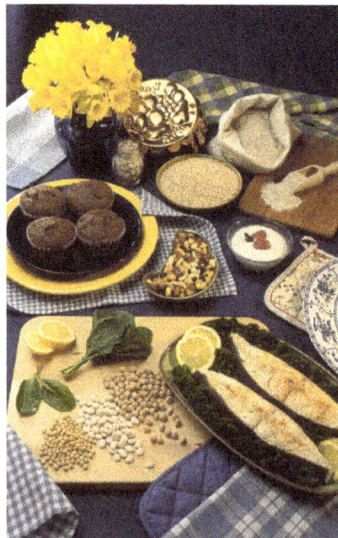

Example of nutrients (in this case for magnesium)

Human nutrition refers to the provision of essential nutrients necessary to support human life and health. Generally, people can survive up to 40 days without food, a period largely depending on the amount of water consumed, stored body fat, muscle mass and genetic factors.

Poor nutrition is a chronic problem often linked to poverty, poor nutrition understanding and practices, and deficient sanitation and food security. Lack of proper nutrition contributes to lower academic performance, lower test scores, and eventually less successful students and a less productive and competitive economy. Malnutrition and its consequences are immense contributors to deaths and disabilities worldwide. Promoting good nutrition helps children grow, promotes human development and advances economic growth and eradication of poverty.

Overview

The human body contains chemical compounds, such as water, carbohydrates (sugar, starch, and fiber), amino acids (in proteins), fatty acids (in lipids), and nucleic acids (DNA and RNA). These compounds consist of elements such as carbon, hydrogen, oxygen, nitrogen, phosphorus, calcium, iron, zinc, magnesium, manganese, and so on. All the chemical compounds and elements contained in the human body occur in various forms and combinations such as hormones, vitamins, phospholipids and hydroxyapatite. These compounds are found in the human body and in the different types of organisms that humans eat.

Any study done to determine nutritional status must take into account the state of the body before and after experiments, as well as the chemical composition of the whole diet and of all the materials excreted and eliminated from the body (including urine and feces). Comparing food to waste material can help determine the specific compounds and elements absorbed and metabolized by the body. The effects of nutrients may only be discernible over an extended period of time, during which all food and waste must be analyzed. The number of variables involved in such experiments is high, making nutritional studies time-consuming and expensive, which explains why the science of human nutrition is still slowly evolving.

Nutrients

The seven major classes of nutrients are: carbohydrates, fats, fiber, minerals, proteins, vitamins, and water. These nutrient classes are categorized as either macronutrients (needed in relatively large amounts) or micronutrients (needed in smaller quantities). The macronutrients are carbohydrates, fats, fiber, proteins, and water. The micronutrients are minerals and vitamins.

The macronutrients (excluding fiber and water) provide structural material (amino acids from which proteins are built, and lipids from which cell membranes and some signaling molecules are built), and energy. Some of the structural material can be used to generate energy internally, and in either case it is measured in Joules or kilocalories (often called "Calories" and written with a capital 'C' to distinguish them from little 'c' calories). Carbohydrates and proteins provide 17 kJ approximately (4 kcal) of energy per gram, while fats provide 37 kJ (9 kcal) per gram, though the net energy from either depends on such factors as absorption and digestive effort, which vary substantially from instance to instance. Vitamins, minerals, fiber, and water do not provide energy, but are required for other reasons. A third class of dietary material, fiber (i.e., nondigestible material such as cellulose), seems also to be required, for both mechanical and biochemical reasons, though the exact reasons remain unclear. For all age groups, males need to consume higher amounts of macronutrients than females. In general, intakes increase with age until the second or third decade of life.

Molecules of carbohydrates and fats consist of carbon, hydrogen, and oxygen atoms. Carbohydrates range from simple monosaccharides (glucose, fructose, galactose) to complex polysaccharides (starch). Fats are triglycerides, made of assorted fatty acid monomers bound to a glycerol backbone. Some fatty acids, but not all, are essential in the diet: they cannot be synthesized in the body. Protein molecules contain nitrogen atoms in addition to carbon, oxygen, and hydrogen. The fundamental components of protein are nitrogen-containing amino acids, some of which are essential in the sense that humans cannot make them internally. Some of the amino acids are convertible (with the expenditure of energy) to glucose and can be used for energy production just as ordinary glucose. By breaking down existing protein, some glucose can be produced internally; the remaining amino acids are discarded, primarily as urea in urine. This occurs naturally when atrophy takes place, or during periods of starvation.

Carbohydrates

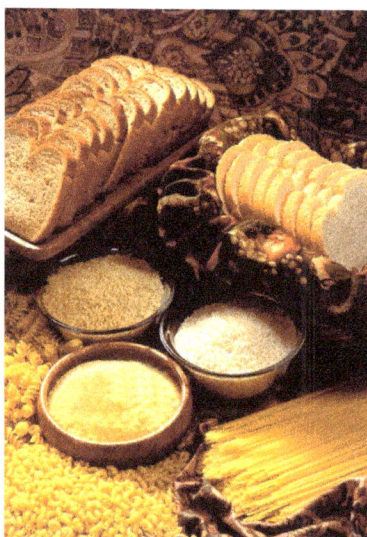

Grain products: rich sources of complex and simple carbohydrates

Carbohydrates may be classified as monosaccharides, disaccharides or polysaccharides depending on the number of monomer (sugar) units they contain. They are a diverse group of substances, with a range of chemical, physical and physiological properties. They make up a large part of foods such as rice, noodles, bread, and other grain-based products.

Monosaccharides contain one sugar unit, disaccharides two, and polysaccharides three or more. Monoscaccharides include glucose, fructose and galactose. Disaccharides include sucrose, lactose, and maltose; purified sucrose, for instance, is used as table sugar. Polysaccharides, which include starch and glycogen, are often referred to as 'complex' carbohydrates because they are typically long multiple-branched chains of sugar units. The difference is that complex carbohydrates take longer to digest and absorb since their sugar units must be separated from the chain before absorption. The spike in blood glucose levels after ingestion of simple sugars is thought to be related to some of the heart and vascular diseases, which have become more common in recent times. Simple sugars form a greater part of modern diets than in the past, perhaps leading to more cardiovascular disease. The degree of causation is still not clear.

Simple carbohydrates are absorbed quickly, and therefore raise blood-sugar levels more rapidly than other nutrients. However, the most important plant carbohydrate nutrient, starch, varies in its absorption. Gelatinized starch (starch heated for a few minutes in the presence of water) is far more digestible than plain starch, and starch which has been divided into fine particles is also more absorbable during digestion. The increased effort and decreased availability reduces the available energy from starchy foods substantially and can be seen experimentally in rats and anecdotally in humans. Additionally, up to a third of dietary starch may be unavailable due to mechanical or chemical difficulty.

Fat

A molecule of dietary fat typically consists of several fatty acids (containing long chains of carbon and hydrogen atoms), bonded to a glycerol. They are typically found as triglycerides (three fatty acids attached to one glycerol backbone). Fats may be classified as saturated or unsaturated depending on the detailed structure of the fatty acids involved. Saturated fats have all of the carbon atoms in their fatty acid chains bonded to hydrogen atoms, whereas unsaturated fats have some of these carbon atoms double-bonded, so their molecules have relatively fewer hydrogen atoms than a saturated fatty acid of the same length. Unsaturated fats may be further classified as monounsaturated (one double-bond) or polyunsaturated (many double-bonds). Furthermore, depending on the location of the double-bond in the fatty acid chain, unsaturated fatty acids are classified as omega-3 or omega-6 fatty acids. Trans fats are a type of unsaturated fat with *trans*-isomer bonds; these are rare in nature and in foods from natural sources; they are typically created in an industrial process called (partial) hydrogenation.

Many studies have shown that consumption of unsaturated fats, particularly monounsaturated fats, is associated with better health in humans. Saturated fats, typically from animal sources, are next in order of preference, while trans fats are associated with a variety of disease and should be avoided. Saturated and some trans fats are typically solid at room temperature (such as butter or lard), while unsaturated fats are typically liquids (such as olive oil or flaxseed oil). Trans fats are very rare in nature, but have properties useful in the food processing industry, such as rancidity resistance.

Most fatty acids are not essential, meaning the body can produce them as needed, generally from other fatty acids and always by expending energy to do so. However, in humans, at least two fatty acids are essential and must be included in the diet. An appropriate balance of essential fatty acids – omega-3 and omega-6 fatty acids – seems also important for health, though definitive experimental demonstration has been elusive. Both of these "omega" long-chain polyunsaturated fatty acids are substrates for a class of eicosanoids known as prostaglandins, which have roles throughout the human body. They are hormones, in some respects. The omega-3 eicosapentaenoic acid (EPA), which can be made in the human body from the omega-3 essential fatty acid alpha-linolenic acid (LNA), or taken in through marine food sources, serves as a building block for series 3 prostaglandins (e.g. weakly inflammatory PGE3). The omega-6 dihomo-gamma-linolenic acid (DGLA) serves as a building block for series 1 prostaglandins (e.g. anti-inflammatory PGE1), whereas arachidonic acid (AA) serves as a building block for series 2 prostaglandins (e.g., pro-inflammatory PGE 2). Both DGLA and AA can be made from the omega-6 linoleic acid (LA) in the human body, or can be taken in directly through food. An appropriately balanced intake of omega-3 and omega-6 partly determines the relative production of different prostaglandins: one reason a balance between omega-3 and omega-6 is believed important for cardiovascular health. In industrialized societies, people typically consume large amounts of processed vegetable oils, which have reduced amounts of the essential fatty acids along with too much of omega-6 fatty acids relative to omega-3 fatty acids.

Fiber

Dietary fiber is a carbohydrate, specifically a polysaccharide, which is incompletely absorbed in humans and in some animals. Like all carbohydrates, when it is metabolized, it can produce four Calories (kilocalories) of energy per gram, but in most circumstances, it accounts for less than that because of its limited absorption and digestibility. The two subcategories are insoluble and soluble fiber. Insoluble dietary fiber consists mainly of cellulose, a large carbohydrate polymer that is indigestible by humans, because humans do not have the required enzymes to break it down, and the human digestive system does not harbor enough of the types of microbes that can do so. Soluble dietary fiber comprises a variety of oligosaccharides, waxes, esters, resistant starches, and other carbohydrates that dissolve or gelatinize in water. Many of these soluble fibers can be fermented or partially fermented by microbes in the human digestive system to produce short-chain fatty acids which are absorbed and therefore introduce some caloric content.

Whole grains, beans and other legumes, fruits (especially plums, prunes, and figs), and vegetables are good sources of dietary fiber. Fiber is important to digestive health and is thought to reduce the risk of colon cancer. For mechanical reasons, fiber can help in alleviating both constipation and diarrhea. Fiber provides bulk to the intestinal contents, and insoluble fiber especially stimulates peristalsis – the rhythmic muscular contractions of the intestines which move digesta along the digestive tract. Some soluble fibers produce a solution of high viscosity; this is essentially a gel, which slows the movement of food through the intestines. Additionally, fiber, perhaps especially that from whole grains, may help lessen insulin spikes and reduce the risk of type 2 diabetes.

Protein

Proteins are the basis of many animal body structures (e.g. muscles, skin, and hair) and form the enzymes which catalyse chemical reactions throughout the body. Each protein molecule is composed of amino acids which contain nitrogen and sometimes sulphur (these components are responsible for the distinctive smell of burning protein, such as the keratin in hair). The body requires amino acids to produce new proteins (protein retention) and to replace damaged proteins (maintenance). Amino acids are soluble in the digestive juices within the small intestine, where they are absorbed into the blood. Once absorbed, they cannot be stored in the body, so they are either metabolized as required or excreted in the urine.

Proteins consist of amino acids in different proportions. The most important aspect and defining characteristic of protein from a nutritional standpoint is its amino acid composition. Amino acids which an animal cannot synthesize on its own from smaller molecules are deemed essential. The synthesis of some amino acids can be limited under special pathophysiological conditions, such as

prematurity in the infant or individuals in severe catabolic distress, and they are called conditionally essential. Foods containing protein can be rated on their relative content of amino acids, for
instance by protein digestibility corrected amino acid score and biological value.

It is a common misconception that a vegetarian diet will be insufficient in essential proteins; both
vegetarians and vegans of any age and gender, with a healthy diet, can flourish throughout all
stages of life, although the latter group typically needs to pay more attention to their nutrition than
the former.

Minerals

Dietary minerals are the chemical elements required by living organisms, other than the four elements carbon, hydrogen, nitrogen, and oxygen that are present in nearly all organic molecules.
The term "mineral" is archaic, since the intent is to describe simply the less common elements in
the diet. Some are heavier than the four just mentioned – including several metals, which often
occur as ions in the body. Some dietitians recommend that these be supplied from foods in which
they occur naturally, or at least as complex compounds, or sometimes even from natural inorganic
sources (such as calcium carbonate from ground oyster shells). Some are absorbed much more
readily in the ionic forms found in such sources. On the other hand, minerals are often artificially
added to the diet as supplements; the most famous is likely iodine in iodized salt which prevents
goiter.

Essential Dietary Minerals

include the following:

- Chlorine as chloride ions; very common electrolyte.

- Magnesium, required for processing ATP and related reactions (builds bone, causes strong
peristalsis, increases flexibility, increases alkalinity). Approximately 50% is in bone, the
remaining 50% is almost all inside body cells, with only about 1% located in extracellular
fluid. Food sources include oats, buckwheat, tofu, nuts, caviar, green leafy vegetables, legumes, and chocolate.

- Phosphorus, required component of bones; essential for energy processing Approximately
80% is found in inorganic portion of bones and teeth. Phosphorus is a component of every
cell, as well as important metabolites, including DNA, RNA, ATP, and phospholipids. Also
important in pH regulation. Food sources include cheese, egg yolk, milk, meat, fish, poultry, whole-grain cereals, and many others.

- Potassium, a very common electrolyte (heart and nerve health). With sodium, potassium
is involved in maintaining normal water balance, osmotic equilibrium, and acid-base balance. In addition to calcium, it is important in the regulation of neuromuscular activity.
Food sources include bananas, avocados, vegetables, potatoes, legumes, fish, and mush-
rooms.

- Sodium, a very common electrolyte; not generally found in dietary supplements, despite
being needed in large quantities, because the ion is very common in food: typically as sodium chloride, or common salt

Trace Minerals

Many elements are required in smaller amounts (microgram quantities), usually because they play a catalytic role in enzymes. Some trace mineral elements (RDA < 200 mg/day) are, in alphabetical order:

- Cobalt required for biosynthesis of vitamin B_{12} family of coenzymes
- Copper required component of many redox enzymes, including cytochrome c oxidase
- Chromium required for sugar metabolism
- Iodine required not only for the biosynthesis of thyroxin, but probably, for other important organs as breast, stomach, salivary glands, thymus etc. For this reason iodine is needed in larger quantities than others in this list, and sometimes classified with the macrominerals
- Iron required for many enzymes, and for hemoglobin and some other proteins
- Manganese (processing of oxygen)
- Molybdenum required for xanthine oxidase and related oxidases
- Nickel present in urease
- Selenium required for peroxidase (antioxidant proteins)
- Zinc required for several enzymes such as carboxypeptidase, liver alcohol dehydrogenase, carbonic anhydrase

Vitamins

As with the minerals discussed above, some vitamins are recognized as essential nutrients, necessary in the diet for good health. (Vitamin D is the exception: it can alternatively be synthesized in the skin, in the presence of UVB radiation.) Certain vitamin-like compounds that are recommended in the diet, such as carnitine, are thought useful for survival and health, but these are not "essential" dietary nutrients because the human body has some capacity to produce them from other compounds. Moreover, thousands of different phytochemicals have recently been discovered in food (particularly in fresh vegetables), which may have desirable properties including antioxidant activity; experimental demonstration has been suggestive but inconclusive. Other essential nutrients not classed as vitamins include essential amino acids, essential fatty acids, and the minerals discussed in the preceding section.

Vitamin deficiencies may result in disease conditions: goiter, scurvy, osteoporosis, impaired immune system, disorders of cell metabolism, certain forms of cancer, symptoms of premature aging, and poor psychological health (including eating disorders), among many others.

Malnutrition

Malnutrition refers to insufficient, excessive, or imbalanced consumption of nutrients. In developed countries, the diseases of malnutrition are most often associated with nutritional imbalances or excessive consumption. Although there are more people in the world who are malnourished due to excessive consumption, according to the United Nations World Health Organization, the greatest challenge in developing nations today is not starvation, but insufficient nutrition – the lack of nutrients necessary for the growth and maintenance of vital functions. The causes of malnutrition are directly linked to inadequate macronutrient consumption and disease, and are indirectly linked to factors like "household food security, maternal and child care, health services, and the environment."

Illnesses

Nutrients*	Deficiency	Excess
Food Energy	starvation, marasmus	obesity, diabetes mellitus, cardiovascular disease
Simple carbohydrates	None.	diabetes mellitus, obesity
Complex carbohydrates	none	obesity
Saturated fat	low sex hormone levels	cardiovascular disease
Trans fat	none	cardiovascular disease
Unsaturated fat	none	obesity
Fat	malabsorption of fat-soluble vitamins, rabbit starvation (if protein intake is high), during development: stunted brain development and reduced brain weight.	cardiovascular disease
Omega-3 fats	cardiovascular disease	bleeding, hemorrhages
Omega-6 fats	none	cardiovascular disease, cancer
Cholesterol	during development: deficiencies in myelinization of the brain.	cardiovascular disease
Protein	kwashiorkor	
Sodium	hyponatremia	hypernatremia, hypertension
Iron	anemia	cirrhosis, cardiovascular disease
Iodine	goiter, hypothyroidism	Iodine toxicity (goiter, hypothyroidism)
Vitamin A	xerophthalmia and night blindness, low testosterone levels	hypervitaminosis A (cirrhosis, hair loss)
Vitamin B$_1$	beriberi	
Vitamin B$_2$	cracking of skin and corneal unclearation	
Niacin	pellagra	dyspepsia, cardiac arrhythmias, birth defects
Vitamin B$_{12}$	pernicious anemia	
Vitamin C	scurvy	diarrhea causing dehydration
Vitamin D	rickets, osteoporosis, balance, immune system, inflammation	hypervitaminosis D (dehydration, vomiting, constipation)
Vitamin E	nervous disorders	hypervitaminosis E (anticoagulant: excessive bleeding)

Vitamin K	hemorrhage	
Calcium	osteoporosis, tetany, carpopedal spasm, laryngospasm, cardiac arrhythmias	fatigue, depression, confusion, anorexia, nausea, vomiting, constipation, pancreatitis, increased urination
Magnesium	hypertension	weakness, nausea, vomiting, impaired breathing, and hypotension
Potassium	hypokalemia, cardiac arrhythmias	hyperkalemia, palpitations

Mental Agility

Research indicates that improving the awareness of nutritious meal choices and establishing long-term habits of healthy eating has a positive effect on a cognitive and spatial memory capacity, potentially increasing a student's potential to process and retain academic information.

Some organizations have begun working with teachers, policymakers, and managed foodservice contractors to mandate improved nutritional content and increased nutritional resources in school cafeterias from primary to university level institutions. Health and nutrition have been proven to have close links with overall educational success. Currently less than 10% of American college students report that they eat the recommended five servings of fruit and vegetables daily. Better nutrition has been shown to affect both cognitive and spatial memory performance; a study showed those with higher blood sugar levels performed better on certain memory tests. In another study, those who consumed yogurt performed better on thinking tasks when compared to those who consumed caffeine free diet soda or confections. Nutritional deficiencies have been shown to have a negative effect on learning behavior in mice as far back as 1951."Better learning performance is associated with diet induced effects on learning and memory ability".

- The "nutrition-learning nexus" demonstrates the correlation between diet and learning and has application in a higher education setting..

- We find that better nourished children perform significantly better in school, partly because they enter school earlier and thus have more time to learn but mostly because of greater learning productivity per year of schooling."

- 91% of college students feel that they are in good health while only 7% eat their recommended daily allowance of fruits and vegetables.

- Nutritional education is an effective and workable model in a higher education setting.

- More "engaged" learning models that encompass nutrition is an idea that is picking up steam at all levels of the learning cycle.

Mental Disorders

Nutritional supplement treatment may be appropriate for major depression, bipolar disorder, schizophrenia, and obsessive compulsive disorder, the four most common mental disorders in developed countries. It is because Lakhan and Vieira mentioned that the supplements possess amino acids that may change into neurotransmitters and improve mental disorders. Supplements that have been studied most for mood elevation and stabilization include eicosapentaenoic acid and docosahexaenoic acid (each of which are an omega-3 fatty acid contained in fish oil, but not in flaxseed oil), vitamin B$_{12}$, folic acid, and inositol.

Cancer

Cancer has become common in developing countries. According to a study by the International Agency for Research on Cancer, "In the developing world, cancers of the liver, stomach and esophagus were more common, often linked to consumption of carcinogenic preserved foods, such as smoked or salted food, and parasitic infections that attack organs." Lung cancer rates are rising rapidly in poorer nations because of increased use of tobacco. Developed countries "tended to have cancers linked to affluence or a 'Western lifestyle' – cancers of the colon, rectum, breast and prostate – that can be caused by obesity, lack of exercise, diet and age."

A comprehensive worldwide report, "Food, Nutrition, Physical Activity and the Prevention of Cancer: a Global Perspective", compiled by the World Cancer Research Fund and the American Institute for Cancer Research, reports that there is a significant relation between lifestyle (including food consumption) and cancer prevention. The same report recommends eating mostly foods of plant origin and aiming to meet nutritional needs through diet alone, while limiting consumption of energy-dense foods, red meat, alcoholic drinks and salt and avoiding sugary drinks, processed meat and moldy cereals (grains) or pulses (legumes). Protein consumption leads to an increase in IGF-1, which plays a role in cancer development.

Metabolic Syndrome and Obesity

Several lines of evidence indicate lifestyle-induced hyperinsulinemia and reduced insulin function (i.e. insulin resistance) as decisive factors in many disease states. For example, hyperinsulinemia and insulin resistance are strongly linked to chronic inflammation, which in turn is strongly linked to a variety of adverse developments such as arterial microinjuries and clot formation (i.e. heart disease) and exaggerated cell division (i.e. cancer). Hyperinsulinemia and insulin resistance (the so-called metabolic syndrome) are characterized by a combination of abdominal obesity, elevated blood sugar, elevated blood pressure, elevated blood triglycerides, and reduced HDL cholesterol.

Obesity can unfavourably alter hormonal and metabolic status via resistance to the hormone leptin, and a vicious cycle may occur in which insulin/leptin resistance and obesity aggravate one another. The vicious cycle is putatively fuelled by continuously high insulin/leptin stimulation and fat storage, as a result of high intake of strongly insulin/leptin stimulating foods and energy. Both insulin and leptin normally function as satiety signals to the hypothalamus in the brain; however, insulin/leptin resistance may reduce this signal and therefore allow continued overfeeding despite large body fat stores.

There is a debate about how and to what extent different dietary factors – such as intake of processed carbohydrates, total protein, fat, and carbohydrate intake, intake of saturated and trans fatty acids, and low intake of vitamins/minerals – contribute to the development of insulin and leptin resistance. Evidence indicates that diets possibly protective against metabolic syndrome include low saturated and trans fat intake and foods rich in dietary fiber, such as high consumption of fruits and vegetables and moderate intake of low-fat dairy products.

Hyponatremia

Excess water intake, without replenishment of sodium and potassium salts, leads to hyponatremia, which can further lead to water intoxication at more dangerous levels. A well-publicized case occurred in 2007, when Jennifer Strange died while participating in a water-drinking contest. More usually, the condition occurs in long-distance endurance events (such as marathon or triathlon competition and training) and causes gradual mental dulling, headache, drowsiness, weakness, and confusion; extreme cases may result in coma, convulsions, and death. The primary damage comes from swelling of the brain, caused by increased osmosis as blood salinity decreases. Effective fluid replacement techniques include Water aid stations during running/cycling races, trainers providing water during team games such as Soccer and devices such as Camel Baks which can provide water for a person without making it too hard to drink the water.

Global Nutrition Challenges

The challenges facing global nutrition are disease, child malnutrition, obesity, and vitamin deficiency.

Disease

The most common non-infectious diseases worldwide, that contribute most to the global mortality rate, are cardiovascular diseases, various cancers, diabetes, and chronic respiratory problems, all of which are linked to poor nutrition. Nutrition and diet are closely associated with the leading causes of death, including cardiovascular disease and cancer. Obesity and high sodium intake can contribute to ischemic heart disease, while consumption of fruits and vegetables can decrease the risk of developing cancer.

Foodborne and infectious diseases can result in malnutrition, and malnutrition exacerbates infectious disease. Poor nutrition leaves children and adults more susceptible to contracting life-threatening diseases such as diarrheal infections and respiratory infections. According to the WHO, in 2011, 6.9 million children died of infectious diseases like pneumonia, diarrhea, malaria, and neonatal conditions, of which at least one third were associated with undernutrition.

Child Malnutrition

According to UNICEF, in 2011, 101 million children across the globe were underweight and one in four children, 165 million, were stunted in growth. Simultaneously, there are 43 million children under five who are overweight or obese. Nearly 20 million children under 5 suffer from severe acute malnutrition, a life-threatening condition requiring urgent treatment. According to estimations at UNICEF, hunger will be responsible for 5.6 million deaths of children under the age of five this year. These all represent significant public health emergencies. This is because proper maternal and child nutrition has immense consequences for survival, acute and chronic disease incidence, normal growth, and economic productivity of individuals.

Childhood malnutrition is common and contributes to the global burden of disease. Childhood is a particularly important time to achieve good nutrition status, because poor nutrition has the capability to lock a child in a vicious cycle of disease susceptibility and recurring sickness, which threatens cognitive and social development. Undernutrition and bias in access to food and health services leaves children less likely to attend or perform well in school.

Under Nutrition

UNICEF defines under nutrition "as the outcome of insufficient food intake (hunger) and repeated infectious diseases. Under nutrition includes being underweight for one's age, too short for one's age (stunted), dangerously thin (wasted), and deficient in vitamins and minerals (micronutrient malnutrient). Under nutrition causes 53% of deaths of children under five across the world. It has been estimated that undernutrition is the underlying cause for 35% of child deaths. The Maternal and Child Nutrition Study Group estimate that under nutrition, "including fetal growth restriction, stunting, wasting, deficiencies of vitamin A and zinc along with suboptimum breastfeeding- is a cause of 3.1 million child deaths and infant mortality, or 45% of all child deaths in 2011".

When humans are undernourished, they no longer maintain normal bodily functions, such as growth, resistance to infection, or have satisfactory performance in school or work. Major causes of under nutrition in young children include lack of proper breast feeding for infants and illnesses such as diarrhea, pneumonia, malaria, and HIV/AIDS. According to UNICEF 146 million children across the globe, that one out of four under the age of five, are underweight. The amount of underweight children has decreased since 1990, from 33 percent to 28 percent between 1990 and 2004. Underweight and stunted children are more susceptible to infection, more likely to fall behind in school, more likely to become overweight and develop non-infectious diseases, and ultimately earn less than their non-stunted coworkers. Therefore, undernutrition can accumulate deficiencies in health which results in less productive individuals and societies

Many children are born with the inherent disadvantage of low birth weight, often caused by intra-uterine growth restriction and poor maternal nutrition, which results in worse growth, development, and health throughout the course of their lifetime. Children born at low birthweight (less than 5.5 pounds), are less likely to be healthy and are more susceptible to disease and early death. Those born at low birthweight also are likely to have a depressed immune system, which can increase their chances of heart disease and diabetes later on in life. Because 96% of low birthweight occurs in the developing world, low birthweight is associated with being born to a mother in poverty with poor nutritional status that has had to perform demanding labor.

Stunting and other forms of undernutrition reduces a child's chance of survival and hinders their optimal growth and health. Stunting has demonstrated association with poor brain development, which reduces cognitive ability, academic performance, and eventually earning potential. Important determinants of stunting include the quality and frequency of infant and child feeding, infectious disease susceptibility, and the mother's nutrition and health status. Undernourished mothers are more likely to birth stunted children, perpetuating a cycle of undernutrition and poverty. Stunted children are more likely to develop obesity and chronic diseases upon reaching adulthood. Therefore, malnutrition resulting in stunting can further worsen the obesity epidemic, especially in low and middle income countries. This creates even new economic and social challenges for vulnerable impoverished groups.

Data on global and regional food supply shows that consumption rose from 2011-2012 in all regions. Diets became more diverse, with a decrease in consumption of cereals and roots and an increase in fruits, vegetables, and meat products. However, this increase masks the discrepancies between nations, where Africa, in particular, saw a decrease in food consumption over the same years. This information is derived from food balance sheets that reflect national food supplies, however, this does not necessarily reflect the distribution of micro and macronutrients. Often inequality in food access leaves distribution which uneven, resulting in undernourishment for some and obesity for others.

Undernourishment, or hunger, according to the FAO, is dietary intake below the minimum daily energy requirement. The amount of undernourishment is calculated utilizing the average amount of food available for consumption, the size of the population, the relative disparities in access to the food, and the minimum calories required for each individual. According to FAO, 868 million people (12% of the global population) were undernourished in 2012. This has decreased across the world since 1990, in all regions except for Africa, where undernourishment has steadily increased. However, the rates of decrease are not sufficient to meet the first Millennium Development Goal of halving hunger between 1990 and 2015. The global financial, economic, and food price crisis in 2008 drove many people to hunger, especially women and children. The spike in food prices prevented many people from escaping poverty, because the poor spend a larger proportion of their income on food and farmers are net consumers of food. High food prices cause consumers to have less purchasing power and to substitute more-nutritious foods with low-cost alternatives.

Adult Overweight and Obesity

Malnutrition in industrialized nations is primarily due to excess calories and non-nutritious carbohydrates, which has contributed to the obesity epidemic affecting both developed and some developing nations. In 2008, 35% of adults above the age of 20 years were overweight (BMI 25 kg/m), a prevalence that has doubled worldwide between 1980 and 2008. Also 10% of men and 14% of women were obese, with an BMI greater than 30. Rates of overweight and obesity vary across the globe, with the highest prevalence in the Americas, followed by European nations, where over 50% of the population is overweight or obese.

Obesity is more prevalent amongst high income and higher middle income groups than lower divisions of income. Women are more likely than men to be obese, where the rate of obesity in women doubled from 8% to 14% between 1980 and 2008. Being overweight as a child has become an increasingly important indicator for later development of obesity and non-infectious diseases such as heart disease. In several western European nations, the prevalence of overweight and obese children rose by 10% from 1980 to 1990, a rate that has begun to accelerate recently.

Vitamin and Mineral Malnutrition

Vitamins and minerals are essential to the proper functioning and maintenance of the human body. Globally, particularly in developing nations, deficiencies in Iodine, Iron and Zinc amog others are said to impair human health when these minerals are not ingested in an adequate quantity. There are 20 trace elements and minerals that are essential in small quantities to body function and overall human health.

Iron deficiency is the most common inadequate nutrient worldwide, affecting approximately 2 billion people. Globally, anemia affects 1.6 billion people, and represents a public health emergency in children under five and mothers. The World Health Organization estimates that there exists 469 million women of reproductive age and approximately 600 million preschool and school-age children worldwide who are anemic. Anemia, especially iron-deficient anemia, is a critical problem for cognitive developments in children, and its presence leads to maternal deaths and poor brain and motor development in children. The development of anemia affects mothers and children more because infants and children have higher iron requirements for growth. Health consequences for iron deficiency in young children include increased perinatal mortality, delayed mental and physical development, negative behavioral consequences, reduced auditory and visual function, and impaired physical performance. The harm caused by iron deficiency during child development cannot be reversed and result in reduced academic performance, poor physical work capacity, and decreased productivity in adulthood. Mothers are also very susceptible to iron-deficient anemia because women lose iron during menstruation, and rarely supplement it in their diet. Maternal iron deficiency anemia increases the chances of maternal mortality, contributing to at least 18% of maternal deaths in low and middle income countries.

Vitamin A plays an essential role in developing the immune system in children, therefore, it is considered an essential micronutrient that can greatly affect health. However, because of the expense of testing for deficiencies, many developing nations have not been able to fully detect and address vitamin A deficiency, leaving vitamin A deficiency considered a silent hunger. According to estimates, subclinical vitamin A deficiency, characterized by low retinol levels, affects 190 million pre-school children and 19 million mothers worldwide. The WHO estimates that 5.2 million of these children under 5 are affected by night blindness, which is considered clinical vitamin A deficiency. Severe vitamin A deficiency (VAD) for developing children can result in visual impairments, anemia and weakened immunity, and increase their risk of morbidity and mortality from infectious disease. This also presents a problem for women, with WHO estimating that 9.8 million women are affected by night blindness. Clinical vitamin A deficiency is particularly common among pregnant women, with prevalence rates as high as 9.8% in South-East Asia.

Estimates say that 28.5% of the global population is iodine deficient, representing 1.88 billion individuals. Although salt iodization programs have reduced the prevalence of iodine deficiency, this is still a public health concern in 32 nations. Moderate deficiencies are common in Europe and Africa, and over consumption is common in the Americas. Iodine-deficient diets can interfere with adequate thyroid hormone production, which is responsible for normal growth in the brain and nervous system. This ultimately leads to poor school performance and impaired intellectual capabilities.

Infant and Young Child Feeding

Improvement of breast feeding practices, like early initiation and exclusive breast feeding for the first two years of life, could save the lives of 1.5 million children annually. Nutrition interventions targeted at infants aged 0–5 months first encourages early initiation of breastfeeding. Though the relationship between early initiation of breast feeding and improved health outcomes has not been formally established, a recent study in Ghana suggests a causal relationship between early initiation and reduced infection-caused neo-natal deaths. Also, experts promote exclusive breastfeeding, rather than using formula, which has shown to promote optimal growth, development, and health of infants. Exclusive breasfeeding often indicates nutritional status because infants that consume breast milk are more likely to receive all adequate nourishment and nutrients that will aid their developing body and immune system. This leaves children less likely to contract diarrheal diseases and respiratory infections.

Besides the quality and frequency of breastfeeding, the nutritional status of mothers affects infant health. When mothers do not receive proper nutrition, it threatens the wellness and potential of their children. Well-nourished women are less likely to experience risks of birth and are more likely to deliver children who will develop well physically and mentally. Maternal undernutrition increases the chances of low-birth weight, which can increase the risk of infections and asphyxia in fetuses, increasing the probability of neonatal deaths. Growth failure during intrauterine conditions, associated with improper mother nutrition, can contribute to lifelong health complications. Approximately 13 million children are born with intrauterine growth restriction annually.

International Food Insecurity and Malnutrition

According to UNICEF, South Asia has the highest levels of underweight children under five, followed by sub-Saharan Africans nations, with Industrialized countries and Latin nations having the lowest rates.

United States

In the United States, 2% of children are underweight, with under 1% stunted and 6% are wasting.

In the US, dietitians are registered (RD) or licensed (LD) with the Commission for Dietetic Registration and the American Dietetic Association, and are only able to use the title "dietitian," as described by the business and professions codes of each respective state, when they have met specific educational and experiential prerequisites and passed a national registration or licensure examination, respectively. In California, registered dietitians must abide by the *"Business and Professions Code of Section 2585-2586.8"*. Anyone may call themselves a nutritionist, including unqualified dietitians, as this term is unregulated. Some states, such as the State of Florida, have begun to include the title "nutritionist" in state licensure requirements. Most governments provide guidance on nutrition, and some also impose mandatory disclosure/labeling requirements for processed food manufacturers and restaurants to assist consumers in complying with such guidance.

In the US, nutritional standards and recommendations are established jointly by the US Department of Agriculture and US Department of Health and Human Services. Dietary and physical activity guidelines from the USDA are presented in the concept of a plate of food which in 2011 superseded the food pyramid that had replaced the Four Food Groups. The Senate committee currently responsible for oversight of the USDA is the *Agriculture, Nutrition and Forestry Committee*. Committee hearings are often televised on C-SPAN. The U.S. Department of Health and Human Services provides a sample week-long menu which fulfills the nutritional recommendations of the government. Canada's Food Guide is another governmental recommendation.

Industrialized Countries

According to UNICEF, the Commonwealth of Independent States has the lowest rates of stunting and wasting, at 14 percent and 3 percent. The nations of Estonia, Finland, Iceland, Lithuania and Sweden have the lowest prevalence of low birthweight children in the world- at 4%. Proper prenatal nutrition is responsible for this small prevalence of low birthweight infants. However, low birthweight rates are increasing, due to the use of fertility drugs, resulting in multiple births, women bearing children at an older age, and the advancement of technology allowing more pre-term infants to survive. Industrialized nations more often face malnutrition in the form of over-nutrition from excess calories and non-nutritious carbohydrates, which has contributed greatly to the public health epidemic of obesity. Disparities, according to gender, geographic location and socio-economic position, both within and between countries, represent the biggest threat to child nutrition in industrialized countries. These disparities are a direct product of social inequalities and social inequalities are rising throughout the industrialized world, particularly in Europe.

South Asia

South Asia has the highest percentage and number of underweight children under five in the world, at approximately 78 million children. Patterns of stunting and wasting are similar, where 44% have not reached optimal height and 15% are wasted, rates much higher than any other regions. This region of the world has extremely high rates of child underweight- 46% of its child population under five is underweight. India, Bangladesh, and Pakistan alone account for half the globe's underweight child population. South Asian nations have made progress towards the MDGs, considering the rate has decreased from 53% since 1990, however, a 1.7% decrease of underweight prevalence per year will not be sufficient to meet the 2015 goal. Some nations, such as Afghanistan, Bangladesh, and Sri Lanka, on the other hand, have made significant improvements, all decreasing their prevalence by half in ten years. While India and Pakistan have made modest improvements, Nepal has made no significant improvement in underweight child prevalence. Other forms of undernutrition have continued to persist with high resistance to improvement, such as the prevalence of stunting and wasting, which has not changed significantly in the past 10 years. Causes of this poor nutrition include energy-insufficient diets, poor sanitation conditions, and the gender disparities in educational and social status. Girls and women face discrimination especially in nutrition status, where South Asia is the only region in the world where girls are more likely to be underweight than boys. In South Asia, 60% of children in the lowest quintile are underweight, compared to only 26% in the highest quintile, and the rate of reduction of underweight is slower amongst the poorest.

Eastern/South Africa

The Eastern and Southern African nations have shown no improvement since 1990 in the rate of underweight children under five. They have also made no progress in halving hunger by 2015, the most prevalent Millennium Development Goal. This is due primarily to the prevalence of famine, declined agricultural productivity, food emergencies, drought, conflict, and increased poverty. This, along with HIV/AIDS, has inhibited the nutrition development of nations such as Lesotho, Malawi, Mozambique, Swaziland, Zambia and Zimbabwe. Botswana has made remarkable achievements in reducing underweight prevalence, dropping 4% in 4 years, despite its place as the second leader in HIV prevalence amongst adults in the globe. South Africa, the wealthiest nation in this region, has the second lowest proportion of underweight children at 12%, but has been steadily increasing in underweight prevalence since 1995. Almost half of Ethiopian children are underweight, and along with Nigeria, they account for almost one-third of the underweight under five in all of Sub-Saharan Africa.

West/Central Africa

West/Central Africa has the highest rate of children under five underweight in the world. Of the countries in this region, the Congo has the lowest rate at 14%, while the nations of Democratic Republic of the Congo, Ghana, Guinea, Mali, Nigeria, Senegal and Togo are improving slowly. In Gambia, rates decreased from 26% to 17% in four years, and their coverage of vitamin A supplementation reaches 91% of vulnerable populations. This region has the next highest proportion of wasted children, with 10% of the population under five not at optimal weight. Little improvement has been made between the years of 1990 and 2004 in reducing the rates of underweight children under five, whose rate stayed approximately the same. Sierra Leone has the highest child under five mortality rate in the world, due predominantly to its extreme infant mortality rate, at 238 deaths per 1000 live births. Other contributing factors include the high rate of low birthweight children (23%) and low levels of exclusive breast feeding (4%). Anemia is prevalent in these nations, with unacceptable rates of iron deficient anemia. The nutritional status of children is further indicated by its high rate of child wasting - 10%. Wasting is a significant problem in Sahelian countries – Burkina Faso, Chad, Mali, Mauritania and Niger – where rates fall between 11% and 19% of under fives, affecting more than 1 million children.

Middle East/North Africa

Six countries in the Middle East and North Africa region are on target to meet goals for reducing underweight children by 2015, and 12 countries have prevalence rates below 10%. However, the nutrition of children in the region as a whole has degraded for the past ten years due to the increasing portion of underweight children in three populous nations – Iraq, Sudan, and Yemen. Forty six percent of all children in Yemen are underweight, a percentage that has worsened by 4% since 1990. In Yemen, 53% of children under five are stunted and 32% are born at low birth weight. Sudan has an underweight prevalence of 41%, and the highest proportion of wasted children in the region at 16%. One percent of households in Sudan consume iodized salt. Iraq has also seen an increase in child underweight since 1990. Djibouti, Jordan, the Occupied Palestinian Territory (OPT), Oman, the Syrian Arab Republic and Tunisia are all projected to meet minimum nutrition goals, with OPT, Syrian AR, and Tunisia the fastest improving regions. This region demonstrates that undernutrition does not always improve with economic prosperity, where the United Arab Emirates, for example, despite being a wealthy nation, has similar child death rates due to malnutrition to those seen in Yemen.

East Asia/Pacific

The East Asia/Pacific region has reached its goals on nutrition, in part due to the improvements contributed by China, the region's most populous country. China has reduced its underweight prevalence from 19 percent to 8 percent between 1990 and 2002. China played the largest role in the world in decreasing the rate of children under five underweight between 1990 and 2004, halving the prevalence. This reduction of underweight prevalence has aided in the lowering of the under 5 mortality rate from 49 to 31 of 1000. They also have a low birthweight rate at 4%, a rate comparable to industrialized countries, and over 90% of households receive adequate iodized salts. However, large disparities exist between children in rural and urban areas, where 5 provinces in China leave 1.5 million children iodine deficient and susceptible to diseases. Singapore, Vietnam, Malaysia, and Indonesia are all projected to reach nutrition MDGs. Singapore has the lowest under five mortality rate of any nation, besides Iceland, in the world, at 3%. Cambodia has the highest rate of child mortality in the region (141 per 1,000 live births), while still its proportion of underweight children increased by 5 percent to 45% in 2000. Further nutrient indicators show that only 12 per cent of Cambodian babies are exclusively breastfed and only 14 per cent of households consume iodized salt.

Latin America/Caribbean

This region has undergone the fastest progress in decreasing poor nutrition status of children in the world. The Latin American region has reduced underweight children prevalence by 3.8% every year between 1990 and 2004, with a current rate of 7% underweight. They also have the lowest rate of child mortality in the developing world, with only 31 per 1000 deaths, and the highest iodine consumption. Cuba has seen improvement from 9 to 4 percent underweight under 5 between 1996 and 2004. The prevalence has also decreased in the Dominican Republic, Jamaica, Peru, and Chile. Chile has a rate of underweight under 5, at merely 1%. The most populous nations, Brazil and Mexico, mostly have relatively low rates of underweight under 5, with only 6% and 8%. Guatemala has the highest percentage of underweight and stunted children in the region, with rates above 45%. There are disparities amongst different populations in this region. For example, children in rural areas have twice the prevalence of underweight at 13%, compared to urban areas at 5%.

Nutrition Access Disparities

Occurring across throughout the world, lack of proper nutrition is both a consequence and cause of poverty. Impoverished individuals are less likely to have access to nutritious food and to escape from poverty than those who have healthy diets. Disparities in socioeconomic status, both between and within nations, provide the largest threat to child nutrition in industrialized nations, where social inequality is on the rise. According to UNICEF, children living in the poorest households are twice as likely to be underweight as those in the richest. Those in the lowest wealth quintile and whose mothers have the least education demonstrate the highest rates of child mortality and stunting. Throughout the developing world, socioeconomic inequality in childhood malnutrition is more severe than in upper income brackets, regardless of the general rate of malnutrition. Concurrently, the greatest increase in childhood obesity has been seen in the lower middle income bracket.

According to UNICEF, children in rural locations are more than twice as likely to be underweight as compared to children under five in urban areas. In Latin American/Caribbean nations, "Children living in rural areas in Bolivia, Honduras, Mexico and Nicaragua are more than twice as likely to be underweight as children living in urban areas. That likelihood doubles to four times in Peru."

In the United States, the incidence of low birthweight is on the rise among all populations, but particularly among minorities.

According to UNICEF, boys and girls have almost identical rates as underweight children under age 5 across the world, except in South Asia.

Nutrition Policy

Nutrition Interventions

Nutrition directly influences progress towards meeting the Millennium Goals of eradicating hunger and poverty through health and education. Therefore, nutrition interventions take a multi-faceted approach to improve the nutrition status of various populations. Policy and programming must target both individual behavioral changes and policy approaches to public health. While most nutrition interventions focus on delivery through the health-sector, non-health sector interventions targeting agriculture, water and sanitation, and education are important as well. Global nutrition micro-nutrient deficiencies often receive large-scale solution approaches by deploying large governmental and non-governmental organizations. For example, in 1990, iodine deficiency was particularly prevalent, with one in five households, or 1.7 billion people, not consuming adequate iodine, leaving them at risk to develop associated diseases. Therefore, a global campaign to iodize salt to eliminate iodine deficiency successfully boosted the rate to 69% of households in the world consuming adequate amounts of iodine.

Emergencies and crises often exacerbate undernutrition, due to the aftermath of crises that include food insecurity, poor health resources, unhealthy environments, and poor healthcare practices. Therefore, the repercussions of natural disasters and other emergencies can exponentially increase the rates of macro and micronutrient deficiencies in populations. Disaster relief interventions often take a multi-faceted public health approach. UNICEF's programming targeting nutrition services amongst disaster settings include nutrition assessments, measles immunization, vitamin A supplementation, provision of fortified foods and micronutrient supplements, support for breastfeeding and complementary feeding for infants and young children, and therapeutic and supplementary feeding. For example, during Nigeria's food crisis of 2005, 300,000 children received therapeutic nutrition feeding programs through the collaboration of UNICEF, the Niger government, the World Food Programme, and 24 NGOs utilizing community and facility based feeding schemes.

Interventions aimed at pregnant women, infants, and children take a behavioral and program-based approach. Behavioral intervention objectives include promoting proper breast-feeding, the immediate initiation of breastfeeding, and its continuation through 2 years and beyond. UNICEF recognizes that to promote these behaviors, healthful environments must be established conducive to promoting these behaviors, like healthy hospital environments, skilled health workers, support in the public and workplace, and removing negative influences. Finally, other interventions include provisions of adequate micro and macro nutrients such as iron, anemia, and vitamin A supplements and vitamin-fortified foods and ready-to-use products. Programs addressing micronutrient deficiencies, such as those aimed at anemia, have attempted to provide iron supplementation to pregnant and lactating women. However, because supplementation often occurs too late, these programs have had little effect. Interventions such as women's nutrition, early and exclusive breastfeeding, appropriate complementary food and micronutrient supplementation have proven to reduce stunting and other manifestations of undernutrition. A Cochrane review of community-based maternal health packages showed that this community-based approach improved the initiation of breastfeeding within one hour of birth. Some programs have had adverse effects. One example is the "Formula for Oil" relief program in Iraq, which resulted in the replacement of breastfeeding for formula, which has negatively affected infant nutrition.

Implementation and Delivery Platforms

In April 2010, the World Bank and the IMF released a policy briefing entitled "Scaling up Nutrition (SUN): A Framework for action" that represented a partnered effort to address the Lancet's Series on under nutrition, and the goals it set out for improving under nutrition. They emphasized the 1000 days after birth as the prime window for effective nutrition intervention, encouraging programming that was cost-effective and showed significant cognitive improvement in populations, as well as enhanced productivity and economic growth. This document was labeled the SUN framework, and was launched by the UN General Assembly in 2010 as a road map encouraging the coherence of stakeholders like governments, academia, UN system organizations and foundations in working towards reducing under nutrition. The SUN framework has initiated a transformation in global nutrition- calling for country-based nutrition programs, increasing evidence based and cost–effective interventions, and "integrating nutrition within national strategies for gender equality, agriculture, food security, social protection, education, water supply, sanitation, and health care". Government often plays a role in implementing nutrition programs through policy. For instance, several East Asian nations have enacted legislation to increase iodization of salt to increase household consumption. Political commitment in the form of evidence-based effective national policies and programs, trained skilled community nutrition workers, and effective communication and advocacy can all work to decrease malnutrition. Market and industrial production can play a role as well. For example, in the Philippines, improved production and market availability of iodized salt increased household consumption. While most nutrition interventions are delivered directly through governments and health services, other sectors, such as agriculture, water and sanitation, and education, are vital for nutrition promotion as well.

Nutrition Education

Nutrition is taught in schools in many countries. In England and Wales the Personal and Social Education and Food Technology curricula include nutrition, stressing the importance of a balanced diet and teaching how to read nutrition labels on packaging. In many schools a Nutrition class will fall within the Family and Consumer Science or Health departments. In some American schools, students are required to take a certain number of FCS or Health related classes. Nutrition is offered at many schools, and if it is not a class of its own, nutrition is included in other FCS or Health classes such as: Life Skills, Independent Living, Single Survival, Freshmen Connection, Health etc. In many Nutrition classes, students learn about the food groups, the food pyramid, Daily Recommended Allowances, calories, vitamins, minerals, malnutrition, physical activity, healthy food choices and how to live a healthy life.

A 1985 US National Research Council report entitled *Nutrition Education in US Medical Schools* concluded that nutrition education in medical schools was inadequate. Only 20% of the schools surveyed taught nutrition as a separate, required course. A 2006 survey found that this number had risen to 30%.

Nutrition for Special Populations

Sports Nutrition

Individuals with highly active lifestyles require more nutrients. Furthermore, recent studies declared that increasing dietary intake of carbohydrates, proteins and Vitamin D may be part of improving athlete's level of performance

Protein

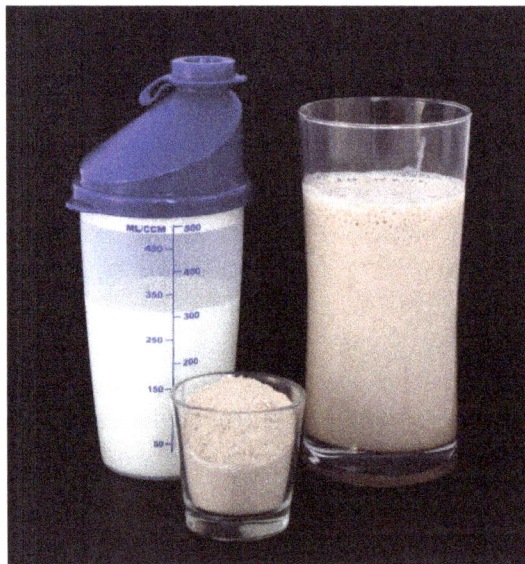

Protein milkshakes, made from protein powder (center) and milk (left), are a common bodybuilding supplement.

Protein is an important component of every cell in the body. Hair and nails are mostly made of protein. The body uses protein to build and repair tissues. Also protein is used to make enzymes, hormones, and other body chemicals. Protein is an important building block of bones, muscles, cartilage, skin, and blood.

The protein requirement for each individual differs, as do opinions about whether and to what extent physically active people require more protein. The 2005 Recommended Dietary Allowances (RDA), aimed at the general healthy adult population, provide for an intake of 0.8 – 1 grams of protein per kilogram of body weight (according to the BMI formula), with the review panel stating that "no additional dietary protein is suggested for healthy adults undertaking resistance or endurance exercise".

Carbohydrates

The main fuel used by the body during exercise is carbohydrates, which is stored in muscle as glycogen – a form of sugar. During exercise, muscle glycogen reserves can be used up, especially when activities last longer than 90 min. Because the amount of glycogen stored in the body is limited, it is important for athletes to replace glycogen by consuming a diet high in carbohydrates. Meeting energy needs can help improve performance during the sport, as well as improve overall strength and endurance..

There are different kinds of carbohydrates: simple (for example from fruits) and complex (for example from grains such as wheat). Simple sugars can be from an unrefined natural source, or may be refined and added to processed food. A typical American consumes about 50% of their carbohydrates as refined sugars. Over the course of a year, the average American consumes 204 litres (54 US gallons @ 3.78l per gallon) of soft drinks, which contain the highest amount of added sugars. Even though carbohydrates are necessary for humans to function, they are not all equally healthful. When machinery has been used to remove bits of high fiber, the carbohydrates are refined. These are the carbohydrates found in white bread and fast food.

Maternal Nutrition

Studies have shown that nutritional status of women pre-conception (specifically body weight) has an influence on foetal growth. However during pregnancy, nutritional intake by the mother is believed not to have any effect during the first and second trimesters, but maternal nutritional intake in the last trimester is widely believed to have some effect on the foetal growth, and therefore maternal nutrition plays a vital role in the development and growth of the foetus.

Paediatric Nutrition

Adequate nutrition is essential for the growth of children from infancy right through until adolescence. Some nutrients are specifically required for growth on top of nutrients required for normal body maintenance, in particular calcium and iron.

Elderly Nutrition

Chwang (2012) reports that malnutrition is higher among the elderly. This article highlights the uneven distribution of nutrients between developed and undeveloped countries. For example, most European countries has a high fat intake; while, the Malaysian elderly were found to have insufficient intake of calcium, thiamine and riboflavin.

History

Humans have evolved as omnivorous hunter-gatherers over the past 250,000 years. The diet of early modern humans varied significantly depending on location and climate. The diet in the tropics tended to depend more heavily on plant foods, while the diet at higher latitudes tended more towards animal products. Analyses of postcranial and cranial remains of humans and animals from the Neolithic, along with detailed bone-modification studies, have shown that cannibalism also occurred among prehistoric humans.

Agriculture developed about 10,000 years ago in multiple locations throughout the world, providing grains (such as wheat, rice and maize) and potatoes; and originating staples such as bread, pasta (attested from 1154), and tortillas. Farming also provided milk and dairy products, and sharply increased the availability of meats and the diversity of vegetables. The importance of food purity was recognized when bulk storage led to infestation and contamination risks.Cooking developed as an often ritualistic activity, due to efficiency and reliability concerns requiring adherence to strict recipes and procedures, and in response to demands for food purity and consistency.

From Antiquity to 1900

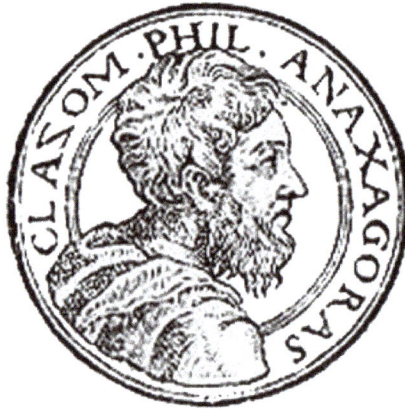

Anaxagoras

Around 3000 BC the Vedic texts made mention of scientific research on nutrition. The Bible's Book of Daniel recounts first recorded nutritional experiment. During an invasion of Judah, King Nebuchadnezzar of Babylon captured Daniel and his friends. Selected as court servants, they were to share in the king's fine foods and wine. But they objected, preferring vegetables (pulses) and water in accordance with their Jewish dietary restrictions. The king's chief steward reluctantly agreed to a trial. Daniel and his friends received their diet for 10 days. On comparison with the king's men, they appeared healthier, and were allowed to continue with their diet. Around 475 BC, Anaxagoras stated that food is absorbed by the human body and therefore contained "homeomerics" (generative components), suggesting the existence of nutrients. Around 400 BC, Hippocrates said: "Let food be your medicine and medicine be your food."

The 16th-century scientist and artist Leonardo da Vinci (1452–1519) compared metabolism to a burning candle. In 1747 Dr. James Lind, a physician in the British navy, performed the first attested scientific nutrition experiment, discovering that lime juice saved sailors who had been at sea for years from scurvy, a deadly and painful bleeding disorder. The discovery was ignored for forty years, but after about 1850 British sailors became known as "limeys". (Scientists would not identify the essential vitamin C within lime juice until the 1930s.)

Around 1770 Antoine Lavoisier, the "Father of Nutrition and Chemistry", discovered the details of metabolism, demonstrating that the oxidation of food is the source of body heat. In 1790 George Fordyce recognized calcium as necessary for fowl survival. In the early 19th century, the elements carbon, nitrogen, hydrogen and oxygen were recognized as the primary components of food, and methods to measure their proportions were developed.

In 1816 François Magendie discovered that dogs fed only carbohydrates and fat lost their body protein and died in a few weeks, but dogs also fed protein survived, identifying protein as an essential dietary component. In 1840, Justus Liebig discovered the chemical makeup of carbohydrates (sugars), fats (fatty acids) and proteins (amino acids). In the 1860s Claude Bernard discovered that body fat can be synthesized from carbohydrate and protein, showing that the energy in blood glucose can be stored as fat or as glycogen.In the early 1880s Kanehiro Takaki observed that Japanese sailors (whose diets consisted almost entirely of white rice) developed beriberi (or endemic neuritis, a disease causing heart problems and paralysis), but British sailors and Japanese naval officers did not. Adding various types of vegetables and meats to the diets of Japanese sailors prevented the disease.

In 1896 Eugen Baumann observed iodine in thyroid glands. In 1897, Christiaan Eijkman worked with natives of Java, who also suffered from beriberi. Eijkman observed that chickens fed the native diet of white rice developed the symptoms of beriberi, but remained healthy when fed unprocessed brown rice with the outer bran intact. Eijkman cured the natives by feeding them brown rice, demonstrating that food can cure disease. Over two decades later, nutritionists learned that the outer rice bran contains vitamin B

From 1900 to the Present

In the early 20th century Carl von Voit and Max Rubner independently measured caloric energy expenditure in different species of animals, applying principles of physics in nutrition. In 1906, Wilcock and Hopkins showed that the amino acid tryptophan was necessary for the survival of rats. He fed them a special mixture of food containing all the nutrients he believed were essential for survival, but the rats died. A second group of rats to which he also fed an amount of milk containing vitamins. Gowland Hopkins recognized "accessory food factors" other than calories, protein and minerals, as organic materials essential to health but which the body cannot synthesize. In 1907 Stephen M. Babcock and Edwin B. Hart conducted the single-grain experiment. This experiment ran through 1911.

In 1912 Casimir Funk coined the term vitamin to label a vital factor in the diet: from the words "vital" and "amine," because these unknown substances preventing scurvy, beriberi, and pellagra, were thought then to derive from ammonia. The vitamins were studied in the first half of the 20th century. In 1913 Elmer McCollum discovered the first vitamins, fat-soluble vitamin A and water-soluble vitamin B (in 1915; later identified as a complex of several water-soluble vitamins) and named vitamin C as the then-unknown substance preventing scurvy. Lafayette Mendel (1872-1935) and Thomas Osborne (1859–1929) also performed pioneering work on vitamins A and B. In 1919 Sir Edward Mellanby incorrectly identified rickets as a vitamin A deficiency, because he could cure it in dogs with cod-liver oil. In 1922 McCollum destroyed the vitamin A in cod liver oil but found it still cured rickets, thus identifying vitamin D. Also in 1922, H.M. Evans and L.S. Bishop discovered vitamin E as essential for rat pregnancy, and originally called it "food factor X" until 1925.

In 1925 Hart discovered that iron absorption requires trace amounts of copper. In 1927 Adolf Otto Reinhold Windaus synthesized vitamin D, for which he won the Nobel Prize in Chemistry in 1928. In 1928 Albert Szent-Györgyi isolated ascorbic acid, and in 1932 proved that it is vitamin C by preventing scurvy. In 1935 he synthesized it, and in 1937 won a Nobel Prize for his efforts. Szent-Györgyi concurrently elucidated much of the citric acid cycle. In the 1930s William Cumming Rose identified essential amino acids, necessary protein components which the body cannot synthesize. In 1935 Eric Underwood and Hedley Marston independently discovered the necessity of cobalt. In

1936 Eugene Floyd Dubois showed that work and school performance relate to caloric intake. In 1938 Erhard Fernholz discovered the chemical structure of vitamin E. It was synthesised by Paul Karrer (1889–1971).

From 1940 rationing in the United Kingdom – during and after World War II – took place according to nutritional principles drawn up by Elsie Widdowson and others. In 1941 the National Research Council established the first Recommended Dietary Allowances (RDAs). In 1992 the U.S. Department of Agriculture introduced the Food Guide Pyramid. In 2002 a Natural Justice study showed a relation between nutrition and violent behavior. In 2005 a study found that in addition to bad nutrition, adenovirus may cause obesity.

Sports Nutrition

Sports Nutrition is the study and practice of nutrition and diet as it relates to athletic performance. It is concerned with the type and quantity of fluid and food taken by an athlete, and deals with nutrients such as vitamins, minerals, supplements and organic substances such as carbohydrates, proteins and fats. Although an important part of many sports training regimens, it is most popular in strength sports (such as weight lifting and bodybuilding) and endurance sports (for example cycling, running, swimming, rowing).

Supplements

All athletes consider taking dietary supplements because they are looking for the "magic ingredient" to increase performance. In the extreme case of performance-enhancing supplements, athletes, particularly bodybuilders may choose to use illegal substances such as anabolic steroids, compounds which are related to the hormone testosterone, which can quickly build mass and strength, but have many adverse effects such as high blood pressure and negative gender specific effects. Blood doping, another illegal ergogenic, was discovered in the 1940s when it was used by World War II pilots.

In the 1940s early results were found regarding consumption of dietary protein for athletes involved in muscle building and resistance and strength training. Protein intake is a part of the nutrient requirements for the regular athlete and is an important component of exercise training, because it can also aid in performance and recovery. Dietary protein intake for well-trained athletes should occur before, during and after physical activity as it is advantageous in gaining muscle mass and strength. However, if too much protein and amino acid supplements are consumed (especially by the average exerciser), it can be more harmful than beneficial; health risks include: "dehydration, gout, calcium loss, liver, and renal damage [and] gastrointestinal side effects include diarrhea, bloating, and water loss" (Lawerence). A bountiful protein diet must be paired with a healthy, well-rounded meal plan and regular resistance exercise. Yet, characteristics such as the type of exercise, intensity, duration, the carbohydrate values of diet, the individual's sex and age and also the amount of background training and training environment.

Creatine may be helpful for well-trained athletes to increase exercise performance and strength in concordance with their dietary regimen. Also, the substance glutamine, found in whey protein supplements, is the most abundant free amino acid found in the human body. For well-trained and well-nourished athletes it is considered that glutamine may have a possible role in stimulated anabolic processes such muscle glycogen and protein synthesis. Other popular supplements studies done include androstenedione, chromium, and ephedra. The findings show that there are no substantial benefits from the extra intake of these supplements, yet higher health risks and costs.

High energy supplements have shown to increase the performance of physical activity. A study done at the University of Texas saw a 4.7% increase of performance in 83% of participants after drinking Red Bull Energy Drink which was more intense than the compared placebo. The energy drink most dominantly increased the epinephrine and noreprinephrine (adrenaline and its precursor) levels and beta-endorphins in the blood than before consumption. Caffeine, carbohydrates and Vitamin B are factors that may have favored performance increase with no change in perceived exertion.

Caffeine has been known since the 1900s and became popularly used since the 1970s when its power of masking fatigue became highly recognized. Similarly, the caffeine found in energy drinks shows an increased reaction performance and increased good feelings of energy, focus and alertness in quickness and reaction anaerobic power tests. In other words, consuming an energy drink with caffeine increases short time/rapid exercise performance (like short full-speed sprints and heavy power weight lifting).

Post-exercise nutrition is just as important, if not more important than pre-exercise nutrition as it pertains to recovery. Traditionally, sports drinks such as Gatorade and Powerade, are consumed during and after exercise because they effectively rehydrate the body by refueling the body with minerals and electrolytes. Gatorade was founded in the 1960s, when the University of Florida, Gainesville Gators improved their performance with "Gator Aid." A drink was made of glucose and sucrose in water and helped the football players' performance. And by the 1970s, many other sports drinks of its kind had been manufactured. However, sports drinks lack protein.

New studies in 2008 have found cow's milk, especially skim milk and chocolate milk may be effective replacements for current sports drink, as milk leads to protein the synthesis which boosts net muscle protein balance. Milk contains many electrolytes, nutrients and other elements that help to make it an effective post-exercise beverage. It is true that chocolate milk has been a proven study that is just as affective of a recovery drink as Gatorade. A recovery drink is supposed to replenish the sugar, and build muscle again so that you are ready for the next workout. Chocolate Milk includes key ingredients such as Vitamin D that helps replace fluids and electrolytes lost after the athlete has worked out.

When compared to plain water or sports drinks, research suggests that chocolate milk is more effective at replacing fluids lost as sweat and maintaining normal body fluid levels. Athletes drinking chocolate milk following exercise-induced dehydration had fluid levels about 2 percent higher (on initial body mass) than those using other post-exercise recovery beverages, allowing for prolonged performance, especially in repeated bouts of exercise or training.

Factors Influencing Nutritional Requirements

Differing conditions and objectives suggest the need for athletes to ensure that their sports nutritional approach is appropriate for their situation. Factors that may affect an athlete's nutritional needs include type of activity (aerobic vs. anaerobic), gender, weight, height, body mass index, workout or activity stage (pre-workout, intra-workout, recovery), and time of day (e.g. some nutrients are utilized by the body more effectively during sleep than while awake). Most culprits that get in the way of performance are fatigue, injury and soreness. A proper diet will reduce these disturbances in performance. The key is to get a variety of food, to get all the macronutrients, vitamins, and minerals. According to Eblere's article (2008), it is optimal to choose raw, unprocessed foods such as oranges instead of orange juice. Eating foods that are natural means the athlete is getting the most nutritional value out of the food. When foods are processed it normally means that nutritional value is reduced.

Anaerobic Exercise

During anaerobic exercise, the process of glycolysis breaks down the sugars from carbohydrates for energy without the use of oxygen. This type of exercise occurs in physical activity such as power sprints, strength resistances and quick explosive movement where the muscles are being used for power and speed, with short-time energy use. After this type of exercise, there is a need to refill glycogen storage sites in the body (the long simple sugar chains in the body that store energy), although they are not likely fully depleted.

To compensate for this glycogen reduction, athletes will often take in a large amount of carbohydrates in the period immediately following exercise. Typically, high-glycemic-index carbohydrates are preferred for their ability to rapidly raise blood glucose levels. For the purpose of protein synthesis, protein or individual amino acids are ingested as well. Branched-chain amino acids are important since they are most responsible for protein synthesis. According to Lemon et al. (1995) female endurance runners have the hardest time getting enough protein in their diet. Endurance athletes in general need more protein in their diet than the sedentary person. Research has shown that endurance athletes are recommended to have 1.2 to 1.4 g of protein per kg of body weight in order to repair damaged tissue. If the athlete consumes too few calories for the body's needs, lean tissue will be broken down for energy and repair. Protein deficiency can cause many problems such as early and extreme fatigue, particularly long recovery, and poor wound healing. Complete proteins such as meat, eggs, and soy provide the athlete with all essential amino acids for synthesising new tissues. However, vegetarian and vegan athletes frequently combine legumes with a whole grain to provide the body with a complete protein across the day's food intake. A popular example is rice and beans.

The following information on the types of carbohydrates comes from Spada's research on endurance sports nutrition (2000). He advises carbohydrates to be unprocessed and/or whole grains for optimal performance while training. This is because these carbohydrates offer the most fuel, nutritional value, and satiety. Fruits and vegetables contribute important carbohydrate foundation for an athlete's diet. They both provide vitamins and minerals that are lost through exercise and need to be replenished. Both fruits and vegetables improve healing, aid in recovery, and reduce risks of cancer, high blood pressure, and constipation. Vegetables offer a little more nutritional value than fruits for the amount of calories, therefore an athlete should strive to eat more vegetables than fruits. It is also important to look at the certain types of vegetables and fruits. Dark-colored vegetables usually have more nutritional value than pale colored ones. A general rule is the darker the color the more nutrient dense it is. Like all foods, it is very important to have a variety. To get the most nutritional value out of fruits and vegetables it is important to eat them in their natural, unprocessed form with no other nutrient (sugar) added.

Often in the continuation of this anaerobic exercise, the product from this metabolic mechanism builds up in what is called lactic acid fermentation. Lactate is produced more quickly than it is being removed and it serves to regenerate NAD^+ to the cells where it's needed. During intense exercise when oxygen is not being used, a high amount of ATP is produced and pH levels fall causing acidosis or more specifically lactic acidosis. Lactic acid build up can be treated by staying well-hydrated throughout and especially after the workout, having good cool down routine and good post-workout stretching.

Intense activity can cause significant damage to bodily tissues. In order to repair, vitamin E and other antioxidants are needed to protect muscle damage. Oxidative damage and muscle tissue breakdown happens all the time in endurance running so athletes need to eat foods high in protein in order to repair these muscle tissues. It is important for female endurance runners to consume proper nutrients in their diet that will repair, fuel, and minimize fatigue and injury. To keep a female runner's body performing at its best, ten nutrients need to be essential in diets.

Nutrition and Pregnancy

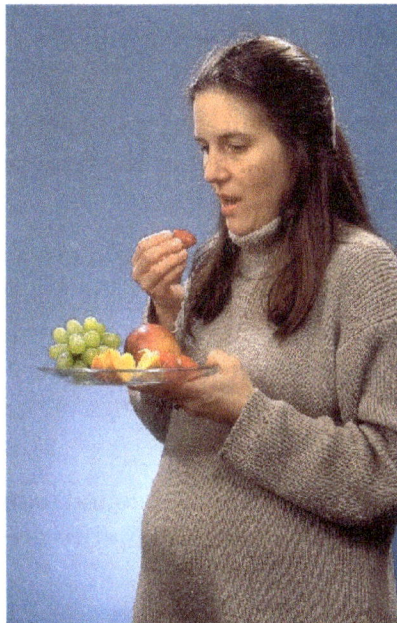

Pregnant woman eating fruit.

Nutrition and pregnancy refers to the nutrient intake, and dietary planning that is undertaken before, during and after pregnancy. Nutrition of the fetus begins at conception. For this reason, the nutrition of the mother is important from before conception (probably several months before) as well as throughout pregnancy and breast feeding. An ever-increasing number of studies have shown that the nutrition of the mother will have an effect on the child, up to and including the risk for cancer, cardiovascular disease, hypertension and diabetes throughout life.

An inadequate or excessive amount of some nutrients may cause malformations or medical problems in the fetus, and neurological disorders and handicaps are a risk that is run by mothers who are malnourished. 23.8% of babies worldwide are estimated to be born with lower than optimal weights at birth due to lack of proper nutrition. Personal habits such as smoking, alcohol, caffeine, using certain medications and street drugs can negatively and irreversibly affect the development of the baby, which happens in the early stages of pregnancy.

Caffeine is sometimes assumed to cause harm to the unborn baby but there is not enough evidence so say if this is true. A recent review showed that more research is needed to show whether caffeine intake effects birth weight, preterm births, gestational diabetes and other outcomes.

Nutrition Before Pregnancy

Beneficial Pre-pregnancy Nutrients

As with most diets, there are chances of over-supplementing, however, as general advice, both state and medical recommendations are that mothers follow instructions listed on particular vitamin packaging as to the correct or recommended daily allowance (RDA). Daily prenatal use of iron substantially improves birth weight, potentially reducing the risk of Low birth weight.

- Folic acid supplementation is recommended prior to conception, to prevent development of spina bifida and other neural tube defects. It should be taken as at least 0.4 mg/day throughout the first trimester of pregnancy, 0.6 mg/day through the pregnancy, and 0.5 mg/day while breastfeeding in addition to eating foods rich in folic acid such as green leafy vegetables.

- Iodine levels are frequently too low in pregnant women, and iodine is necessary for normal thyroid function and mental development of the fetus, even cretinism. Pregnant women should take prenatal vitamins containing iodine.

- Vitamin D levels vary with exposure to sunlight. While it was assumed that supplementation was necessary only in areas of high latitudes, recent studies of Vitamin D levels throughout the United States and many other countries have shown a large number of women with low levels. For this reason, there is a growing movement to recommend supplementation with 1000 mg of Vitamin D daily throughout pregnancy, vitamin D is necessary to prevent rickets, a disease causing weak bones.

- A large number of pregnant women have been found to have low levels of vitamin B12, but supplementation has not yet been shown to improve pregnancy outcome or the health of the newborn, although there are suspicions.

- Polyunsaturated fatty acids, specifically docosahexaenoic acid (DHA) and eicosapentaenoic acid (EPA) are very beneficial for fetal development. Several studies have shown a small drop in preterm delivery and in low birth weight in mothers with higher intakes. The best dietary source of omega-3 fatty acids is oily fish. Some other omega-3 fatty acids not found in fish can be found in foods such as flaxseeds, walnuts, pumpkin seeds, and enriched eggs.

- Iron is needed for the healthy growth of the fetus and placenta, especially during the second and third trimesters. It is also essential before pregnancy for the production of hemoglobin.

There is no evidence that a hemoglobin level of 7 grams/100 ml or higher is detrimental to pregnancy, but it must be acknowledged that maternal hemorrhage is a major source of maternal mortality worldwide, and a reserve capacity to carry oxygen is desirable. Evidence shows that giving 100 mg of elemental iron three times weekly is adequate during pregnancy.

Nutrition During Pregnancy

During the early stages of pregnancy, since the placenta is not yet formed, there is no mechanism to protect the embryo from the deficiencies which may be inherent in the mother's circulation. Thus, it is critical that an adequate amount of nutrients and energy is consumed.

Multiple micronutrient supplements taken with iron and folic acid can improve birth outcomes for women in low income countries. These supplements reduce numbers of low birth weight babies, small for gestational age babies and stillbirths in women who may not have many micronutrients in their usual diets. Undernourished women can benefit from having dietary education sessions and, balanced energy and protein supplements.

A review showed that dietary education increased the mother's protein intake and helped the baby grow more inside the womb. The balanced protein and energy supplement lowered risk of stillbirth and small babies and increased weight gain for both the mother and baby. Although more research is needed into the longer term effects on the mothers' and infants' health, the short term effects look promising.

Supplementing one's diet with foods rich in folic acid, such as oranges and dark green leafy vegetables, helps to prevent neural tube birth defects in the fetus. In addition, prenatal vitamins typically contain increased amounts of folic acid, iodine, iron, vitamin A, vitamin D, zinc, and calcium over the amounts found in standard multi-vitamins.

Zinc supplements have reduced preterm births by around 14% mainly in low income countries. No other benefits were seen4. The World Health Organisation does not routinely recommend zinc supplementation for pregnant women because there is not enough good quality evidence.

For women with low calcium diets, taking calcium supplementation can reduce their risk of pre-eclampsia. It has also been suggested that calcium can reduce numbers of births that happen before the 37th week of pregnancy (preterm birth). However a more recent review looking into other benefits of calcium supplementation did not find any improvement in numbers of preterm or low birth weight babies. There is not enough good quality to research to suggest best doses and timing of calcium supplementation.

Pregnant women are advised to pay attention to the foods they eat during pregnancy, such as soft cheese and certain fish, in order to reduce the risk of exposure to substances or bacteria that may be harmful to the developing fetus. This can include food pathogens and toxic food components, alcohol, and dietary supplements such as vitamin A and potentially harmful pathogens such as listeria, toxoplasmosis, and salmonella. Dietary vitamin A is obtained in two forms which contain the preformed vitamin (retinol), that can be found in some animal products such as liver and fish liver oils, and as a vitamin A precursor in the form of carotene, which can be found in many fruits and vegetables. Intake of large amounts or, conversely, a deficiency, of retinol has been linked to birth defects and abnormalities. It is noted that a 100 g serving of liver may contain a large amount of retinol, so it is best that it is not eaten daily during pregnancy. Excessive amounts of alcohol have been proven to cause fetal alcohol syndrome. The World Health Organization recommends that alcohol should be avoided entirely during pregnancy, given the relatively unknown effects of even small amounts of alcohol during pregnancy. Although seafood contains high levels of Omega-3 fatty acids which are beneficial for both mother and the baby, but there is no consensus on consuming seafood during pregnancy. Pregnant women are advised to eat seafood in moderation.

Folic Acid

Folic acid, which is the synthetic form of the vitamin folate, is critical both in pre-and peri-conception. Deficiencies in folic acid may cause neural tube defects; women who had 0.4 mg of folic acid in their systems due to supplementing 3 months before childbirth significantly reduced the risk of NTD within the fetus. The development of every human cell is dependent on an adequate supply of folic acid. Folic acid governs the synthesis of the precursors of DNA, which is the nucleic acid that gives each cell life and character. Folic acid deficiency results in defective cellular growth and the effects are most obvious on those tissues which grow most rapidly.

Water

During pregnancy, one's mass increases by about 12 kg. Most of this added weight (6 to 9 L) is water because the plasma volume increases, 85% of the placenta is water and the fetus itself is 70-90% water. This means that hydration is an important aspect of nutrition throughout pregnancy. The European Food Safety Authority recommends an increase of 300 mL per day compared to the normal intake for non-pregnant women, taking the total adequate water intake (from food and fluids) to 2,300 mL, or approximately 1,850 mL/ day from fluids alone

Nutrition after Pregnancy

Proper nutrition is important after delivery to help the mother recover, and to provide enough food energy and nutrients for a woman to breastfeed her child. Women having serum ferritin less than 70 µg/L may need iron supplements to prevent iron deficiency anaemia during pregnancy and postpartum.

During lactation, water intake may need to be increased. Human milk is made of 88% water, and the IOM recommends that breastfeeding women increase their water intake by about 300 mL/ day to a total volume of 3000 mL/day (from food and drink); approximately 2,400 mL/day from fluids.

References

- Whitney, Ellie; Rolfes, Sharon Rady (2013). Understanding Nutrition (13 ed.). Wadsworth, Cengage Learning. pp. 667, 670. ISBN 978-1133587521.

- Payne-Palacio, June R.; Canter, Deborah D. (2014). The Profession of Dietetics. Jones & Bartlett Learning. pp. 3, 4. ISBN 978-1-284-02608-5.

- Willett, Walter C. with Skerrett, Patrick J. (2005) [2001]. Eat, Drink, and be Healthy: The Harvard Medical School Guide To Healthy Eating. Free Press (Simon & Schuster). p. 183. ISBN 0-684-86337-5.

- Silberberg, Martin S. (2009). Chemistry: The Molecular Nature of Matter and Change (5 ed.). McGraw-Hill. p. 44. ISBN 978-0-07-304859-8.

- Semenza, G., ed. (2012). Comprehensive Biochemistry: Selected Topics in the History of Biochemistry: Personal Recollections, Part 1. 35. Elsevier via Google Books. p. 117. ISBN 0444598200. Retrieved March 15, 2016.

- Nestle, Marion (2013) [2002]. Food Politics: How the Food Industry Influences Nutrition and Health. University of California Press. p. 413. ISBN 978-0-520-27596-6.

- Nelson, D. L.; Cox, M. M. (2000). Lehninger Principles of Biochemistry (3rd ed.). New York: Worth Publishing. ISBN 1-57259-153-6.

- Corbridge, D. E. C. (1995). Phosphorus: An Outline of its Chemistry, Biochemistry, and Technology (5th ed.). Amsterdam: Elsevier. ISBN 0-444-89307-5.

- Lippard, S. J.; Berg, J. M. (1994). Principles of Bioinorganic Chemistry. Mill Valley, CA: University Science Books. ISBN 0935702725.

- Shils, M. S.; et al., eds. (2005). Modern Nutrition in Health and Disease. Lippincott Williams and Wilkins. ISBN 0-7817-4133-5.

- World Health Organization, Food and Agricultural Organization of the United Nations (2004). Vitamin and mineral requirements in human nutrition (2. ed.). Geneva [u.a.]: World Health Organization. ISBN 9241546123.

- Berg J, Tymoczko JL, Stryer L (2002). Biochemistry (5th ed.). San Francisco: W.H. Freeman. p. 603. ISBN 0-7167-4684-0.

- D. E. C. Corbridge (1995). Phosphorus: An Outline of its Chemistry, Biochemistry, and Technology (5th ed.). Amsterdam: Elsevier. ISBN 0-444-89307-5.

- Lippard, S. J.; Berg, J. M. (1994). Principles of Bioinorganic Chemistry. Mill Valley, CA: University Science Books. ISBN 0-935702-73-3.

- Di Pasquale, Mauro G. (2008). "Utilization of Proteins in Energy Metabolism". In Ira Wolinsky, Judy A. Driskell. Sports Nutrition: Energy metabolism and exercise. CRC Press. p. 73. ISBN 978-0-8493-7950-5.

- William D. McArdle; Frank I. Katch; Victor L. Katch (2006). Exercise Physiology: Energy, Nutrition, and Human Performance. Lippincott Williams & Wilkins. ISBN 0-8121-0682-2.

- Wahlqvist, M. L. (2011). Food and Nutrition: Food and Health Systems in Australia and New Zealand (3rd ed.). NSW, Australia: Allen & Unwin. pp. 429–441. ISBN 978 1 74175 897 9.

- Laura Riley. Stephanie Karpinske, ed. Pregnancy: The Ultimate Week-by-Week Pregnancy Guide. Meredith Books. pp. 21–22. ISBN 0-696-22221-3.

- Schaefer, Christof (2001). Drugs During Pregnancy and Lactation: Handbook of Prescription Drugs and Comparative Risk Assessment. Gulf Professional Publishing. ISBN 9780444507631. Retrieved 2015-05-13.

- Shils, Maurice Edward; Shike, Moshe (2006). Modern Nutrition in Health and Disease. Lippincott Williams & Wilkins. ISBN 9780781741330. Retrieved 2015-05-13.

- Briggs, Gerald G.; Freeman, Roger K.; Yaffe, Sumner J. (2011). Drugs in Pregnancy and Lactation: A Reference Guide to Fetal and Neonatal Risk. Lippincott Williams & Wilkins. ISBN 9781608317080. Retrieved 2015-05-13.

- Laura Riley (2006-02-02). Stephanie Karpinske, ed. Pregnancy: The Ultimate Week-by-Week Pregnancy Guide. Meredith Books. pp. 21–22. ISBN 0-696-22221-3.

- L. Kathleen Mahan; Janice L. Raymond; Sylvia Escott-Stump (2012). Krausw's Food and the Nutrition Care Process (13th ed.). St. Louis: Elsevier. ISBN 978-1-4377-2233-8.

Introduction to Metabolism

Metabolism has three purposes which are the conversion of food to energy to run cellular processes, the conversion of fuel to building blocks for proteins and some carbohydrates and the elimination of nitrogenous wastes. This chapter discusses the process of metabolism and provides with key analysis to the subject matter by explaining digestion, microbial metabolism and the basal metabolic rate briefly.

Metabolism

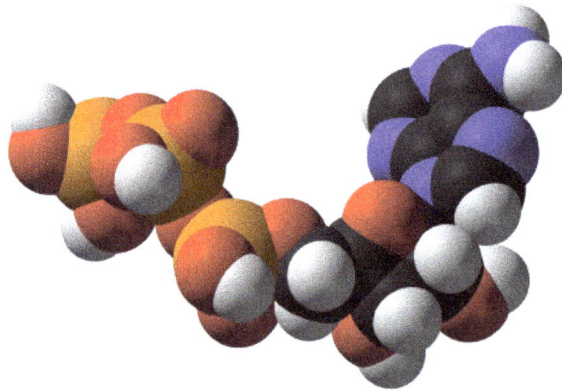

Structure of adenosine triphosphate (ATP), a central intermediate in energy metabolism

Metabolism is the set of life-sustaining chemical transformations within the cells of living organisms. The three main purposes of metabolism are the conversion of food/fuel to energy to run cellular processes, the conversion of food/fuel to building blocks for proteins, lipids, nucleic acids, and some carbohydrates, and the elimination of nitrogenous wastes. These enzyme-catalyzed reactions allow organisms to grow and reproduce, maintain their structures, and respond to their environments. The word metabolism can also refer to the sum of all chemical reactions that occur in living organisms, including digestion and the transport of substances into and between different cells, in which case the set of reactions within the cells is called intermediary metabolism or intermediate metabolism.

Metabolism is usually divided into two categories: catabolism, the *breaking down* of organic matter, for example, by cellular respiration, and anabolism, the *building up* of components of cells such as proteins and nucleic acids. Usually, breaking down releases energy and building up consumes energy.

The chemical reactions of metabolism are organized into metabolic pathways, in which one chemical is transformed through a series of steps into another chemical, by a sequence of enzymes.

Enzymes are crucial to metabolism because they allow organisms to drive desirable reactions that require energy that will not occur by themselves, by coupling them to spontaneous reactions that release energy. Enzymes act as catalysts that allow the reactions to proceed more rapidly. Enzymes also allow the regulation of metabolic pathways in response to changes in the cell's environment or to signals from other cells.

The metabolic system of a particular organism determines which substances it will find nutritious and which poisonous. For example, some prokaryotes use hydrogen sulfide as a nutrient, yet this gas is poisonous to animals. The speed of metabolism, the metabolic rate, influences how much food an organism will require, and also affects how it is able to obtain that food.

A striking feature of metabolism is the similarity of the basic metabolic pathways and components between even vastly different species. For example, the set of carboxylic acids that are best known as the intermediates in the citric acid cycle are present in all known organisms, being found in species as diverse as the unicellular bacterium *Escherichia coli* and huge multicellular organisms like elephants. These striking similarities in metabolic pathways are likely due to their early appearance in evolutionary history, and their retention because of their efficacy.

Key Biochemicals

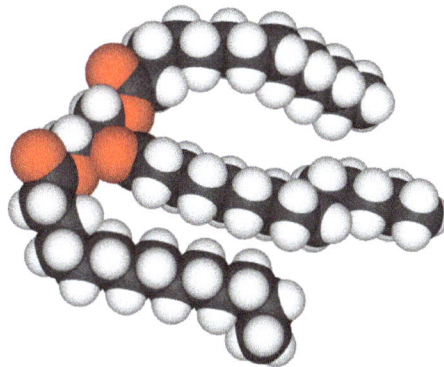

Structure of a triacylglycerol lipid

Most of the structures that make up animals, plants and microbes are made from three basic classes of molecule: amino acids, carbohydrates and lipids (often called fats). As these molecules are vital for life, metabolic reactions either focus on making these molecules during the construction of cells and tissues, or by breaking them down and using them as a source of energy, by their digestion. These biochemicals can be joined together to make polymers such as DNA and proteins, essential macromolecules of life.

Type of molecule	Name of monomer forms	Name of polymer forms	Examples of polymer forms
Amino acids	Amino acids	Proteins (made of polypeptides)	Fibrous proteins and globular proteins
Carbohydrates	Monosaccharides	Polysaccharides	Starch, glycogen and cellulose
Nucleic acids	Nucleotides	Polynucleotides	DNA and RNA

Amino Acids and Proteins

Proteins are made of amino acids arranged in a linear chain joined together by peptide bonds. Many proteins are enzymes that catalyze the chemical reactions in metabolism. Other proteins have structural or mechanical functions, such as those that form the cytoskeleton, a system of scaffolding that maintains the cell shape. Proteins are also important in cell signaling, immune responses, cell adhesion, active transport across membranes, and the cell cycle. Amino acids also contribute to cellular energy metabolism by providing a carbon source for entry into the citric acid cycle (tricarboxylic acid cycle), especially when a primary source of energy, such as glucose, is scarce, or when cells undergo metabolic stress.

Lipids

Lipids are the most diverse group of biochemicals. Their main structural uses are as part of biological membranes both internal and external, such as the cell membrane, or as a source of energy. Lipids are usually defined as hydrophobic or amphipathic biological molecules but will dissolve in organic solvents such as benzene or chloroform. The fats are a large group of compounds that contain fatty acids and glycerol; a glycerol molecule attached to three fatty acid esters is called a triacylglyceride. Several variations on this basic structure exist, including alternate backbones such as sphingosine in the sphingolipids, and hydrophilic groups such as phosphate as in phospholipids. Steroids such as cholesterol are another major class of lipids.

Carbohydrates

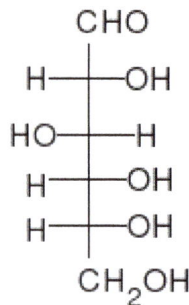

Glucose can exist in both a straight-chain and ring form.

Carbohydrates are aldehydes or ketones, with many hydroxyl groups attached, that can exist as straight chains or rings. Carbohydrates are the most abundant biological molecules, and fill numerous roles, such as the storage and transport of energy (starch, glycogen) and structural components (cellulose in plants, chitin in animals). The basic carbohydrate units are called monosaccharides and include galactose, fructose, and most importantly glucose. Monosaccharides can be linked together to form polysaccharides in almost limitless ways.

Nucleotides

The two nucleic acids, DNA and RNA, are polymers of nucleotides. Each nucleotide is composed of a phosphate attached to a ribose or deoxyribose sugar group which is attached to a nitrogenous base. Nucleic acids are critical for the storage and use of genetic information, and its interpretation through the processes of transcription and protein biosynthesis. This information is protected by DNA repair mechanisms and propagated through DNA replication. Many viruses have an RNA genome, such as HIV, which uses reverse transcription to create a DNA template from its viral RNA genome. RNA in ribozymes such as spliceosomes and ribosomes is similar to enzymes as it can catalyze chemical reactions. Individual nucleosides are made by attaching a nucleobase to a ribose sugar. These bases are heterocyclic rings containing nitrogen, classified as purines or pyrimidines. Nucleotides also act as coenzymes in metabolic-group-transfer reactions.

Coenzymes

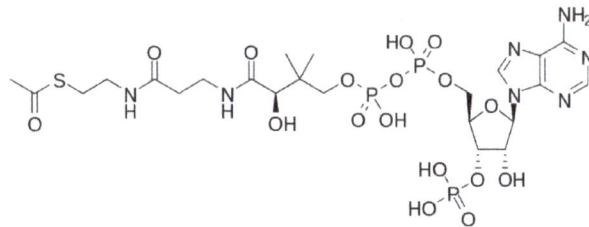

Structure of the coenzyme acetyl-CoA. The transferable acetyl group is bonded to the sulfur atom at the extreme left.

Metabolism involves a vast array of chemical reactions, but most fall under a few basic types of reactions that involve the transfer of functional groups of atoms and their bonds within molecules. This common chemistry allows cells to use a small set of metabolic intermediates to carry chemical groups between different reactions. These group-transfer intermediates are called coenzymes. Each class of group-transfer reactions is carried out by a particular coenzyme, which is the substrate for a set of enzymes that produce it, and a set of enzymes that consume it. These coenzymes are therefore continuously made, consumed and then recycled.

One central coenzyme is adenosine triphosphate (ATP), the universal energy currency of cells. This nucleotide is used to transfer chemical energy between different chemical reactions. There is only a small amount of ATP in cells, but as it is continuously regenerated, the human body can use about its own weight in ATP per day. ATP acts as a bridge between catabolism and anabolism. Catabolism breaks down molecules and anabolism puts them together. Catabolic reactions generate ATP and anabolic reactions consume it. It also serves as a carrier of phosphate groups in phosphorylation reactions.

A vitamin is an organic compound needed in small quantities that cannot be made in cells. In human nutrition, most vitamins function as coenzymes after modification; for example, all water-soluble vitamins are phosphorylated or are coupled to nucleotides when they are used in cells. Nicotinamide adenine dinucleotide (NAD^+), a derivative of vitamin B_3 (niacin), is an important coenzyme that acts as a hydrogen acceptor. Hundreds of separate types of dehydrogenases remove electrons from their substrates and reduce NAD^+ into NADH. This reduced form of the coenzyme is then a substrate for any of the reductases in the cell that need to reduce their substrates. Nicotinamide adenine dinucleotide exists in two related forms in the cell, NADH and NADPH. The NAD^+/NADH form is more important in catabolic reactions, while $NADP^+$/NADPH is used in anabolic reactions.

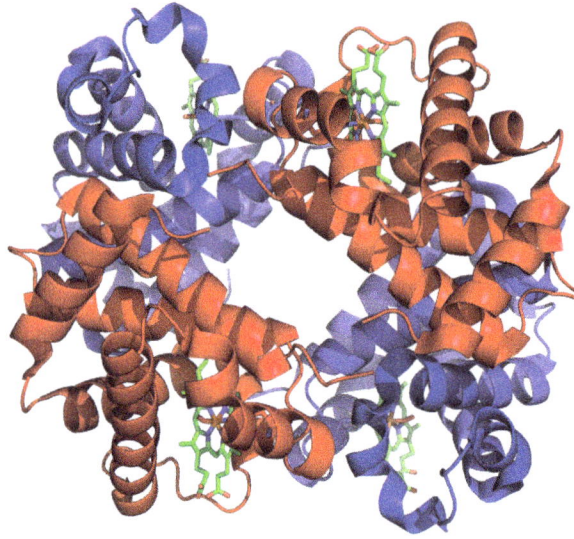

Structure of hemoglobin. The protein subunits are in red and blue, and the iron-containing heme groups in green. From PDB: 1GZX.

Minerals and Cofactors

Inorganic elements play critical roles in metabolism; some are abundant (e.g. sodium and potassium) while others function at minute concentrations. About 99% of a mammal's mass is made up of the elements carbon, nitrogen, calcium, sodium, chlorine, potassium, hydrogen, phosphorus, oxygen and sulfur. Organic compounds (proteins, lipids and carbohydrates) contain the majority of the carbon and nitrogen; most of the oxygen and hydrogen is present as water.

The abundant inorganic elements act as ionic electrolytes. The most important ions are sodium, potassium, calcium, magnesium, chloride, phosphate and the organic ion bicarbonate. The maintenance of precise ion gradients across cell membranes maintains osmotic pressure and pH. Ions are also critical for nerve and muscle function, as action potentials in these tissues are produced by the exchange of electrolytes between the extracellular fluid and the cell's fluid, the cytosol. Electrolytes enter and leave cells through proteins in the cell membrane called ion channels. For example, muscle contraction depends upon the movement of calcium, sodium and potassium through ion channels in the cell membrane and T-tubules.

Transition metals are usually present as trace elements in organisms, with zinc and iron being most abundant of those. These metals are used in some proteins as cofactors and are essential for the activity of enzymes such as catalase and oxygen-carrier proteins such as hemoglobin. Metal cofactors are bound tightly to specific sites in proteins; although enzyme cofactors can be modified during catalysis, they always return to their original state by the end of the reaction catalyzed. Metal micronutrients are taken up into organisms by specific transporters and bind to storage proteins such as ferritin or metallothionein when not in use.

Catabolism

Catabolism is the set of metabolic processes that break down large molecules. These include breaking down and oxidizing food molecules. The purpose of the catabolic reactions is to provide the energy and components needed by anabolic reactions. The exact nature of these catabolic reactions differ from organism to organism and organisms can be classified based on their sources of energy and carbon (their primary nutritional groups), as shown in the table below. Organic molecules are used as a source of energy by organotrophs, while lithotrophs use inorganic substrates and phototrophs capture sunlight as chemical energy. However, all these different forms of metabolism depend on redox reactions that involve the transfer of electrons from reduced donor molecules such as organic molecules, water, ammonia, hydrogen sulfide or ferrous ions to acceptor molecules such as oxygen, nitrate or sulfate. In animals these reactions involve complex organic molecules that are broken down to simpler molecules, such as carbon dioxide and water. In photosynthetic organisms such as plants and cyanobacteria, these electron-transfer reactions do not release energy, but are used as a way of storing energy absorbed from sunlight.

Classification of organisms based on their metabolism					
Energy source	sunlight	photo-			
Energy source	Preformed molecules	chemo-			
Electron donor	organic compound		organo-		-troph
Electron donor	inorganic compound		litho-		-troph
Carbon source	organic compound			hetero-	-troph
Carbon source	inorganic compound	auto-			-troph

The most common set of catabolic reactions in animals can be separated into three main stages. In the first, large organic molecules such as proteins, polysaccharides or lipids are digested into their smaller components outside cells. Next, these smaller molecules are taken up by cells and converted to yet smaller molecules, usually acetyl coenzyme A (acetyl-CoA), which releases some energy. Finally, the acetyl group on the CoA is oxidised to water and carbon dioxide in the citric acid cycle and electron transport chain, releasing the energy that is stored by reducing the coenzyme nicotinamide adenine dinucleotide (NAD^+) into NADH.

Digestion

Macromolecules such as starch, cellulose or proteins cannot be rapidly taken up by cells and must be broken into their smaller units before they can be used in cell metabolism. Several common classes of enzymes digest these polymers. These digestive enzymes include proteases that digest proteins into amino acids, as well as glycoside hydrolases that digest polysaccharides into simple sugars known as monosaccharides.

Microbes simply secrete digestive enzymes into their surroundings, while animals only secrete these enzymes from specialized cells in their guts. The amino acids or sugars released by these extracellular enzymes are then pumped into cells by active transport proteins.

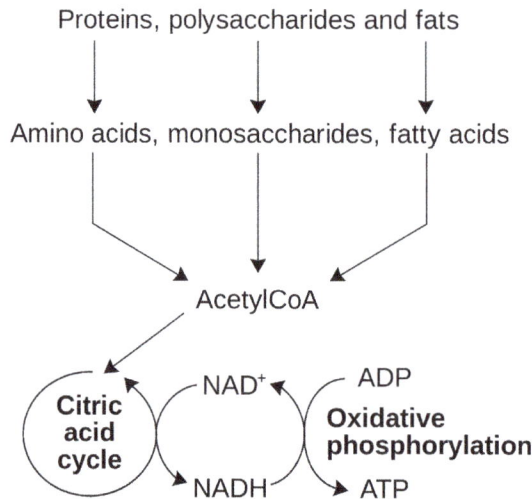

A simplified outline of the catabolism of proteins, carbohydrates and fats

Energy From Organic Compounds

Carbohydrate catabolism is the breakdown of carbohydrates into smaller units. Carbohydrates are usually taken into cells once they have been digested into monosaccharides. Once inside, the major route of breakdown is glycolysis, where sugars such as glucose and fructose are converted into pyruvate and some ATP is generated. Pyruvate is an intermediate in several metabolic pathways, but the majority is converted to acetyl-CoA and fed into the citric acid cycle. Although some more ATP is generated in the citric acid cycle, the most important product is NADH, which is made from NAD^+ as the acetyl-CoA is oxidized. This oxidation releases carbon dioxide as a waste product. In anaerobic conditions, glycolysis produces lactate, through the enzyme lactate dehydrogenase re-oxidizing NADH to NAD+ for re-use in glycolysis. An alternative route for glucose breakdown is the pentose phosphate pathway, which reduces the coenzyme NADPH and produces pentose sugars such as ribose, the sugar component of nucleic acids.

Fats are catabolised by hydrolysis to free fatty acids and glycerol. The glycerol enters glycolysis and the fatty acids are broken down by beta oxidation to release acetyl-CoA, which then is fed into the citric acid cycle. Fatty acids release more energy upon oxidation than carbohydrates because carbohydrates contain more oxygen in their structures. Steroids are also broken down by some bacteria in a process similar to beta oxidation, and this breakdown process involves the release of significant amounts of acetyl-CoA, propionyl-CoA, and pyruvate, which can all be used by the cell for energy. *M. tuberculosis* can also grow on the lipid cholesterol as a sole source of carbon, and genes involved in the cholesterol use pathway(s) have been validated as important during various stages of the infection lifecycle of *M. tuberculosis*.

Amino acids are either used to synthesize proteins and other biomolecules, or oxidized to urea and carbon dioxide as a source of energy. The oxidation pathway starts with the removal of the amino group by a transaminase. The amino group is fed into the urea cycle, leaving a deaminated carbon skeleton in the form of a keto acid. Several of these keto acids are intermediates in the citric acid cycle, for example the deamination of glutamate forms α-ketoglutarate. The glucogenic amino acids can also be converted into glucose, through gluconeogenesis (discussed below).

Energy Transformations

Oxidative Phosphorylation

In oxidative phosphorylation, the electrons removed from organic molecules in areas such as the protagon acid cycle are transferred to oxygen and the energy released is used to make ATP. This is done in eukaryotes by a series of proteins in the membranes of mitochondria called the electron transport chain. In prokaryotes, these proteins are found in the cell's inner membrane. These proteins use the energy released from passing electrons from reduced molecules like NADH onto oxygen to pump protons across a membrane.

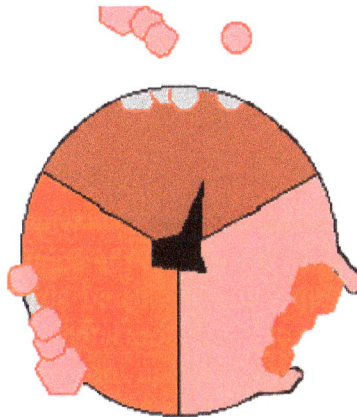

Mechanism of ATP synthase. ATP is shown in red, ADP and phosphate in pink and the rotating stalk subunit in black.

Pumping protons out of the mitochondria creates a proton concentration difference across the membrane and generates an electrochemical gradient. This force drives protons back into the mitochondrion through the base of an enzyme called ATP synthase. The flow of protons makes the stalk subunit rotate, causing the active site of the synthase domain to change shape and phosphorylate adenosine diphosphate – turning it into ATP.

Energy From Inorganic Compounds

Chemolithotrophy is a type of metabolism found in prokaryotes where energy is obtained from the oxidation of inorganic compounds. These organisms can use hydrogen, reduced sulfur compounds (such as sulfide, hydrogen sulfide and thiosulfate), ferrous iron (FeII) or ammonia as sources of reducing power and they gain energy from the oxidation of these compounds with electron acceptors such as oxygen or nitrite. These microbial processes are important in global biogeochemical cycles such as acetogenesis, nitrification and denitrification and are critical for soil fertility.

Energy From Light

The energy in sunlight is captured by plants, cyanobacteria, purple bacteria, green sulfur bacteria and some protists. This process is often coupled to the conversion of carbon dioxide into organic compounds, as part of photosynthesis, which is discussed below. The energy capture and carbon fixation systems can however operate separately in prokaryotes, as purple bacteria and green sulfur bacteria can use sunlight as a source of energy, while switching between carbon fixation and the fermentation of organic compounds.

In many organisms the capture of solar energy is similar in principle to oxidative phosphorylation, as it involves the storage of energy as a proton concentration gradient. This proton motive force then drives ATP synthesis. The electrons needed to drive this electron transport chain come from light-gathering proteins called photosynthetic reaction centres or rhodopsins. Reaction centers are classed into two types depending on the type of photosynthetic pigment present, with most photosynthetic bacteria only having one type, while plants and cyanobacteria have two.

In plants, algae, and cyanobacteria, photosystem II uses light energy to remove electrons from water, releasing oxygen as a waste product. The electrons then flow to the cytochrome b6f complex, which uses their energy to pump protons across the thylakoid membrane in the chloroplast. These protons move back through the membrane as they drive the ATP synthase, as before. The electrons then flow through photosystem I and can then either be used to reduce the coenzyme $NADP^+$, for use in the Calvin cycle, which is discussed below, or recycled for further ATP generation.

Anabolism

Anabolism is the set of constructive metabolic processes where the energy released by catabolism is used to synthesize complex molecules. In general, the complex molecules that make up cellular structures are constructed step-by-step from small and simple precursors. Anabolism involves three basic stages. First, the production of precursors such as amino acids, monosaccharides, isoprenoids and nucleotides, secondly, their activation into reactive forms using energy from ATP, and thirdly, the assembly of these precursors into complex molecules such as proteins, polysaccharides, lipids and nucleic acids.

Organisms differ in how many of the molecules in their cells they can construct for themselves. Autotrophs such as plants can construct the complex organic molecules in cells such as polysaccharides and proteins from simple molecules like carbon dioxide and water. Heterotrophs, on the other hand, require a source of more complex substances, such as monosaccharides and amino acids, to produce these complex molecules. Organisms can be further classified by ultimate source of their energy: photoautotrophs and photoheterotrophs obtain energy from light, whereas chemoautotrophs and chemoheterotrophs obtain energy from inorganic oxidation reactions.

Carbon Fixation

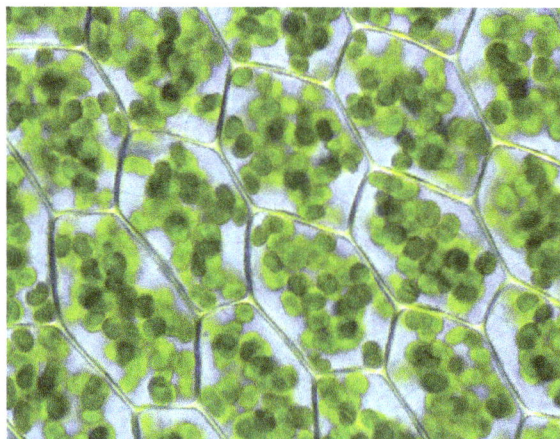

Plant cells (bounded by purple walls) filled with chloroplasts (green), which are the site of photosynthesis

Photosynthesis is the synthesis of carbohydrates from sunlight and carbon dioxide (CO_2). In plants, cyanobacteria and algae, oxygenic photosynthesis splits water, with oxygen produced as a waste product. This process uses the ATP and NADPH produced by the photosynthetic reaction centres, as described above, to convert CO_2 into glycerate 3-phosphate, which can then be converted into glucose. This carbon-fixation reaction is carried out by the enzyme RuBisCO as part of the Calvin – Benson cycle. Three types of photosynthesis occur in plants, C3 carbon fixation, C4 carbon fixation and CAM photosynthesis. These differ by the route that carbon dioxide takes to the Calvin cycle, with C3 plants fixing CO_2 directly, while C4 and CAM photosynthesis incorporate the CO_2 into other compounds first, as adaptations to deal with intense sunlight and dry conditions.

In photosynthetic prokaryotes the mechanisms of carbon fixation are more diverse. Here, carbon dioxide can be fixed by the Calvin – Benson cycle, a reversed citric acid cycle, or the carboxylation of acetyl-CoA. Prokaryotic chemoautotrophs also fix CO_2 through the Calvin – Benson cycle, but use energy from inorganic compounds to drive the reaction.

Carbohydrates and Glycans

In carbohydrate anabolism, simple organic acids can be converted into monosaccharides such as glucose and then used to assemble polysaccharides such as starch. The generation of glucose from compounds like pyruvate, lactate, glycerol, glycerate 3-phosphate and amino acids is called gluconeogenesis. Gluconeogenesis converts pyruvate to glucose-6-phosphate through a series of intermediates, many of which are shared with glycolysis. However, this pathway is not simply glycolysis run in reverse, as several steps are catalyzed by non-glycolytic enzymes. This is important as it allows the formation and breakdown of glucose to be regulated separately, and prevents both pathways from running simultaneously in a futile cycle.

Although fat is a common way of storing energy, in vertebrates such as humans the fatty acids in these stores cannot be converted to glucose through gluconeogenesis as these organisms cannot convert acetyl-CoA into pyruvate; plants do, but animals do not, have the necessary enzymatic machinery. As a result, after long-term starvation, vertebrates need to produce ketone bodies from fatty acids to replace glucose in tissues such as the brain that cannot metabolize fatty acids. In other organisms such as plants and bacteria, this metabolic problem is solved using the glyoxylate cycle, which bypasses the decarboxylation step in the citric acid cycle and allows the transformation of acetyl-CoA to oxaloacetate, where it can be used for the production of glucose.

Polysaccharides and glycans are made by the sequential addition of monosaccharides by glycosyltransferase from a reactive sugar-phosphate donor such as uridine diphosphate glucose (UDP-glucose) to an acceptor hydroxyl group on the growing polysaccharide. As any of the hydroxyl groups on the ring of the substrate can be acceptors, the polysaccharides produced can have straight or branched structures. The polysaccharides produced can have structural or metabolic functions themselves, or be transferred to lipids and proteins by enzymes called oligosaccharyltransferases.

Fatty Acids, Isoprenoids and Steroids

Fatty acids are made by fatty acid synthases that polymerize and then reduce acetyl-CoA units. The acyl chains in the fatty acids are extended by a cycle of reactions that add the acyl group, reduce it to an alcohol, dehydrate it to an alkene group and then reduce it again to an alkane group. The enzymes of fatty acid biosynthesis are divided into two groups: in animals and fungi, all these fatty acid synthase reactions are carried out by a single multifunctional type I protein, while in plant plastids and bacteria separate type II enzymes perform each step in the pathway.

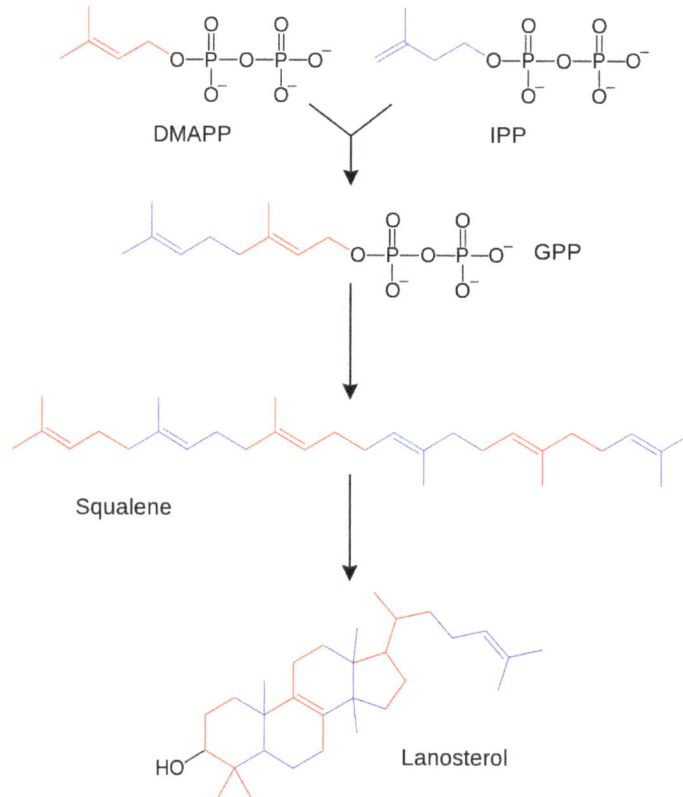

Simplified version of the steroid synthesis pathway with the intermediates isopentenyl pyrophosphate (IPP), dimethylallyl pyrophosphate (DMAPP), geranyl pyrophosphate (GPP) and squalene shown. Some intermediates are omitted for clarity.

Terpenes and isoprenoids are a large class of lipids that include the carotenoids and form the largest class of plant natural products. These compounds are made by the assembly and modification of isoprene units donated from the reactive precursors isopentenyl pyrophosphate and dimethylallyl pyrophosphate. These precursors can be made in different ways. In animals and archaea, the mevalonate pathway produces these compounds from acetyl-CoA, while in plants and bacteria the non-mevalonate pathway uses pyruvate and glyceraldehyde 3-phosphate as substrates. One important reaction that uses these activated isoprene donors is steroid biosynthesis. Here, the isoprene units are joined together to make squalene and then folded up and formed into a set of rings to make lanosterol. Lanosterol can then be converted into other steroids such as cholesterol and ergosterol.

Proteins

Organisms vary in their ability to synthesize the 20 common amino acids. Most bacteria and plants can synthesize all twenty, but mammals can only synthesize eleven nonessential amino acids, so nine essential amino acids must be obtained from food. Some simple parasites, such as the bacteria

Mycoplasma pneumoniae, lack all amino acid synthesis and take their amino acids directly from their hosts. All amino acids are synthesized from intermediates in glycolysis, the citric acid cycle, or the pentose phosphate pathway. Nitrogen is provided by glutamate and glutamine. Amino acid synthesis depends on the formation of the appropriate alpha-keto acid, which is then transaminated to form an amino acid.

Amino acids are made into proteins by being joined together in a chain of peptide bonds. Each different protein has a unique sequence of amino acid residues: this is its primary structure. Just as the letters of the alphabet can be combined to form an almost endless variety of words, amino acids can be linked in varying sequences to form a huge variety of proteins. Proteins are made from amino acids that have been activated by attachment to a transfer RNA molecule through an ester bond. This aminoacyl-tRNA precursor is produced in an ATP-dependent reaction carried out by an aminoacyl tRNA synthetase. This aminoacyl-tRNA is then a substrate for the ribosome, which joins the amino acid onto the elongating protein chain, using the sequence information in a messenger RNA.

Nucleotide Synthesis and Salvage

Nucleotides are made from amino acids, carbon dioxide and formic acid in pathways that require large amounts of metabolic energy. Consequently, most organisms have efficient systems to salvage preformed nucleotides. Purines are synthesized as nucleosides (bases attached to ribose). Both adenine and guanine are made from the precursor nucleoside inosine monophosphate, which is synthesized using atoms from the amino acids glycine, glutamine, and aspartic acid, as well as formate transferred from the coenzyme tetrahydrofolate. Pyrimidines, on the other hand, are synthesized from the base orotate, which is formed from glutamine and aspartate.

Xenobiotics and Redox Metabolism

All organisms are constantly exposed to compounds that they cannot use as foods and would be harmful if they accumulated in cells, as they have no metabolic function. These potentially damaging compounds are called xenobiotics. Xenobiotics such as synthetic drugs, natural poisons and antibiotics are detoxified by a set of xenobiotic-metabolizing enzymes. In humans, these include cytochrome P450 oxidases, UDP-glucuronosyltransferases, and glutathione *S*-transferases. This system of enzymes acts in three stages to firstly oxidize the xenobiotic (phase I) and then conjugate water-soluble groups onto the molecule (phase II). The modified water-soluble xenobiotic can then be pumped out of cells and in multicellular organisms may be further metabolized before being excreted (phase III). In ecology, these reactions are particularly important in microbial biodegradation of pollutants and the bioremediation of contaminated land and oil spills. Many of these microbial reactions are shared with multicellular organisms, but due to the incredible diversity of types of microbes these organisms are able to deal with a far wider range of xenobiotics than multicellular organisms, and can degrade even persistent organic pollutants such as organochloride compounds.

A related problem for aerobic organisms is oxidative stress. Here, processes including oxidative phosphorylation and the formation of disulfide bonds during protein folding produce reactive oxygen species such as hydrogen peroxide. These damaging oxidants are removed by antioxidant metabolites such as glutathione and enzymes such as catalases and peroxidases.

Thermodynamics of Living Organisms

Living organisms must obey the laws of thermodynamics, which describe the transfer of heat and work. The second law of thermodynamics states that in any closed system, the amount of entropy (disorder) cannot decrease. Although living organisms' amazing complexity appears to contradict this law, life is possible as all organisms are open systems that exchange matter and energy with their surroundings. Thus living systems are not in equilibrium, but instead are dissipative systems that maintain their state of high complexity by causing a larger increase in the entropy of their environments. The metabolism of a cell achieves this by coupling the spontaneous processes of catabolism to the non-spontaneous processes of anabolism. In thermodynamic terms, metabolism maintains order by creating disorder.

Regulation and Control

As the environments of most organisms are constantly changing, the reactions of metabolism must be finely regulated to maintain a constant set of conditions within cells, a condition called homeostasis. Metabolic regulation also allows organisms to respond to signals and interact actively with their environments. Two closely linked concepts are important for understanding how metabolic pathways are controlled. Firstly, the *regulation* of an enzyme in a pathway is how its activity is increased and decreased in response to signals. Secondly, the *control* exerted by this enzyme is the effect that these changes in its activity have on the overall rate of the pathway (the flux through the pathway). For example, an enzyme may show large changes in activity (*i.e.* it is highly regulated) but if these changes have little effect on the flux of a metabolic pathway, then this enzyme is not involved in the control of the pathway.

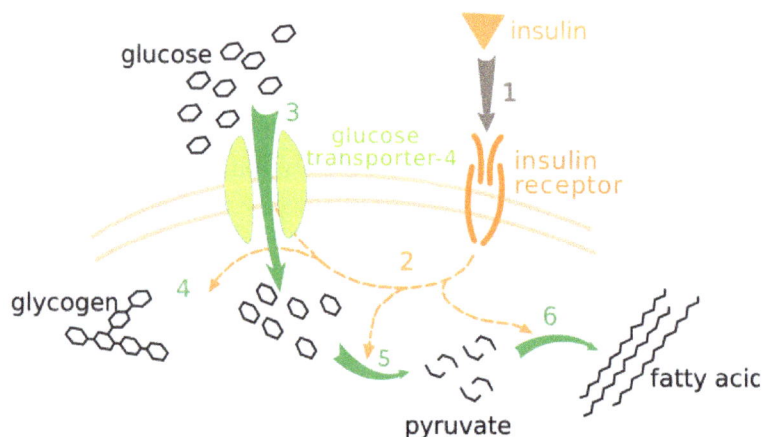

Effect of insulin on glucose uptake and metabolism. Insulin binds to its receptor (1), which in turn starts many protein activation cascades (2). These include: translocation of Glut-4 transporter to the plasma membrane and influx of glucose (3), glycogen synthesis (4), glycolysis (5) and fatty acid synthesis (6).

There are multiple levels of metabolic regulation. In intrinsic regulation, the metabolic pathway self-regulates to respond to changes in the levels of substrates or products; for example, a decrease in the amount of product can increase the flux through the pathway to compensate. This type of regulation often involves allosteric regulation of the activities of multiple enzymes in the pathway. Extrinsic control involves a cell in a multicellular organism changing its metabolism in response to signals from other cells. These signals are usually in the form of soluble messengers such as hormones and growth factors and are detected by specific receptors on the cell surface. These signals are then transmitted inside the cell by second messenger systems that often involved the phosphorylation of proteins.

A very well understood example of extrinsic control is the regulation of glucose metabolism by the hormone insulin. Insulin is produced in response to rises in blood glucose levels. Binding of the hormone to insulin receptors on cells then activates a cascade of protein kinases that cause the cells to take up glucose and convert it into storage molecules such as fatty acids and glycogen. The metabolism of glycogen is controlled by activity of phosphorylase, the enzyme that breaks down glycogen, and glycogen synthase, the enzyme that makes it. These enzymes are regulated in a reciprocal fashion, with phosphorylation inhibiting glycogen synthase, but activating phosphorylase. Insulin causes glycogen synthesis by activating protein phosphatases and producing a decrease in the phosphorylation of these enzymes.

Evolution

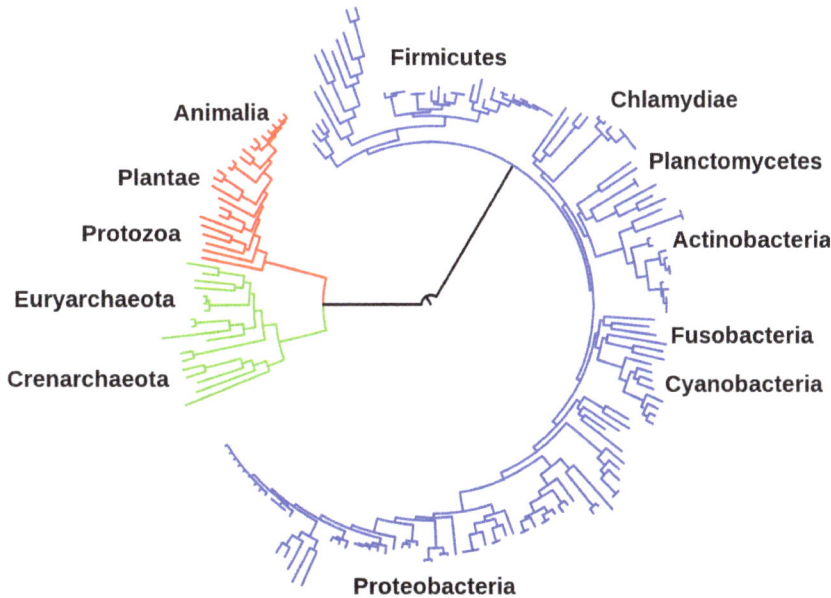

Evolutionary tree showing the common ancestry of organisms from all three domains of life. Bacteria are colored blue, eukaryotes red, and archaea green. Relative positions of some of the phyla included are shown around the tree.

The central pathways of metabolism described above, such as glycolysis and the citric acid cycle, are present in all three domains of living things and were present in the last universal ancestor. This universal ancestral cell was prokaryotic and probably a methanogen that had extensive amino acid, nucleotide, carbohydrate and lipid metabolism. The retention of these ancient pathways during later evolution may be the result of these reactions having been an optimal solution to their particular metabolic problems, with pathways such as glycolysis and the citric acid cycle producing their end products highly efficiently and in a minimal number of steps. The first pathways of enzyme-based metabolism may have been parts of purine nucleotide metabolism, while previous metabolic pathways were a part of the ancient RNA world.

Many models have been proposed to describe the mechanisms by which novel metabolic pathways evolve. These include the sequential addition of novel enzymes to a short ancestral pathway, the duplication and then divergence of entire pathways as well as the recruitment of pre-existing enzymes and their assembly into a novel reaction pathway. The relative importance of these mechanisms is unclear, but genomic studies have shown that enzymes in a pathway are likely to have a shared ancestry, suggesting that many pathways have evolved in a step-by-step fashion with novel functions created from pre-existing steps in the pathway. An alternative model comes from studies that trace the evolution of proteins' structures in metabolic networks, this has suggested that enzymes are pervasively recruited, borrowing enzymes to perform similar functions in different metabolic pathways (evident in the MANET database) These recruitment processes result in an evolutionary enzymatic mosaic. A third possibility is that some parts of metabolism might exist as "modules" that can be reused in different pathways and perform similar functions on different molecules.

As well as the evolution of new metabolic pathways, evolution can also cause the loss of metabolic functions. For example, in some parasites metabolic processes that are not essential for survival are lost and preformed amino acids, nucleotides and carbohydrates may instead be scavenged from the host. Similar reduced metabolic capabilities are seen in endosymbiotic organisms.

Investigation and Manipulation

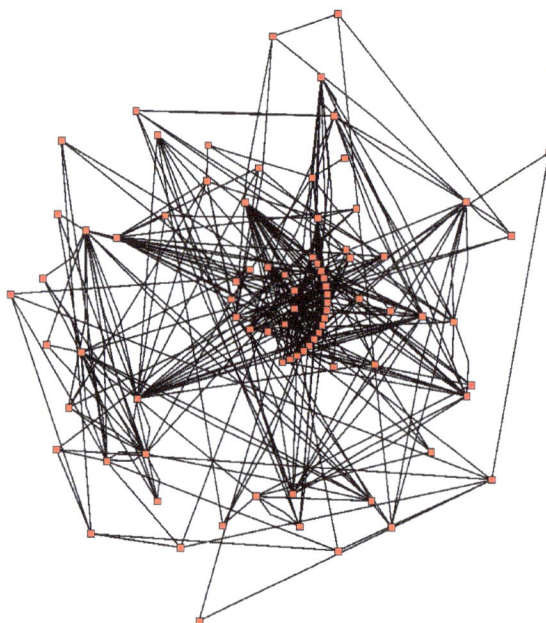

Metabolic network of the *Arabidopsis thaliana* citric acid cycle. Enzymes and metabolites are shown as red squares and the interactions between them as black lines.

Classically, metabolism is studied by a reductionist approach that focuses on a single metabolic pathway. Particularly valuable is the use of radioactive tracers at the whole-organism, tissue and cellular levels, which define the paths from precursors to final products by identifying radioactively labelled intermediates and products. The enzymes that catalyze these chemical reactions can then be purified and their kinetics and responses to inhibitors investigated. A parallel approach is to identify the small molecules in a cell or tissue; the complete set of these molecules is called the metabolome. Overall, these studies give a good view of the structure and function of simple metabolic pathways, but are inadequate when applied to more complex systems such as the metabolism of a complete cell.

An idea of the complexity of the metabolic networks in cells that contain thousands of different enzymes is given by the figure showing the interactions between just 43 proteins and 40 metabolites to the right: the sequences of genomes provide lists containing anything up to 45,000 genes. However, it is now possible to use this genomic data to reconstruct complete networks of biochemical reactions and produce more holistic mathematical models that may explain and predict their behavior. These models are especially powerful when used to integrate the pathway and metabolite data obtained through classical methods with data on gene expression from proteomic and DNA microarray studies. Using these techniques, a model of human metabolism has now been produced, which will guide future drug discovery and biochemical research. These models are now used in network analysis, to classify human diseases into groups that share common proteins or metabolites.

Bacterial metabolic networks are a striking example of bow-tie organization, an architecture able to input a wide range of nutrients and produce a large variety of products and complex macromolecules using a relatively few intermediate common currencies.

A major technological application of this information is metabolic engineering. Here, organisms such as yeast, plants or bacteria are genetically modified to make them more useful in biotechnology and aid the production of drugs such as antibiotics or industrial chemicals such as 1,3-propanediol and shikimic acid. These genetic modifications usually aim to reduce the amount of energy used to produce the product, increase yields and reduce the production of wastes.

History

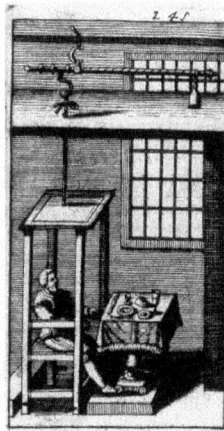

Santorio Santorio in his steelyard balance, from *Ars de statica medicina*, first published 1614

The first documented references of metabolism were made by Ibn al-Nafis in his 1260 AD work titled Al-Risalah al-Kamiliyyah fil Siera al-Nabawiyyah (The Treatise of Kamil on the Prophet's Biography) which included the following phrase "Both the body and its parts are in a continuous state of dissolution and nourishment, so they are inevitably undergoing permanent change." The history of the scientific study of metabolism spans several centuries and has moved from examining whole animals in early studies, to examining individual metabolic reactions in modern biochemistry. The first controlled experiments in human metabolism were published by Santorio Santorio in 1614 in his book *Ars de statica medicina*. He described how he weighed himself before and after eating, sleep, working, sex, fasting, drinking, and excreting. He found that most of the food he took in was lost through what he called "insensible perspiration".

In these early studies, the mechanisms of these metabolic processes had not been identified and a vital force was thought to animate living tissue. In the 19th century, when studying the fermentation of sugar to alcohol by yeast, Louis Pasteur concluded that fermentation was catalyzed by substances within the yeast cells he called "ferments". He wrote that "alcoholic fermentation is an act correlated with the life and organization of the yeast cells, not with the death or putrefaction of the cells." This discovery, along with the publication by Friedrich Wöhler in 1828 of a paper on the chemical synthesis of urea, and is notable for being the first organic compound prepared from wholly inorganic precursors. This proved that the organic compounds and chemical reactions found in cells were no different in principle than any other part of chemistry.

It was the discovery of enzymes at the beginning of the 20th century by Eduard Buchner that separated the study of the chemical reactions of metabolism from the biological study of cells, and marked the beginnings of biochemistry. The mass of biochemical knowledge grew rapidly throughout the early 20th century. One of the most prolific of these modern biochemists was Hans Krebs who made huge contributions to the study of metabolism. He discovered the urea cycle and later, working with Hans Kornberg, the citric acid cycle and the glyoxylate cycle. Modern biochemical research has been greatly aided by the development of new techniques such as chromatography, X-ray diffraction, NMR spectroscopy, radioisotopic labelling, electron microscopy and molecular dynamics simulations. These techniques have allowed the discovery and detailed analysis of the many molecules and metabolic pathways in cells.

Digestion

Digestion is the breakdown of large insoluble food molecules into small water-soluble food molecules so that they can be absorbed into the watery blood plasma. In certain organisms, these smaller substances are absorbed through the small intestine into the blood stream. Digestion is a form of catabolism that is often divided into two processes based on how food is broken down: mechanical and chemical digestion. The term mechanical digestion refers to the physical breakdown of large pieces of food into smaller pieces which can subsequently be accessed by digestive enzymes. In chemical digestion, enzymes break down food into the small molecules the body can use.

In the human digestive system, food enters the mouth and mechanical digestion of the food starts by the action of mastication (chewing), a form of mechanical digestion, and the wetting contact of saliva. Saliva, a liquid secreted by the salivary glands, contains salivary amylase, an enzyme which starts the digestion of starch in the food; the saliva also contains mucus, which lubricates the food, and hydrogen carbonate, which provides the ideal conditions of pH (alkaline) for amylase to work. After undergoing mastication and starch digestion, the food will be in the form of a small, round slurry mass called a bolus. It will then travel down the esophagus and into the stomach by the action of peristalsis. Gastric juice in the stomach starts protein digestion. Gastric juice mainly contains hydrochloric acid and pepsin. As these two chemicals may damage the stomach wall, mucus is secreted by the stomach, providing a slimy layer that acts as a shield against the damaging effects of the chemicals. At the same time protein digestion is occurring, mechanical mixing occurs by peristalsis, which is waves of muscular contractions that move along the stomach wall. This allows the mass of food to further mix with the digestive enzymes.

After some time (typically 1–2 hours in humans, 4–6 hours in dogs, 3–4 hours in house cats), the resulting thick liquid is called chyme. When the pyloric sphincter valve opens, chyme enters the duodenum where it mixes with digestive enzymes from the pancreas and bile juice from the liver and then passes through the small intestine, in which digestion continues. When the chyme is fully digested, it is absorbed into the blood. 95% of absorption of nutrients occurs in the small intestine. Water and minerals are reabsorbed back into the blood in the colon (large intestine) where the pH is slightly acidic about 5.6 ~ 6.9. Some vitamins, such as biotin and vitamin K (K_2MK7) produced by bacteria in the colon are also absorbed into the blood in the colon. Waste material is eliminated from the rectum during defecation.

Digestive System

Digestive systems take many forms. There is a fundamental distinction between internal and external digestion. External digestion developed earlier in evolutionary history, and most fungi still rely on it. In this process, enzymes are secreted into the environment surrounding the organism, where they break down an organic material, and some of the products diffuse back to the organism. Animals have a tube (gastrointestinal tract) in which internal digestion occurs, which is more efficient because more of the broken down products can be captured, and the internal chemical environment can be more efficiently controlled.

Some organisms, including nearly all spiders, simply secrete biotoxins and digestive chemicals (e.g., enzymes) into the extracellular environment prior to ingestion of the consequent "soup". In others, once potential nutrients or food is inside the organism, digestion can be conducted to a vesicle or a sac-like structure, through a tube, or through several specialized organs aimed at making the absorption of nutrients more efficient.

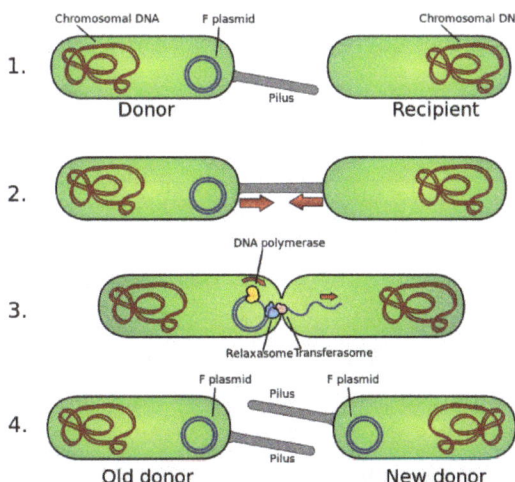

Schematic drawing of bacterial conjugation. 1- Donor cell produces pilus. 2- Pilus attaches to recipient cell, bringing the two cells together. 3- The mobile plasmid is nicked and a single strand of DNA is transferred to the recipient cell. 4- Both cells recircularize their plasmids, synthesize second strands, and reproduce pili; both cells are now viable donors.

Secretion Systems

Bacteria use several systems to obtain nutrients from other organisms in the environments.

Channel Transport System

In a channel transupport system, several proteins form a contiguous channel traversing the inner and outer membranes of the bacteria. It is a simple system, which consists of only three protein subunits: the ABC protein, membrane fusion protein (MFP), and outer membrane protein (OMP). This secretion system transports various molecules, from ions, drugs, to proteins of various sizes (20 – 900 kDa). The molecules secreted vary in size from the small *Escherichia coli* peptide colicin V, (10 kDa) to the *Pseudomonas fluorescens* cell adhesion protein LapA of 900 kDa.

Molecular Syringe

One molecular syringe is used through which a bacterium (e.g. certain types of *Salmonella*, *Shigella*, *Yersinia*) can inject nutrients into protist cells. One such mechanism was first discovered in *Y. pestis* and showed that toxins could be injected directly from the bacterial cytoplasm into the cytoplasm of its host's cells rather than simply be secreted into the extracellular medium.

Conjugation Machinery

The conjugation machinery of some bacteria (and archaeal flagella) is capable of transporting both DNA and proteins. It was discovered in *Agrobacterium tumefaciens*, which uses this system to introduce the Ti plasmid and proteins into the host, which develops the crown gall (tumor). The VirB complex of *Agrobacterium tumefaciens* is the prototypic system.

The nitrogen fixing *Rhizobia* are an interesting case, wherein conjugative elements naturally engage in inter-kingdom conjugation. Such elements as the *Agrobacterium* Ti or Ri plasmids contain elements that can transfer to plant cells. Transferred genes enter the plant cell nucleus and effectively transform the plant cells into factories for the production of opines, which the bacteria use as carbon and energy sources. Infected plant cells form crown gall or root tumors. The Ti and Ri plasmids are thus endosymbionts of the bacteria, which are in turn endosymbionts (or parasites) of the infected plant.

The Ti and Ri plasmids are themselves conjugative. Ti and Ri transfer between bacteria uses an independent system (the *tra*, or transfer, operon) from that for inter-kingdom transfer (the *vir*, or virulence, operon). Such transfer creates virulent strains from previously avirulent *Agrobacteria*.

Release of Outer Membrane Vesicles

In addition to the use of the multiprotein complexes listed above, Gram-negative bacteria possess another method for release of material: the formation of outer membrane vesicles. Portions of the outer membrane pinch off, forming spherical structures made of a lipid bilayer enclosing periplasmic materials. Vesicles from a number of bacterial species have been found to contain virulence factors, some have immunomodulatory effects, and some can directly adhere to and intoxicate host cells. While release of vesicles has been demonstrated as a general response to stress conditions, the process of loading cargo proteins seems to be selective.

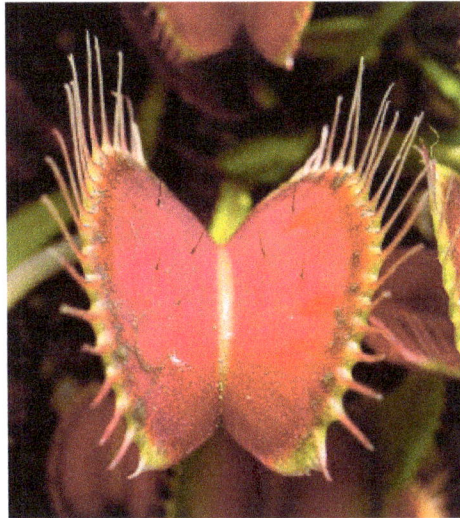

Venus Flytrap (*Dionaea muscipula*) leaf

Gastrovascular Cavity

The gastrovascular cavity functions as a stomach in both digestion and the distribution of nutrients to all parts of the body. Extracellular digestion takes place within this central cavity, which is lined with the gastrodermis, the internal layer of epithelium. This cavity has only one opening to the outside that functions as both a mouth and an anus: waste and undigested matter is excreted through the mouth/anus, which can be described as an incomplete gut.

In a plant such as the Venus Flytrap that can make its own food through photosynthesis, it does not eat and digest its prey for the traditional objectives of harvesting energy and carbon, but mines prey primarily for essential nutrients (nitrogen and phosphorus in particular) that are in short supply in its boggy, acidic habitat.

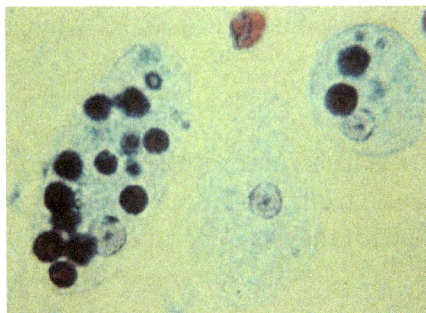

Trophozoites of *Entamoeba histolytica* with ingested erythrocytes

Phagosome

A phagosome is a vacuole formed around a particle absorbed by phagocytosis. The vacuole is formed by the fusion of the cell membrane around the particle. A phagosome is a cellular compartment in which pathogenic microorganisms can be killed and digested. Phagosomes fuse with lysosomes in their maturation process, forming phagolysosomes. In humans, *Entamoeba histolytica* can phagocytose red blood cells.

Specialised Organs and Behaviours

To aid in the digestion of their food animals evolved organs such as beaks, tongues, teeth, a crop, gizzard, and others.

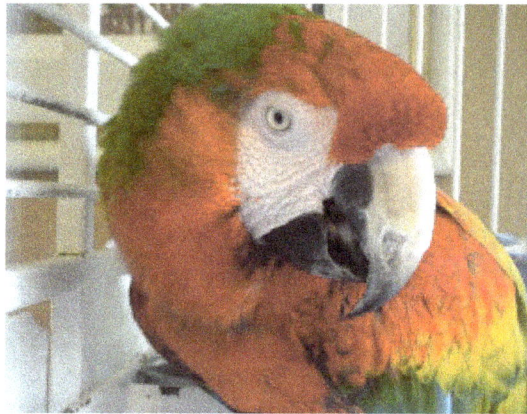

A Catalina Macaw's seed-shearing beak

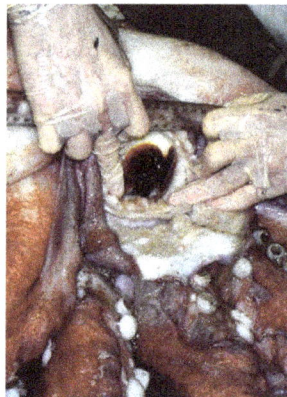

Squid beak with ruler for size comparison

Beaks

Birds have bony beaks that are specialised according to the bird's ecological niche. For example, macaws primarily eat seeds, nuts, and fruit, using their impressive beaks to open even the toughest seed. First they scratch a thin line with the sharp point of the beak, then they shear the seed open with the sides of the beak.

The mouth of the squid is equipped with a sharp horny beak mainly made of cross-linked proteins. It is used to kill and tear prey into manageable pieces. The beak is very robust, but does not contain any minerals, unlike the teeth and jaws of many other organisms, including marine species. The beak is the only indigestible part of the squid.

Tongue

The tongue is skeletal muscle on the floor of the mouth that manipulates food for chewing (mastication) and swallowing (deglutition). It is sensitive and kept moist by saliva. The underside of the tongue is covered with a smooth mucous membrane. The tongue also has a touch sense for locating and positioning food particles that require further chewing. The tongue is utilized to roll food particles into a bolus before being transported down the esophagus through peristalsis.

The sublingual region underneath the front of the tongue is a location where the oral mucosa is very thin, and underlain by a plexus of veins. This is an ideal location for introducing certain medications to the body. The sublingual route takes advantage of the highly vascular quality of the oral cavity, and allows for the speedy application of medication into the cardiovascular system, bypassing the gastrointestinal tract.

Teeth

Teeth (singular tooth) are small whitish structures found in the jaws (or mouths) of many vertebrates that are used to tear, scrape, milk and chew food. Teeth are not made of bone, but rather of tissues of varying density and hardness, such as enamel, dentine and cementum. Human teeth have a blood and nerve supply which enables proprioception. This is the ability of sensation when chewing, for example if we were to bite into something too hard for our teeth, such as a chipped plate mixed in food, our teeth send a message to our brain and we realise that it cannot be chewed, so we stop trying.

The shapes, sizes and numbers of types of animals' teeth are related to their diets. For example, herbivores have a number of molars which are used to grind plant matter, which is difficult to digest. Carnivores have canine teeth which are used to kill and tear meat.

Crop

A crop, or croup, is a thin-walled expanded portion of the alimentary tract used for the storage of food prior to digestion. In some birds it is an expanded, muscular pouch near the gullet or throat. In adult doves and pigeons, the crop can produce crop milk to feed newly hatched birds.

Certain insects may have a crop or enlarged esophagus.

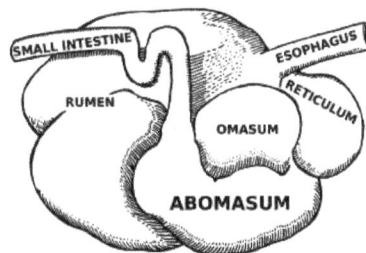

Rough illustration of a ruminant digestive system

Abomasum

Herbivores have evolved cecums (or an abomasum in the case of ruminants). Ruminants have a fore-stomach with four chambers. These are the rumen, reticulum, omasum, and abomasum. In the first two chambers, the rumen and the reticulum, the food is mixed with saliva and separates into layers of solid and liquid material. Solids clump together to form the cud (or bolus). The cud is then regurgitated, chewed slowly to completely mix it with saliva and to break down the particle size.

Fibre, especially cellulose and hemi-cellulose, is primarily broken down into the volatile fatty acids, acetic acid, propionic acid and butyric acid in these chambers (the reticulo-rumen) by microbes: (bacteria, protozoa, and fungi). In the omasum, water and many of the inorganic mineral elements are absorbed into the blood stream.

The abomasum is the fourth and final stomach compartment in ruminants. It is a close equivalent of a monogastric stomach (e.g., those in humans or pigs), and digesta is processed here in much the same way. It serves primarily as a site for acid hydrolysis of microbial and dietary protein, preparing these protein sources for further digestion and absorption in the small intestine. Digesta is finally moved into the small intestine, where the digestion and absorption of nutrients occurs. Microbes produced in the reticulo-rumen are also digested in the small intestine.

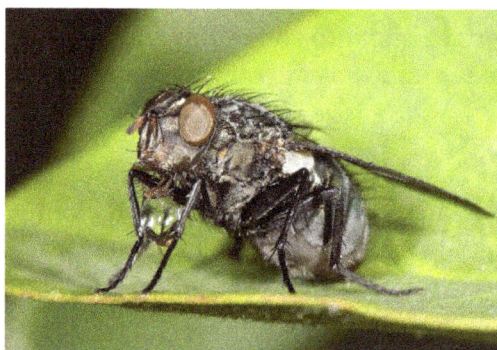

A flesh fly "blowing a bubble", possibly to concentrate its food by evaporating water

Specialised Behaviours

Regurgitation has been mentioned above under abomasum and crop, referring to crop milk, a secretion from the lining of the crop of pigeons and doves with which the parents feed their young by regurgitation.

Many sharks have the ability to turn their stomachs inside out and evert it out of their mouths in order to get rid of unwanted contents (perhaps developed as a way to reduce exposure to toxins).

Other animals, such as rabbits and rodents, practise coprophagia behaviours – eating specialised faeces in order to re-digest food, especially in the case of roughage. Capybara, rabbits, hamsters and other related species do not have a complex digestive system as do, for example, ruminants. Instead they extract more nutrition from grass by giving their food a second pass through the gut. Soft faecal pellets of partially digested food are excreted and generally consumed immediately. They also produce normal droppings, which are not eaten.

Young elephants, pandas, koalas, and hippos eat the faeces of their mother, probably to obtain the bacteria required to properly digest vegetation. When they are born, their intestines do not contain these bacteria (they are completely sterile). Without them, they would be unable to get any nutritional value from many plant components.

In earthworms

An earthworm's digestive system consists of a mouth, pharynx, esophagus, crop, gizzard, and intestine. The mouth is surrounded by strong lips, which act like a hand to grab pieces of dead grass, leaves, and weeds, with bits of soil to help chew. The lips break the food down into smaller pieces. In the pharynx, the food is lubricated by mucus secretions for easier passage. The esophagus adds calcium carbonate to neutralize the acids formed by food matter decay. Temporary storage occurs in the crop where food and calcium carbonate are mixed. The powerful muscles of the gizzard churn and mix the mass of food and dirt. When the churning is complete, the glands in the walls of the gizzard add enzymes to the thick paste, which helps chemically breakdown the organic matter. By peristalsis, the mixture is sent to the intestine where friendly bacteria continue chemical breakdown. This releases carbohydrates, protein, fat, and various vitamins and minerals for absorption into the body.

Overview of Vertebrate Digestion

In most vertebrates, digestion is a multistage process in the digestive system, starting from ingestion of raw materials, most often other organisms. Ingestion usually involves some type of mechanical and chemical processing. Digestion is separated into four steps:

1. Ingestion: placing food into the mouth (entry of food in the digestive system),

2. Mechanical and chemical breakdown: mastication and the mixing of the resulting bolus with water, acids, bile and enzymes in the stomach and intestine to break down complex molecules into simple structures,

3. Absorption: of nutrients from the digestive system to the circulatory and lymphatic capillaries through osmosis, active transport, and diffusion, and

4. Egestion (Excretion): Removal of undigested materials from the digestive tract through defecation.

Underlying the process is muscle movement throughout the system through swallowing and peristalsis. Each step in digestion requires energy, and thus imposes an "overhead charge" on the energy made available from absorbed substances. Differences in that overhead cost are important influences on lifestyle, behavior, and even physical structures. Examples may be seen in humans, who differ considerably from other hominids (lack of hair, smaller jaws and musculature, different dentition, length of intestines, cooking, etc.).

The major part of digestion takes place in the small intestine. The large intestine primarily serves as a site for fermentation of indigestible matter by gut bacteria and for resorption of water from digests before excretion.

In mammals, preparation for digestion begins with the cephalic phase in which saliva is produced in the mouth and digestive enzymes are produced in the stomach. Mechanical and chemical digestion begin in the mouth where food is chewed, and mixed with saliva to begin enzymatic processing of starches. The stomach continues to break food down mechanically and chemically through churning and mixing with both acids and enzymes. Absorption occurs in the stomach and gastrointestinal tract, and the process finishes with defecation.

Human Digestion Process

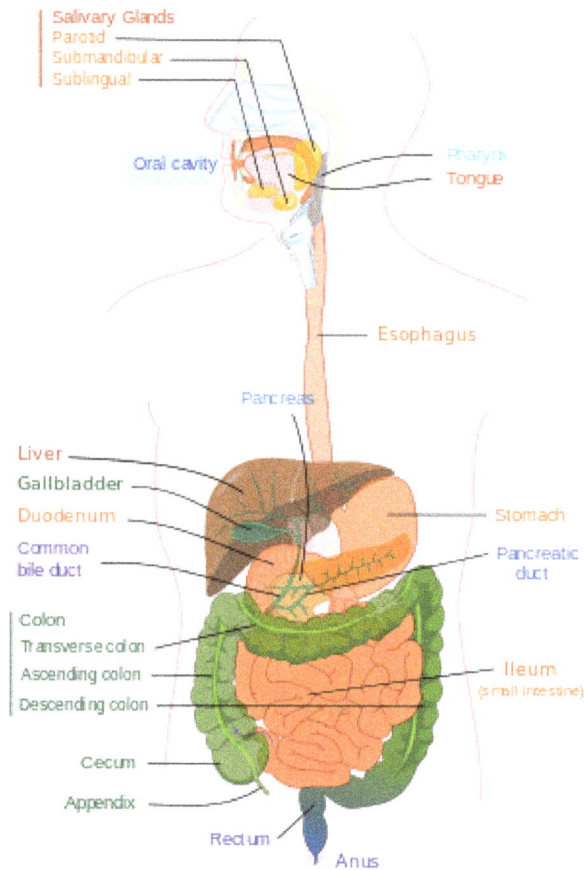

Upper and Lower human gastrointestinal tract

The human gastrointestinal tract is around 9 meters long. Food digestion physiology varies between individuals and upon other factors such as the characteristics of the food and size of the meal, and the process of digestion normally takes between 24 and 72 hours.

Different phases of digestion take place including: the cephalic phase , gastric phase, and intestinal phase. The cephalic phase occurs at the sight, thought and smell of food, which stimulate the cerebral cortex. Taste and smell stimuli are sent to the hypothalamus and medulla oblongata. After this it is routed through the vagus nerve and release of acetylcholine. Gastric secretion at this phase rises to 40% of maximum rate. Acidity in the stomach is not buffered by food at this point and thus acts to inhibit parietal (secretes acid) and G cell (secretes gastrin) activity via D cell secretion of somatostatin. The gastric phase takes 3 to 4 hours. It is stimulated by distension of the stomach, presence of food in stomach and decrease in pH. Distention activates long and myenteric reflexes. This activates the release of acetylcholine, which stimulates the release of more gastric juices. As protein enters the stomach, it binds to hydrogen ions, which raises the pH of the stomach. Inhibition of gastrin and gastric acid secretion is lifted. This triggers G cells to release gastrin, which in turn stimulates parietal cells to secrete gastric acid. Gastric acid is about 0.5% hydrochloric acid (HCl), which lowers the pH to the desired pH of 1-3. Acid release is also triggered by acetylcholine and histamine. The intestinal phase has two parts, the excitatory and the inhibitory. Partially digested food fills the duodenum. This triggers intestinal gastrin to be released. Enterogastric reflex inhibits vagal nuclei, activating sympathetic fibers causing the pyloric sphincter to tighten to prevent more food from entering, and inhibits local reflexes.

Digestion begins in the mouth with the secretion of saliva and its digestive enzymes. Food is formed into a bolus by the mechanical mastication and swallowed into the esophagus from where it enters the stomach through the action of peristalsis. Gastric juice contains hydrochloric acid and pepsin which would damage the walls of the stomach and mucus is secreted for protection. In the stomach further release of enzymes break down the food further and this is combined with the churning action of the stomach. The partially digested food enters the duodenum as a thick semi-liquid chyme. In the small intestine, the larger part of digestion takes place and this is helped by the secretions of bile, pancreatic juice and intestinal juice. The intestinal walls are lined with villi, and their epithelial cells is covered with numerous microvilli to improve the absorption of nutrients by increasing the surface area of the intestine.

In the large intestine the passage of food is slower to enable fermentation by the gut flora to take place. Here water is absorbed and waste material stored as feces to be removed by defecation via the anal canal and anus.

Breakdown Into Nutrients

Protein Digestion

Protein digestion occurs in the stomach and duodenum in which 3 main enzymes, pepsin secreted by the stomach and trypsin and chymotrypsin secreted by the pancreas, break down food proteins into polypeptides that are then broken down by various exopeptidases and dipeptidases into amino acids. The digestive enzymes however are mostly secreted as their inactive precursors, the zymogens. For example, trypsin is secreted by pancreas in the form of trypsinogen, which is activated in the duodenum by enterokinase to form trypsin. Trypsin then cleaves proteins to smaller polypeptides.

Fat Digestion

Digestion of some fats can begin in the mouth where lingual lipase breaks down some short chain lipids into diglycerides. However fats are mainly digested in the small intestine. The presence of fat in the small intestine produces hormones that stimulate the release of pancreatic lipase from the pancreas and bile from the liver which helps in the emulsification of fats for absorption of fatty acids. Complete digestion of one molecule of fat (a triglyceride) results a mixture of fatty acids, mono- and di-glycerides, as well as some undigested triglycerides, but no free glycerol molecules.

Carbohydrate Digestion

In humans, dietary starches are composed of glucose units arranged in long chains called amylose, a polysaccharide. During digestion, bonds between glucose molecules are broken by salivary and pancreatic amylase, resulting in progressively smaller chains of glucose. This results in simple sugars glucose and maltose (2 glucose molecules) that can be absorbed by the small intestine.

Lactase is an enzyme that breaks down the disaccharide lactose to its component parts, glucose and galactose. Glucose and galactose can be absorbed by the small intestine. Approximately 65 percent of the adult population produce only small amounts of lactase and are unable to eat unfermented milk-based foods. This is commonly known as lactose intolerance. Lactose intolerance varies widely by ethnic heritage; more than 90 percent of peoples of east Asian descent are lactose intolerant, in contrast to about 5 percent of people of northern European descent.

Sucrase is an enzyme that breaks down the disaccharide sucrose, commonly known as table sugar, cane sugar, or beet sugar. Sucrose digestion yields the sugars fructose and glucose which are readily absorbed by the small intestine.

DNA and RNA Digestion

DNA and RNA are broken down into mononucleotides by the nucleases deoxyribonuclease and ribonuclease (DNase and RNase) from the pancreas.

Non-destructive Digestion

Some nutrients are complex molecules (for example vitamin B_{12}) which would be destroyed if they were broken down into their functional groups. To digest vitamin B_{12} non-destructively, haptocorrin in saliva strongly binds and protects the B_{12} molecules from stomach acid as they enter the stomach and are cleaved from their protein complexes.

After the B_{12}-haptocorrin complexes pass from the stomach via the pylorus to the duodenum, pancreatic proteases cleave haptocorrin from the B_{12} molecules which rebind to intrinsic factor (IF). These B_{12}-IF complexes travel to the ileum portion of the small intestine where cubilin receptors enable assimilation and circulation of B_{12}-IF complexes in the blood.

Digestive Hormones

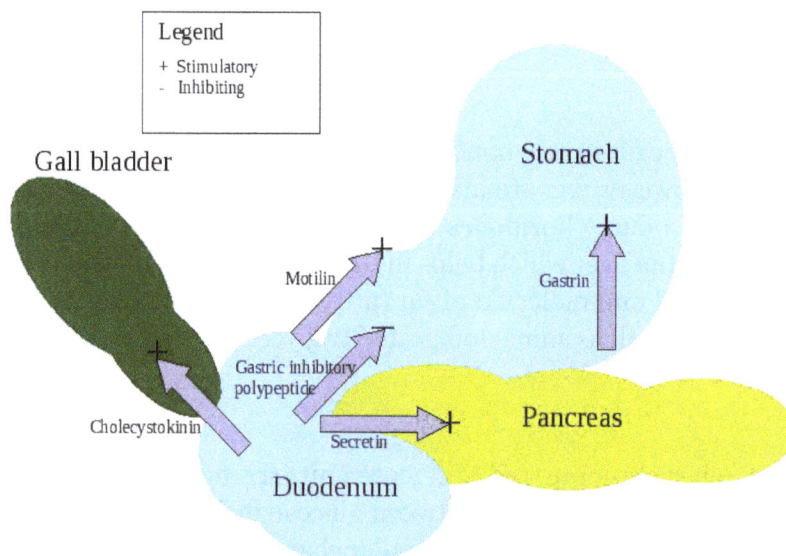

Action of the major digestive hormones

There are at least five hormones that aid and regulate the digestive system in mammals. There are variations across the vertebrates, as for instance in birds. Arrangements are complex and additional details are regularly discovered. For instance, more connections to metabolic control (largely the glucose-insulin system) have been uncovered in recent years.

- Gastrin – is in the stomach and stimulates the gastric glands to secrete pepsinogen (an inactive form of the enzyme pepsin) and hydrochloric acid. Secretion of gastrin is stimulated by food arriving in stomach. The secretion is inhibited by low pH.

- Secretin – is in the duodenum and signals the secretion of sodium bicarbonate in the pancreas and it stimulates the bile secretion in the liver. This hormone responds to the acidity of the chyme.

- Cholecystokinin (CCK) – is in the duodenum and stimulates the release of digestive enzymes in the pancreas and stimulates the emptying of bile in the gall bladder. This hormone is secreted in response to fat in chyme.

- Gastric inhibitory peptide (GIP) – is in the duodenum and decreases the stomach churning in turn slowing the emptying in the stomach. Another function is to induce insulin secretion.

- Motilin – is in the duodenum and increases the migrating myoelectric complex component of gastrointestinal motility and stimulates the production of pepsin.

Significance of pH

Digestion is a complex process controlled by several factors. pH plays a crucial role in a normally functioning digestive tract. In the mouth, pharynx and esophagus, pH is typically about 6.8, very weakly acidic. Saliva controls pH in this region of the digestive tract. Salivary amylase is contained in saliva and starts the breakdown of carbohydrates into monosaccharides. Most digestive enzymes are sensitive to pH and will denature in a high or low pH environment.

The stomach's high acidity inhibits the breakdown of carbohydrates within it. This acidity confers two benefits: it denatures proteins for further digestion in the small intestines, and provides non-specific immunity, damaging or eliminating various pathogens.

In the small intestines, the duodenum provides critical pH balancing to activate digestive enzymes. The liver secretes bile into the duodenum to neutralize the acidic conditions from the stomach, and the pancreatic duct empties into the duodenum, adding bicarbonate to neutralize the acidic chyme, thus creating a neutral environment. The mucosal tissue of the small intestines is alkaline with a pH of about 8.5.

Microbial Metabolism

Microbial metabolism is the means by which a microbe obtains the energy and nutrients (e.g. carbon) it needs to live and reproduce. Microbes use many different types of metabolic strategies and species can often be differentiated from each other based on metabolic characteristics. The specific metabolic properties of a microbe are the major factors in determining that microbe's ecological niche, and often allow for that microbe to be useful in industrial processes or responsible for bio-geochemical cycles.

Types of Microbial Metabolism

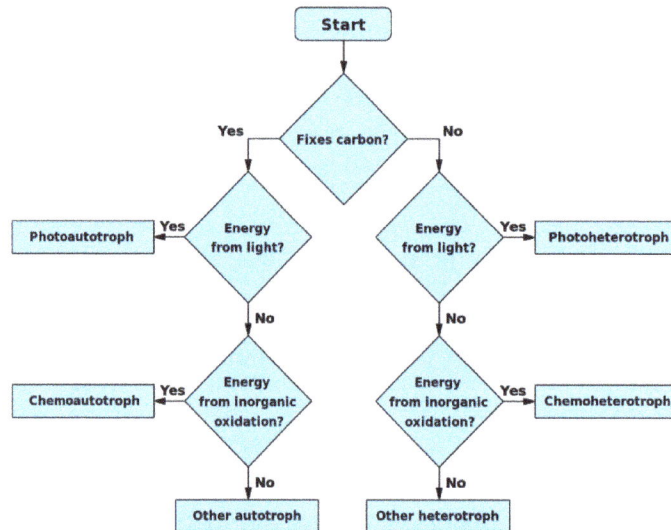

Flow chart to determine the metabolic characteristics of microorganisms

All microbial metabolisms can be arranged according to three principles:

1. How the organism obtains carbon for synthesising cell mass:

    *   autotrophic – carbon is obtained from carbon dioxide (CO_2)
    *   heterotrophic – carbon is obtained from organic compounds
    *   mixotrophic – carbon is obtained from both organic compounds and by fixing carbon dioxide

2. How the organism obtains reducing equivalents used either in energy conservation or in biosynthetic reactions:

    *   lithotrophic – reducing equivalents are obtained from inorganic compounds
    *   organotrophic – reducing equivalents are obtained from organic compounds

3. How the organism obtains energy for living and growing:

    *   chemotrophic – energy is obtained from external chemical compounds
    *   phototrophic – energy is obtained from light

In practice, these terms are almost freely combined. Typical examples are as follows:

*   chemolithoautotrophs obtain energy from the oxidation of inorganic compounds and carbon from the fixation of carbon dioxide. Examples: Nitrifying bacteria, Sulfur-oxidizing bacteria, Iron-oxidizing bacteria, Knallgas-bacteria

- photolithoautotrophs obtain energy from light and carbon from the fixation of carbon di-oxide, using reducing equivalents from inorganic compounds. Examples: Cyanobacteria (water (H_2O) as reducing equivalent donor), Chlorobiaceae, Chromatiaceae (hydrogen sul-fide (H_2S) as reducing equivalent donor), *Chloroflexus* (hydrogen (H2) as reducing equiva-lent donor)

- chemolithoheterotrophs obtain energy from the oxidation of inorganic compounds, but cannot fix carbon dioxide (CO_2). Examples: some *Thiobacilus*, some *Beggiatoa*, some *Ni-trobacter* spp., *Wolinella* (with H2 as reducing equivalent donor), some Knallgas-bacteria, some sulfate-reducing bacteria

- chemoorganoheterotrophs obtain energy, carbon, and reducing equivalents for biosyn-thetic reactions from organic compounds. Examples: most bacteria, e. g. *Escherichia coli*, *Bacillus* spp., *Actinobacteria*

- photoorganoheterotrophs obtain energy from light, carbon and reducing equivalents for biosynthetic reactions from organic compounds. Some species are strictly heterotrophic, many others can also fix carbon dioxide and are mixotrophic. Examples: *Rhodobacter*, *Rhodopseudomonas*, *Rhodospirillum*, *Rhodomicrobium*, *Rhodocyclus*, *Heliobacterium*, *Chloroflexus* (alternatively to photolithoautotrophy with hydrogen)

Heterotrophic Microbial Metabolism

Some microbes are heterotrophic (more precisely chemoorganoheterotrophic), using organic compounds as both carbon and energy sources. Heterotrophic microbes live off of nutrients that they scavenge from living hosts (as commensals or parasites) or find in dead organic mat-ter of all kind (saprophages). Microbial metabolism is the main contribution for the bodily decay of all organisms after death. Many eukaryotic microorganisms are heterotrophic by predation or parasitism, properties also found in some bacteria such as *Bdellovibrio* (an in-tracellular parasite of other bacteria, causing death of its victims) and Myxobacteria such as *Myxococcus* (predators of other bacteria which are killed and lysed by cooperating swarms of many single cells of Myxobacteria). Most pathogenic bacteria can be viewed as heterotrophic parasites of humans or the other eukaryotic species they affect. Heterotrophic microbes are extremely abundant in nature and are responsible for the breakdown of large organic polymers such as cellulose, chitin or lignin which are generally indigestible to larger animals. Generally, the breakdown of large polymers to carbon dioxide (mineralization) requires several different organisms, with one breaking down the polymer into its constituent monomers, one able to use the monomers and excreting simpler waste compounds as by-products, and one able to use the excreted wastes. There are many variations on this theme, as different organisms are able to degrade different polymers and secrete different waste products. Some organisms are even able to degrade more recalcitrant compounds such as petroleum compounds or pesticides, making them useful in bioremediation.

Biochemically, prokaryotic heterotrophic metabolism is much more versatile than that of eukary-otic organisms, although many prokaryotes share the most basic metabolic models with eukary-otes, e. g. using glycolysis (also called EMP pathway) for sugar metabolism and the citric acid cycle to degrade acetate, producing energy in the form of ATP and reducing power in the form of NADH or quinols. These basic pathways are well conserved because they are also involved in biosynthesis of many conserved building blocks needed for cell growth (sometimes in reverse direction). However, many bacteria and archaea utilize alternative metabolic pathways other than glycolysis and the citric acid cycle. A well-studied example is sugar metabolism via the keto-deoxy-phosphogluconate pathway (also called ED pathway) in *Pseudomonas*. Moreover, there is a third alternative sugar-catabolic pathway used by some bacteria, the pentose phosphate pathway. The metabolic diversity and ability of prokaryotes to use a large variety of organic compounds arises from the much deeper evolutionary history and diversity of prokaryotes, as compared to eukaryotes. It is also noteworthy that the mitochondrion, the small membrane-bound intracellular organelle that is the site of eukaryotic energy metabolism, arose from the endosymbiosis of a bacterium related to obligate intracellular *Rickettsia*, and also to plant-associated *Rhizobium* or *Agrobacterium*. Therefore, it is not surprising that all mitrochondriate eukaryotes share metabolic properties with these Proteobacteria. Most microbes respire (use an electron transport chain), although oxygen is not the only terminal electron acceptor that may be used. As discussed below, the use of terminal electron acceptors other than oxygen has important biogeochemical consequences.

Fermentation

Fermentation is a specific type of heterotrophic metabolism that uses organic carbon instead of oxygen as a terminal electron acceptor. This means that these organisms do not use an electron transport chain to oxidize NADH to NAD+ and therefore must have an alternative method of using this reducing power and maintaining a supply of NAD+ for the proper functioning of normal metabolic pathways (e.g. glycolysis). As oxygen is not required, fermentative organisms are anaerobic. Many organisms can use fermentation under anaerobic conditions and aerobic respiration when oxygen is present. These organisms are facultative anaerobes. To avoid the overproduction of NADH, obligately fermentative organisms usually do not have a complete citric acid cycle. Instead of using an ATP synthase as in respiration, ATP in fermentative organisms is produced by substrate-level phosphorylation where a phosphate group is transferred from a high-energy organic compound to ADP to form ATP. As a result of the need to produce high energy phosphate-containing organic compounds (generally in the form of Coenzyme A-esters) fermentative organisms use NADH and other cofactors to produce many different reduced metabolic by-products, often including hydrogen gas (H_2). These reduced organic compounds are generally small organic acids and alcohols derived from pyruvate, the end product of glycolysis. Examples include ethanol, acetate, lactate, and butyrate. Fermentative organisms are very important industrially and are used to make many different types of food products. The different metabolic end products produced by each specific bacterial species are responsible for the different tastes and properties of each food.

Not all fermentative organisms use substrate-level phosphorylation. Instead, some organisms are able to couple the oxidation of low-energy organic compounds directly to the formation of a proton (or sodium) motive force and therefore ATP synthesis. Examples of these unusual forms of fermentation include succinate fermentation by *Propionigenium modestum* and oxalate fermentation by *Oxalobacter formigenes*. These reactions are extremely low-energy yielding. Humans and other higher animals also use fermentation to produce lactate from excess NADH, although this is not the major form of metabolism as it is in fermentative microorganisms.

Special Metabolic Properties

Methylotrophy

Methylotrophy refers to the ability of an organism to use C1-compounds as energy sources. These compounds include methanol, methyl amines, formaldehyde, and formate. Several other less common substrates may also be used for metabolism, all of which lack carbon-carbon bonds. Examples of methylotrophs include the bacteria *Methylomonas* and *Methylobacter*. Methanotrophs are a specific type of methylotroph that are also able to use methane (CH_4) as a carbon source by oxidizing it sequentially to methanol (CH_3OH), formaldehyde (CH_2O), formate ($HCOO-$), and carbon dioxide CO_2 initially using the enzyme methane monooxygenase. As oxygen is required for this process, all (conventional) methanotrophs are obligate aerobes. Reducing power in the form of quinones and NADH is produced during these oxidations to produce a proton motive force and therefore ATP generation. Methylotrophs and methanotrophs are not considered as autotrophic, because they are able to incorporate some of the oxidized methane (or other metabolites) into cellular carbon before it is completely oxidized to CO_2 (at the level of formaldehyde), using either the serine pathway (*Methylosinus*, *Methylocystis*) or the ribulose monophosphate pathway (*Methylococcus*), depending on the species of methylotroph.

In addition to aerobic methylotrophy, methane can also be oxidized anaerobically. This occurs by a consortium of sulfate-reducing bacteria and relatives of methanogenic Archaea working syntrophically. Little is currently known about the biochemistry and ecology of this process.

Methanogenesis is the biological production of methane. It is carried out by methanogens, strictly anaerobic Archaea such as *Methanococcus*, *Methanocaldococcus*, *Methanobacterium*, *Methanothermus*, *Methanosarcina*, *Methanosaeta* and *Methanopyrus*. The biochemistry of methanogenesis is unique in nature in its use of a number of unusual cofactors to sequentially reduce methanogenic substrates to methane, such as coenzyme M and methanofuran. These cofactors are responsible (among other things) for the establishment of a proton gradient across the outer membrane thereby driving ATP synthesis. Several types of methanogenesis occur, differing in the starting compounds oxidized. Some methanogens reduce carbon dioxide (CO_2) to methane (CH_4) using electrons (most often) from hydrogen gas (H_2) chemolithoautotrophically. These methanogens can often be found in environments containing fermentative organisms. The tight association of methanogens and fermentative bacteria can be considered to be syntrophic because the methanogens, which rely on the fermentors for hydrogen, relieve feedback inhibition of the fermentors by the build-up of excess hydrogen that would otherwise inhibit their growth. This type of syntrophic relationship is specifically known as interspecies hydrogen transfer. A second group of methanogens use methanol (CH_3OH) as a substrate for methanogenesis. These are chemoorganotrophic, but still autotrophic in using CO_2 as only carbon source. The biochemistry of this process is quite different from that of the carbon dioxide-reducing methanogens. Lastly, a third group of methanogens produce both methane and carbon dioxide from acetate (CH_3COO-) with the acetate being split between the two carbons. These acetate-cleaving organisms are the only chemoorganoheterotrophic methanogens. All autotrophic methanogens use a variation of the reductive acetyl-CoA pathway to fix CO_2 and obtain cellular carbon.

Syntrophy

Syntrophy, in the context of microbial metabolism, refers to the pairing of multiple species to achieve a chemical reaction that, on its own, would be energetically unfavorable. The best studied example of this process is the oxidation of fermentative end products (such as acetate, ethanol and butyrate) by organisms such as *Syntrophomonas*. Alone, the oxidation of butyrate to acetate and hydrogen gas is energetically unfavorable. However, when a hydrogenotrophic (hydrogen-using) methanogen is present the use of the hydrogen gas will significantly lower the concentration of hydrogen (down to 10^{-5} atm) and thereby shift the equilibrium of the butyrate oxidation reaction under standard conditions ($\Delta G^{0'}$) to non-standard conditions ($\Delta G'$). Because the concentration of one product is lowered, the reaction is "pulled" towards the products and shifted towards net energetically favorable conditions (for butyrate oxidation: $\Delta G^{0'}= +48.2$ kJ/mol, but $\Delta G' = -8.9$ kJ/mol at 10^{-5} atm hydrogen and even lower if also the initially produced acetate is further metabolized by methanogens). Conversely, the available free energy from methanogenesis is lowered from $\Delta G^{0'}= -131$ kJ/mol under standard conditions to $\Delta G' = -17$ kJ/mol at 10^{-5} atm hydrogen. This is an example of intraspecies hydrogen transfer. In this way, low energy-yielding carbon sources can be used by a consortium of organisms to achieve further degradation and eventual mineralization of these compounds. These reactions help prevent the excess sequestration of carbon over geologic time scales, releasing it back to the biosphere in usable forms such as methane and CO_2.

Anaerobic Respiration

While aerobic organisms during respiration use oxygen as a terminal electron acceptor, anaerobic organisms use other electron acceptors. These inorganic compounds have a lower reduction potential than oxygen, meaning that respiration is less efficient in these organisms and leads to slower growth rates than aerobes. Many facultative anaerobes can use either oxygen or alternative terminal electron acceptors for respiration depending on the environmental conditions.

Most respiring anaerobes are heterotrophs, although some do live autotrophically. All of the processes described below are dissimilative, meaning that they are used during energy production and not to provide nutrients for the cell (assimilative). Assimilative pathways for many forms of anaerobic respiration are also known.

Denitrification — Nitrate as Electron Acceptor

Denitrification is the utilization of nitrate (NO_3^-) as a terminal electron acceptor. It is a widespread process that is used by many members of the Proteobacteria. Many facultative anaerobes use denitrification because nitrate, like oxygen, has a high reduction potential. Many denitrifying bacteria can also use ferric iron (Fe^{3+}) and some organic electron acceptors. Denitrification involves the stepwise reduction of nitrate to nitrite (NO_2^-), nitric oxide (NO), nitrous oxide (N_2O), and dinitrogen (N_2) by the enzymes nitrate reductase, nitrite reductase, nitric oxide reductase, and nitrous oxide reductase, respectively. Protons are transported across the membrane by the initial NADH reductase, quinones, and nitrous oxide reductase to produce the electrochemical gradient critical for respiration. Some organisms (e.g. *E. coli*) only produce nitrate reductase and therefore can accomplish only the first reduction leading to the accumulation of nitrite. Others (e.g. *Paracoccus denitrificans* or *Pseudomonas stutzeri*) reduce nitrate completely. Complete denitrification is an environmentally significant process because some intermediates of denitrification (nitric oxide and nitrous oxide) are important greenhouse gases that react with sunlight and ozone to produce nitric acid, a component of acid rain. Denitrification is also important in biological wastewater treatment where it is used to reduce the amount of nitrogen released into the environment thereby reducing eutrophication.

Sulfate Reduction — Sulfate as Electron Acceptor

Dissimilatory sulfate reduction is a relatively energetically poor process used by many Gram negative bacteria found within the δ-Proteobacteria, Gram-positive organisms relating to *Desulfotomaculum* or the archaeon *Archaeoglobus*. Hydrogen sulfide (H_2S) is produced as a metabolic end product. For sulfate reduction electron donors and energy are needed.

Electron Donors

Many sulfate reducers are organotrophic, using carbon compounds such as lactate and pyruvate (among many others) as electron donors, while others are lithotrophic, using hydrogen gas (H_2) as an electron donor. Some unusual autotrophic sulfate-reducing bacteria (e.g. *Desulfotignum phosphitoxidans*) can use phosphite (HPO_3^-) as an electron donor whereas others (e.g. *Desulfovibrio sulfodismutans*, *Desulfocapsa thiozymogenes*, *Desulfocapsa sulfoexigens*) are capable of sulfur disproportionation (splitting one compound into two different compounds, in this case an electron donor and an electron acceptor) using elemental sulfur (S^o), sulfite (SO_3^{2-}), and thiosulfate ($S_2O_3^{2-}$) to produce both hydrogen sulfide (H_2S) and sulfate (SO_4^{2-}).

Energy for Reduction

All sulfate-reducing organisms are strict anaerobes. Because sulfate is energetically stable, before it can be metabolized it must first be activated by adenylation to form APS (adenosine 5'-phosphosulfate) thereby consuming ATP. The APS is then reduced by the enzyme APS reductase to form sulfite (SO_3^{2-}) and AMP. In organisms that use carbon compounds as electron donors, the ATP consumed is accounted for by fermentation of the carbon substrate. The hydrogen produced during fermentation is actually what drives respiration during sulfate reduction.

Acetogenesis — Carbon Dioxide as Electron Acceptor

Acetogenesis is a type of microbial metabolism that uses hydrogen (H_2) as an electron donor and carbon dioxide (CO_2) as an electron acceptor to produce acetate, the same electron donors and acceptors used in methanogenesis. Bacteria that can autotrophically synthesize acetate are called homoacetogens. Carbon dioxide reduction in all homoacetogens occurs by the acetyl-CoA pathway. This pathway is also used for carbon fixation by autotrophic sulfate-reducing bacteria and hydrogenotrophic methanogens. Often homoacetogens can also be fermentative, using the hydrogen and carbon dioxide produced as a result of fermentation to produce acetate, which is secreted as an end product.

Other Inorganic Electron Acceptors

Ferric iron (Fe_{3+}) is a widespread anaerobic terminal electron acceptor both for autotrophic and heterotrophic organisms. Electron flow in these organisms is similar to those in electron transport, ending in oxygen or nitrate, except that in ferric iron-reducing organisms the final enzyme in this system is a ferric iron reductase. Model organisms include *Shewanella putrefaciens* and *Geobacter metallireducens*. Since some ferric iron-reducing bacteria (e.g. *G. metallireducens*) can use toxic hydrocarbons such as toluene as a carbon source, there is significant interest in using these organisms as bioremediation agents in ferric iron-rich contaminated aquifers.

Although ferric iron is the most prevalent inorganic electron acceptor, a number of organisms (including the iron-reducing bacteria mentioned above) can use other inorganic ions in anaerobic respiration. While these processes may often be less significant ecologically, they are of considerable interest for bioremediation, especially when heavy metals or radionuclides are used as electron acceptors. Examples include:

- Manganic ion (Mn_{4+}) reduction to manganous ion (Mn_{2+})
- Selenate (SeO_{2-4}) reduction to selenite (SeO_{2-3}) and selenite reduction to inorganic selenium (Se^o)
- Arsenate (AsO_{3-4}) reduction to arsenite (AsO_{3-3})
- Uranyl ion ion (UO_{2+2}) reduction to uranium dioxide (UO_2)

Organic Terminal Electron Acceptors

A number of organisms, instead of using inorganic compounds as terminal electron acceptors, are able to use organic compounds to accept electrons from respiration. Examples include:

- Fumarate reduction to succinate
- Trimethylamine *N*-oxide (TMAO) reduction to trimethylamine (TMA)
- Dimethyl sulfoxide (DMSO) reduction to Dimethyl sulfide (DMS)
- Reductive dechlorination

TMAO is a chemical commonly produced by fish, and when reduced to TMA produces a strong odor. DMSO is a common marine and freshwater chemical which is also odiferous when reduced to DMS. Reductive dechlorination is the process by which chlorinated organic compounds are reduced to form their non-chlorinated endproducts. As chlorinated organic compounds are often important (and difficult to degrade) environmental pollutants, reductive dechlorination is an important process in bioremediation.

Chemolithotrophy

Chemolithotrophy is a type of metabolism where energy is obtained from the oxidation of inorganic compounds. Most chemolithotrophic organisms are also autotrophic. There are two major objectives to chemolithotrophy: the generation of energy (ATP) and the generation of reducing power (NADH).

Hydrogen Oxidation

Many organisms are capable of using hydrogen (H_2) as a source of energy. While several mechanisms of anaerobic hydrogen oxidation have been mentioned previously (e.g. sulfate reducing- and acetogenic bacteria), hydrogen can also be used as an energy source aerobically. In these organisms, hydrogen is oxidized by a membrane-bound hydrogenase causing proton pumping via electron transfer to various quinones and cytochromes. In many organisms, a second cytoplasmic hydrogenase is used to generate reducing power in the form of NADH, which is subsequently used to fix carbon dioxide via the Calvin cycle. Hydrogen-oxidizing organisms, such as *Cupriavidus necator* (formerly *Ralstonia eutropha*), often inhabit oxic-anoxic interfaces in nature to take advantage of the hydrogen produced by anaerobic fermentative organisms while still maintaining a supply of oxygen.

Sulfur Oxidation

Sulfur oxidation involves the oxidation of reduced sulfur compounds (such as sulfide H_2S), inorganic sulfur (S), and thiosulfate ($S_2O_2{-}3$) to form sulfuric acid (H_2SO_4). A classic example of a sulfur-oxidizing bacterium is *Beggiatoa*, a microbe originally described by Sergei Winogradsky, one of the founders of environmental microbiology. Another example is *Paracoccus*. Generally, the oxidation of sulfide occurs in stages, with inorganic sulfur being stored either inside or outside of the cell until needed. This two step process occurs because energetically sulfide is a better electron donor than inorganic sulfur or thiosulfate, allowing for a greater number of protons to be translocated across the membrane. Sulfur-oxidizing organisms generate reducing power for carbon dioxide fixation via the Calvin cycle using reverse electron flow, an energy-requiring process that pushes the electrons against their thermodynamic gradient to produce NADH. Biochemically, reduced sulfur compounds are converted to sulfite ($SO_2{-}3$) and subsequently converted to sulfate ($SO_2{-}4$) by the enzyme sulfite oxidase. Some organisms, however, accomplish the same oxidation using a reversal of the APS reductase system used by sulfate-reducing bacteria. In all cases the energy liberated is transferred to the electron transport chain for ATP and NADH production. In addition to aerobic sulfur oxidation, some organisms (e.g. *Thiobacillus denitrificans*) use nitrate ($NO{-}3$) as a terminal electron acceptor and therefore grow anaerobically.

Ferrous iron (Fe2+) Oxidation

Ferrous iron is a soluble form of iron that is stable at extremely low pHs or under anaerobic conditions. Under aerobic, moderate pH conditions ferrous iron is oxidized spontaneously to the ferric ($Fe_{3}+$) form and is hydrolyzed abiotically to insoluble ferric hydroxide ($Fe(OH)_3$). There are three distinct types of ferrous iron-oxidizing microbes. The first are acidophiles, such as the bacteria *Acidithiobacillus ferrooxidans* and *Leptospirillum ferrooxidans*, as well as the archaeon *Ferroplasma*. These microbes oxidize iron in environments that have a very low pH and are important in acid mine drainage. The second type of microbes oxidize ferrous iron at cirum-neutral pH. These micro-organisms (for example *Gallionella ferruginea*, *Leptothrix ochracea*, or *Mariprofundus ferrooxydans*) live at the oxic-anoxic interfaces and are microaerophiles. The third type of iron-oxidizing microbes are anaerobic photosynthetic bacteria such as Rhodopseudomonas, which use ferrous iron to produce NADH for autotrophic carbon dioxide fixation. Biochemically, aerobic iron oxidation is a very energetically poor process which therefore requires large amounts of iron to be oxidized by the enzyme rusticyanin to facilitate the formation of proton motive force. Like sulfur oxidation, reverse electron flow must be used to form the NADH used for carbon dioxide fixation via the Calvin cycle.

Nitrification

Nitrification is the process by which ammonia (NH_3) is converted to nitrate (NO_3^-). Nitrification is actually the net result of two distinct processes: oxidation of ammonia to nitrite (NO_2^-) by nitrosifying bacteria (e.g. *Nitrosomonas*) and oxidation of nitrite to nitrate by the nitrite-oxidizing bacteria (e.g. *Nitrobacter*). Both of these processes are extremely energetically poor leading to very slow growth rates for both types of organisms. Biochemically, ammonia oxidation occurs by the stepwise oxidation of ammonia to hydroxylamine (NH_2OH) by the enzyme ammonia monooxygenase in the cytoplasm, followed by the oxidation of hydroxylamine to nitrite by the enzyme hydroxylamine oxidoreductase in the periplasm.

Electron and proton cycling are very complex but as a net result only one proton is translocated across the membrane per molecule of ammonia oxidized. Nitrite reduction is much simpler, with nitrite being oxidized by the enzyme nitrite oxidoreductase coupled to proton translocation by a very short electron transport chain, again leading to very low growth rates for these organisms. Oxygen is required in both ammonia and nitrite oxidation, meaning that both nitrosifying and nitrite-oxidizing bacteria are aerobes. As in sulfur and iron oxidation, NADH for carbon dioxide fixation using the Calvin cycle is generated by reverse electron flow, thereby placing a further metabolic burden on an already energy-poor process.

In 2015, two groups independently showed the microbial genus *Nitrospira* is capable of complete nitrification (Comammox).

Anammox

Anammox stands for anaerobic ammonia oxidation and the organisms responsible were relatively recently discovered, in the late 1990s. This form of metabolism occurs in members of the Planctomycetes (e.g. Candidatus *Brocadia anammoxidans*) and involves the coupling of ammonia oxidation to nitrite reduction. As oxygen is not required for this process, these organisms are strict anaerobes. Amazingly, hydrazine (N_2H_4 — rocket fuel) is produced as an intermediate during anammox metabolism. To deal with the high toxicity of hydrazine, anammox bacteria contain a hydrazine-containing intracellular organelle called the anammoxasome, surrounded by highly compact (and unusual) ladderane lipid membrane. These lipids are unique in nature, as is the use of hydrazine as a metabolic intermediate. Anammox organisms are autotrophs although the mechanism for carbon dioxide fixation is unclear. Because of this property, these organisms could be used to remove nitrogen in industrial wastewater treatment processes. Anammox has also been shown have widespread occurrence in anaerobic aquatic systems and has been speculated to account for approximately 50% of nitrogen gas production in the ocean.

Phototrophy

Many microbes (phototrophs) are capable of using light as a source of energy to produce ATP and organic compounds such as carbohydrates, lipids, and proteins. Of these, algae are particularly significant because they are oxygenic, using water as an electron donor for electron transfer during photosynthesis. Phototrophic bacteria are found in the phyla Cyanobacteria, Chlorobi, Proteobacteria, Chloroflexi, and Firmicutes. Along with plants these microbes are responsible for all biological generation of oxygen gas on Earth. Because chloroplasts were derived from a lineage of the Cyanobacteria, the general principles of metabolism in these endosymbionts can also be applied to chloroplasts. In addition to oxygenic photosynthesis, many bacteria can also photosynthesize anaerobically, typically using sulfide (H_2S) as an electron donor to produce sulfate. Inorganic sulfur (S_0), thiosulfate (S_2O_{2-3}) and ferrous iron (Fe^{2+}) can also be used by some organisms. Phylogenetically, all oxygenic photosynthetic bacteria are Cyanobacteria, while anoxygenic photosynthetic bacteria belong to the purple bacteria (Proteobacteria), Green sulfur bacteria (e.g. Chlorobium), Green non-sulfur bacteria (e.g. Chloroflexus), or the heliobacteria (Low %G+C Gram positives). In addition to these organisms, some microbes (e.g. the Archaeon *Halobacterium* or the bacterium *Roseobacter*, among others) can utilize light to produce energy using the enzyme bacteriorhodopsin, a light-driven proton pump. However, there are no known Archaea that carry out photosynthesis.

As befits the large diversity of photosynthetic bacteria, there are many different mechanisms by which light is converted into energy for metabolism. All photosynthetic organisms locate their photosynthetic reaction centers within a membrane, which may be invaginations of the cytoplasmic membrane (Proteobacteria), thylakoid membranes (Cyanobacteria), specialized antenna structures called chlorosomes (Green sulfur and non-sulfur bacteria), or the cytoplasmic membrane itself (heliobacteria). Different photosynthetic bacteria also contain different photosynthetic pigments, such as chlorophylls and carotenoids, allowing them to take advantage of different portions of the electromagnetic spectrum and thereby inhabit different niches. Some groups of organisms contain more specialized light-harvesting structures (e.g. phycobilisomes in Cyanobacteria and chlorosomes in Green sulfur and non-sulfur bacteria), allowing for increased efficiency in light utilization.

Biochemically, anoxygenic photosynthesis is very different from oxygenic photosynthesis. Cyanobacteria (and by extension, chloroplasts) use the Z scheme of electron flow in which electrons eventually are used to form NADH. Two different reaction centers (photosystems) are used and proton motive force is generated both by using cyclic electron flow and the quinone pool. In anoxygenic photosynthetic bacteria, electron flow is cyclic, with all electrons used in photosynthesis eventually being transferred back to the single reaction center. A proton motive force is generated using only the quinone pool. In heliobacteria, Green sulfur, and Green non-sulfur bacteria, NADH is formed using the protein ferredoxin, an energetically favorable reaction. In purple bacteria, NADH is formed by reverse electron flow due to the lower chemical potential of this reaction center. In all cases, however, a proton motive force is generated and used to drive ATP production via an ATPase.

Most photosynthetic microbes are autotrophic, fixing carbon dioxide via the Calvin cycle. Some photosynthetic bacteria (e.g. Chloroflexus) are photoheterotrophs, meaning that they use organic carbon compounds as a carbon source for growth. Some photosynthetic organisms also fix nitrogen.

Nitrogen Fixation

Nitrogen is an element required for growth by all biological systems. While extremely common (80% by volume) in the atmosphere, dinitrogen gas (N_2) is generally biologically inaccessible due to its high activation energy. Throughout all of nature, only specialized bacteria and Archaea are capable of nitrogen fixation, converting dinitrogen gas into ammonia (NH3), which is easily assimilated by all organisms. These prokaryotes, therefore, are very important ecologically and are often essential for the survival of entire ecosystems. This is especially true in the ocean, where nitrogen-fixing cyanobacteria are often the only sources of fixed nitrogen, and in soils, where specialized symbioses exist between legumes and their nitrogen-fixing partners to provide the nitrogen needed by these plants for growth.

Nitrogen fixation can be found distributed throughout nearly all bacterial lineages and physiological classes but is not a universal property. Because the enzyme nitrogenase, responsible for nitrogen fixation, is very sensitive to oxygen which will inhibit it irreversibly, all nitrogen-fixing organisms must possess some mechanism to keep the concentration of oxygen low. Examples include:

- heterocyst formation (cyanobacteria e.g. *Anabaena*) where one cell does not photosynthesize but instead fixes nitrogen for its neighbors which in turn provide it with energy

- root nodule symbioses (e.g. *Rhizobium*) with plants that supply oxygen to the bacteria bound to molecules of leghaemoglobin

- anaerobic lifestyle (e.g. *Clostridium pasteurianum*)

- very fast metabolism (e.g. *Azotobacter vinelandii*)

The production and activity of nitrogenases is very highly regulated, both because nitrogen fixation is an extremely energetically expensive process (16–24 ATP are used per N 2 fixed) and due to the extreme sensitivity of the nitrogenase to oxygen.

Basal Metabolic Rate

Basal metabolic rate (BMR) is the minimal rate of energy expenditure per unit time by endothermic animals at rest. It is reported in energy units per unit time ranging from watt (joule/second) to ml O_2/min or joule per hour per kg body mass J/(h·kg)). Proper measurement requires a strict set of criteria be met. These criteria include being in a physically and psychologically undisturbed state, in a thermally neutral environment, while in the post-absorptive state (i.e., not actively digesting food). In bradymetabolic animals, such as fish and reptiles, the equivalent term standard metabolic rate (SMR) is used. It follows the same criteria as BMR, but requires the documentation of the temperature at which the metabolic rate was measured. This makes BMR a variant of standard metabolic rate measurement that excludes the temperature data, a practice that has led to problems in defining "standard" rates of metabolism for many mammals.

Metabolism refers to the processes that the body needs to function. Basal Metabolic Rate is the amount of energy expressed in calories that a person needs to keep the body functioning at rest. Some of those processes are breathing, blood circulation, controlling body temperature, cell growth, brain and nerve function, and contraction of muscles. Basal metabolic rate (BMR) affects the rate that a person burns calories and ultimately whether that individual maintains, gains, or loses weight. The basal metabolic rate accounts for about 60 to 75% of the daily calorie expenditure by individuals. It is influenced by several factors. BMR typically declines by 1-2% per decade after age 20, mostly due to loss of fat-free mass, although the variability between individuals is high.

Description

The body's generation of heat is known as thermogenesis and it can be measured to determine the amount of energy expended. BMR generally decreases with age and with the decrease in lean body mass (as may happen with aging). Increasing muscle mass has the effect of increasing BMR. Aerobic (resistance) fitness level, a product of cardiovascular exercise, while previously thought to have effect on BMR, has been shown in the 1990s not to correlate with BMR when adjusted for fat-free body mass. But anaerobic exercise does increase resting energy consumption. Illness, previously consumed food and beverages, environmental temperature, and stress levels can affect one's overall energy expenditure as well as one's BMR.

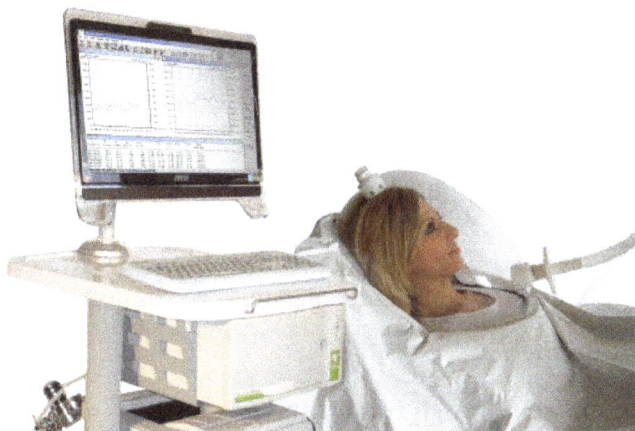

Indirect calorimetry laboratory with canopy hood (dilution technique)

BMR is measured under very restrictive circumstances when a person is awake. An accurate BMR measurement requires that the person's sympathetic nervous system not be stimulated, a condition which requires complete rest. A more common measurement, which uses less strict criteria, is resting metabolic rate (RMR).

BMR may be measured by gas analysis through either direct or Indirect Calorimetry, though a rough estimation can be acquired through an equation using age, sex, height, and weight. Studies of energy metabolism using both methods provide convincing evidence for the validity of the respiratory quotient (R.Q.), which measures the inherent composition and utilization of carbohydrates, fats and proteins as they are converted to energy substrate units that can be used by the body as energy.

Nutrition and Dietary Considerations

Basal metabolism is usually by far the largest component of total caloric expenditure. However, the Harris–Benedict equations are only approximate and variation in BMR (reflecting varying body composition), in physical activity levels, and in energy expended in thermogenesis make it difficult to estimate the dietary consumption any particular individual needs in order to maintain body weight.

Physiology

The early work of the scientists J. Arthur Harris and Francis G. Benedict showed that approximate values for BMR could be derived using body surface area (computed from height and weight), age, and sex, along with the oxygen and carbon dioxide measures taken from calorimetry. Studies also showed that by eliminating the sex differences that occur with the accumulation of adipose tissue by expressing metabolic rate per unit of "fat-free" or lean body mass, the values between sexes for basal metabolism are essentially the same. Exercise physiology textbooks have tables to show the conversion of height and body surface area as they relate to weight and basal metabolic values.

The primary organ responsible for regulating metabolism is the hypothalamus. The hypothalamus is located on the diencephalon and forms the floor and part of the lateral walls of the third ventricle of the cerebrum. The chief functions of the hypothalamus are:

1. control and integration of activities of the autonomic nervous system (ANS)

    o   The ANS regulates contraction of smooth muscle and cardiac muscle, along with secretions of many endocrine organs such as the thyroid gland (associated with many metabolic disorders).

    o   Through the ANS, the hypothalamus is the main regulator of visceral activities, such as heart rate, movement of food through the gastrointestinal tract, and contraction of the urinary bladder.

2. production and regulation of feelings of rage and aggression

3. regulation of body temperature

4. regulation of food intake, through two centers:

    o   The feeding center or hunger center is responsible for the sensations that cause us to seek food. When sufficient food or substrates have been received and leptin is high, then the satiety center is stimulated and sends impulses that inhibit the feeding center. When insufficient food is present in the stomach and ghrelin levels are high, receptors in the hypothalamus initiate the sense of hunger.

    o   The thirst center operates similarly when certain cells in the hypothalamus are stimulated by the rising osmotic pressure of the extracellular fluid. If thirst is satisfied, osmotic pressure decreases.

All of these functions taken together form a survival mechanism that causes us to sustain the body processes that BMR measures.

Bmr Estimation Formulas

Several prediction equations exist. Historically, the most notable one was the Harris-Benedict equation, which was created in 1919.

In each of the formulas:

- P   is total heat production at complete rest,

- m   is mass (kg),

- h   is height (cm), and

- a   is age (years),

The Original Harris-Benedict Equation:

- for men,

- for women,

The difference in BMR for men and women is mainly due to differences in body weight.

In 1984, the original Harris-Benedict equations were revised using new data. In comparisons with actual expenditure, the revised equations were found to be more accurate.

The Revised Harris-Benedict Equation:

- for men,

- for women,

It was the best prediction equation until 1990, when Mifflin *et al.* introduced the equation:

The Mifflin St Jeor Equation:

- , where *s* is +5 for males and −161 for females.

According to this formula, the woman in the example above has a BMR of 1204 kcal per day. During the last 100 years, lifestyles have changed and Frankenfield *et al.* showed it to be about 5% more accurate.

These formulas are based on body weight, which does not take into account the difference in metabolic activity between lean body mass and body fat. Other formulas exist which take into account lean body mass, two of which are the Katch-McArdle formula, and Cunningham formula. The Katch-McArdle formula is used to predict Resting Daily Energy Expenditure (RDEE). The Cunningham formula is commonly attributed as being used to predict RMR instead of BMR, however the formulas provided by Katch-McArdle and Cunningham are the same.

The Katch-McArdle Formula (Resting Daily Energy Expenditure):

- , where *LBM* is the lean body mass in kg.

According to this formula, if the woman in the example has a body fat percentage of 30%, her RDEE (the authors use the term of basal and resting metabolism interchangeably) would be 1263 kcal per day.

Causes of individual Differences in BMR

The basal metabolic rate varies between individuals. One study of 150 adults representative of the population in Scotland reported basal metabolic rates from as low as 1027 kcal per day (4301 kJ/

day) to as high as 2499 kcal/day (10455 kJ/day); with a mean BMR of 1500 kcal/day (6279 kJ/day). Statistically, the researchers calculated that 62.3% of this variation was explained by differences in fat free mass. Other factors explaining the variation included fat mass (6.7%), age (1.7%), and experimental error including within-subject difference (2%). The rest of the variation (26.7%) was unexplained. This remaining difference was not explained by sex nor by differing tissue size of highly energetic organs such as the brain.

Differences in BMR have been observed when comparing subjects with *the same* lean body mass. In one study, when comparing individuals with the same lean body mass, the top 5% of BMRs are 28-32% higher than the lowest 5% BMR. Additionally, this study reports a case where two individuals with the same lean body mass of 43 kg had BMRs of 1075 kcal/day (4.5 MJ/day) and 1790 kcal/day (7.5 MJ/day). This difference of 715 kcal/day (67%) is equivalent to one of the individuals completing a 10 kilometer run every day. However, this study did not account for the sex, height, fasting-state, or body fat percentage of the subjects.

Biochemistry

Energy expenditure breakdown	
Liver	27%
Brain	19%
Skeletal Muscle	18%
Kidneys	10%
Heart	7%
Other organs	19%

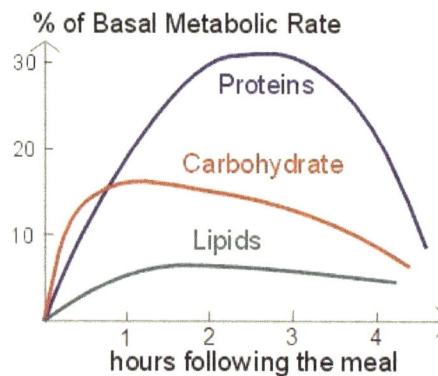

Postprandial thermogenesis increases in basal metabolic rate occur at different degrees depending on consumed food composition.

About 70% of a human's total energy expenditure is due to the basal life processes within the organs of the body (see table). About 20% of one's energy expenditure comes from physical activity and another 10% from thermogenesis, or digestion of food (*postprandial thermogenesis*). All of these processes require an intake of oxygen along with coenzymes to provide energy for survival (usually from macronutrients like carbohydrates, fats, and proteins) and expel carbon dioxide, due to processing by the Krebs cycle.

For the BMR, most of the energy is consumed in maintaining fluid levels in tissues through osmo-regulation, and only about one-tenth is consumed for mechanical work, such as digestion, heart-beat, and breathing.

What enables the Krebs cycle to perform metabolic changes to fats, carbohydrates, and proteins is energy, which can be defined as the ability or capacity to do work. The breakdown of large mol-ecules into smaller molecules—associated with release of energy—is catabolism. The building up process is termed anabolism. The breakdown of proteins into amino acids is an example of catabo-lism, while the formation of proteins from amino acids is an anabolic process.

Exergonic reactions are energy-releasing reactions and are generally catabolic. Endergonic reac-tions require energy and include anabolic reactions and the contraction of muscle. Metabolism is the total of all catabolic, exergonic, anabolic, endergonic reactions.

Adenosine Triphosphate (ATP) is the intermediate molecule that drives the exergonic transfer of energy to switch to endergonic anabolic reactions used in muscle contraction. This is what causes muscles to work which can require a breakdown, and also to build in the rest period, which oc-curs during the strengthening phase associated with muscular contraction. ATP is composed of adenine, a nitrogen containing base, ribose, a five carbon sugar (collectively called adenosine), and three phosphate groups. ATP is a high energy molecule because it stores large amounts of energy in the chemical bonds of the two terminal phosphate groups. The breaking of these chemical bonds in the Krebs Cycle provides the energy needed for muscular contraction.

Glucose

Because the ratio of hydrogen to oxygen atoms in all carbohydrates is always the same as that in water—that is, 2 to 1—all of the oxygen consumed by the cells is used to oxidize the carbon in the carbohydrate molecule to form carbon dioxide. Consequently, during the complete oxidation of a glucose molecule, six molecules of carbon dioxide and six molecules of water are produced and six molecules of oxygen are consumed.

The overall equation for this reaction is:

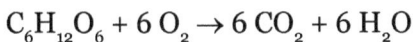

$$C_6H_{12}O_6 + 6\ O_2 \rightarrow 6\ CO_2 + 6\ H_2O$$

(38 ATP molecules)

Because the gas exchange in this reaction is equal, the respiratory quotient (R.Q.) for carbohydrate is unity or 1.0:

$$R.Q. = 6\ CO_2\ /\ 6\ O_2 = 1.0$$

Fats

The chemical composition for fats differs from that of carbohydrates in that fats contain consider-ably fewer oxygen atoms in proportion to atoms of carbon and hydrogen. When listed on nutri-tional information tables, fats are generally divided into six categories: total fats, saturated fatty acid, polyunsaturated fatty acid, monounsaturated fatty acid, dietary cholesterol, and trans fatty acid. From a basal metabolic or resting metabolic perspective, more energy is needed to burn a saturated fatty acid than an unsaturated fatty acid. The fatty acid molecule is broken down and categorized based on the number of carbon atoms in its molecular structure. The chemical equation for metabolism of the twelve to sixteen carbon atoms in a saturated fatty acid molecule shows the difference between metabolism of carbohydrates and fatty acids. Palmitic acid is a commonly studied example of the saturated fatty acid molecule.

The overall equation for the substrate utilization of palmitic acid is:

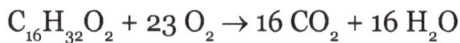

$$C_{16}H_{32}O_2 + 23\ O_2 \rightarrow 16\ CO_2 + 16\ H_2O$$

Thus the R.Q. for palmitic acid is 0.696:

$$R.Q. = 16\ CO_2\ /\ 23\ O_2 = 0.696$$

Proteins

Proteins are composed of carbon, hydrogen, oxygen, and nitrogen arranged in a variety of ways to form a large combination of amino acids. Unlike fat the body has no storage deposits of protein. All of it is contained in the body as important parts of tissues, blood hormones, and enzymes. The structural components of the body that contain these amino acids are continually undergoing a process of breakdown and replacement. The respiratory quotient for protein metabolism can be demonstrated by the chemical equation for oxidation of albumin:

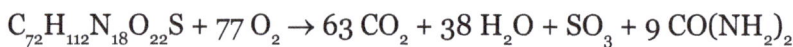

$$C_{72}H_{112}N_{18}O_{22}S + 77\ O_2 \rightarrow 63\ CO_2 + 38\ H_2O + SO_3 + 9\ CO(NH_2)_2$$

The R.Q. for albumin is 63 CO_2/ 77 O_2 = 0.818

The reason this is important in the process of understanding protein metabolism is that the body can blend the three macronutrients and based on the mitochondrial density, a preferred ratio can be established which determines how much fuel is utilized in which packets for work accomplished by the muscles. Protein catabolism (breakdown) has been estimated to supply 10% to 15% of the total energy requirement during a two-hour aerobic training session. This process could severely degrade the protein structures needed to maintain survival such as contractile properties of proteins in the heart, cellular mitochondria, myoglobin storage, and metabolic enzymes within muscles.

The oxidative system (aerobic) is the primary source of ATP supplied to the body at rest and during low intensity activities and uses primarily carbohydrates and fats as substrates. Protein is not normally metabolized significantly, except during long term starvation and long bouts of exercise (greater than 90 minutes.) At rest approximately 70% of the ATP produced is derived from fats and 30% from carbohydrates. Following the onset of activity, as the intensity of the exercise increases, there is a shift in substrate preference from fats to carbohydrates. During high intensity aerobic exercise, almost 100% of the energy is derived from carbohydrates, if an adequate supply is available.

Aerobic vs. Anaerobic Exercise

Studies published in 1992 and 1997 indicate that the level of aerobic fitness of an individual does not have any correlation with the level of resting metabolism. Both studies find that aerobic fitness levels do not improve the predictive power of fat free mass for resting metabolic rate.

Anaerobic exercise, such as weight lifting, builds additional muscle mass. Muscle contributes to the fat-free mass of an individual and therefore effective results from anaerobic exercise will increase BMR. However, the actual effect on BMR is controversial and difficult to enumerate. Various studies suggest that the resting metabolic rate of trained muscle is around 55kJ per kilogram, per day. Even a substantial increase in muscle mass, say 5 kg, would make only a minor impact on BMR.

Longevity

In 1926, Raymond Pearl proposed that longevity varies inversely with basal metabolic rate (the "rate of living hypothesis"). Support for this hypothesis comes from the fact that mammals with larger body size have longer maximum life spans (large animals do have higher total metabolic rates, but the metabolic rate at the cellular level is much lower, and the breathing rate and heartbeat are slower in larger animals) and the fact that the longevity of fruit flies varies inversely with ambient temperature. Additionally, the life span of houseflies can be extended by preventing physical activity. This theory has been bolstered by several new studies linking lower basal metabolic rate to increased life expectancy, across the animal kingdom—including humans. Calorie restriction and reduced thyroid hormone levels, both of which decrease the metabolic rate, have been associated with higher longevity in animals.

However, the ratio of total daily energy expenditure to resting metabolic rate can vary between 1.6 and 8.0 between species of mammals. Animals also vary in the degree of coupling between oxidative phosphorylation and ATP production, the amount of saturated fat in mitochondrial membranes, the amount of DNA repair, and many other factors that affect maximum life span.

Organism Longevity and Basal Metabolic Rate

In allometric scaling, maximum potential life span (MPLS) is directly related to metabolic rate (MR), where MR is the recharge rate of a biomass made up of covalent bonds. That biomass (W) is subjected to deterioration over time from thermodynamic, entropic pressure. Metabolism is essentially understood as redox coupling, and has nothing to do with thermogenesis. Metabolic efficiency (ME) is then expressed as the efficiency of this coupling, a ratio of amperes captured and used by biomass, to the amperes available for that purpose. MR is measured in watts, W is measured in grams. These factors are combined in a power law, an elaboration on Kleiber's law relating MR to W and MPLS, that appears as $MR = W^{(4ME-1)/4ME}$. When ME is 100%, $MR = W^{3/4}$; this is popularly known as quarter power scaling, a version of allometric scaling that is premised upon unrealistic estimates of biological efficiency.

The equation reveals that as ME drops below 20%, for W < one gram, MR/MPLS increases so dramatically as to endow W with virtual immortality by 16%. The smaller W is to begin with, the more dramatic is the increase in MR as ME diminishes. All of the cells of an organism fit into this range, i.e., less than one gram, and so this MR will be referred to as BMR.

But the equation reveals that as ME increases over 25%, BMR approaches zero. The equation also shows that for all W > one gram, where W is the organization of all of the BMRs of the organism's structure, but also includes the activity of the structure, as ME increases over 25%, MR/MPLS increases rather than decreases, as it does for BMR. An MR made up of an organization of BMRs will be referred to as an FMR. As ME decreases below 25%, FMR diminishes rather than increases as it does for BMR.

The antagonism between FMR and BMR is what marks the process of aging of biomass W in energetic terms. The ME for the organism is the same as that for the cells, such that the success of the organism's ability to find food (and lower its ME), is key to maintaining the BMR of the cells driven, otherwise, by starvation, to approaching zero; while at the same time a lower ME diminishes the FMR/MPLS of the organism.

Medical Considerations

A person's metabolism varies with their physical condition and activity. Weight training can have a longer impact on metabolism than aerobic training, but there are no known mathematical formulas that can exactly predict the length and duration of a raised metabolism from trophic changes with anabolic neuromuscular training.

A decrease in food intake will typically lower the metabolic rate as the body tries to conserve energy. Researcher Gary Foster, Ph.D., estimates that a very low calorie diet of fewer than 800 calories a day would reduce the metabolic rate by more than 10 percent.

The metabolic rate can be affected by some drugs, such as antithyroid agents, drugs used to treat hyperthyroidism, such as propylthiouracil and methimazole, bring the metabolic rate down to normal and restore euthyroidism. Some research has focused on developing antiobesity drugs to raise the metabolic rate, such as drugs to stimulate thermogenesis in skeletal muscle.

The metabolic rate may be elevated in stress, illness, and diabetes. Menopause may also affect metabolism.

Cardiovascular Implications

Heart rate is determined by the medulla oblongata and part of the pons, two organs located inferior to the hypothalamus on the brain stem. Heart rate is important for basal metabolic rate and resting metabolic rate because it drives the blood supply, stimulating the Krebs cycle. During exercise that achieves the anaerobic threshold, it is possible to deliver substrates that are desired for optimal energy utilization. The anaerobic threshold is defined as the energy utilization level of heart rate exertion that occurs without oxygen during a standardized test with a specific protocol for accuracy of measurement, such as the Bruce Treadmill protocol. With four to six weeks of targeted training the body systems can adapt to a higher perfusion of mitochondrial density for increased oxygen availability for the Krebs cycle, or tricarboxylic cycle, or the glycolitic cycle. This in turn leads to a lower resting heart rate, lower blood pressure, and increased resting or basal metabolic rate.

By measuring heart rate we can then derive estimations of what level of substrate utilization is actually causing biochemical metabolism in our bodies at rest or in activity. This in turn can help a person to maintain an appropriate level of consumption and utilization by studying a graphical representation of the anaerobic threshold. This can be confirmed by blood tests and gas analysis using either direct or indirect calorimetry to show the effect of substrate utilization. The measures of basal metabolic rate and resting metabolic rate are becoming essential tools for maintaining a healthy body weight.

References

- Friedrich C (1998). "Physiology and genetics of sulfur-oxidizing bacteria". Adv Microb Physiol. Advances in Microbial Physiology. 39: 235–89. doi:10.1016/S0065-2911(08)60018-1. ISBN 978-0-12-027739-1.

- Nelson, David L.; Michael M. Cox (2005). Lehninger Principles of Biochemistry. New York: W. H. Freeman and company. p. 841. ISBN 0-7167-4339-6.

- Koch A (1998). "How did bacteria come to be?". Adv Microb Physiol. Advances in Microbial Physiology. 40: 353–99. doi:10.1016/S0065-2911(08)60135-6. ISBN 978-0-12-027740-7.

- Zhu G, Peng Y, Li B, Guo J, Yang Q, Wang S (2008). "Biological removal of nitrogen from wastewater". Rev Environ Contam Toxicol. Reviews of Environmental Contamination and Toxicology. 192: 159–95. doi:10.1007/978-0-387-71724-1_5. ISBN 978-0-387-71723-4.

- McArdle, W (2006). Essentials of Exercise Physiology. Lippincott Williams & Wilkins. p. 266. ISBN 9780495014836.

- Lisa Gordon-Davis (2004). Hospitality Industry Handbook on Nutrition and Menu Planning. Juta and Company Ltd. p. 112. ISBN 978-0-7021-5578-9.

- Maton, Anthea; Jean Hopkins; Charles William McLaughlin; Susan Johnson; Maryanna Quon Warner; David LaHart; Jill D. Wright (1993). Human Biology and Health. Englewood Cliffs, New Jersey, USA: Prentice Hall. ISBN 0-13-981176-1. OCLC 32308337.

- Wooldridge K (editor) (2009). Bacterial Secreted Proteins: Secretory Mechanisms and Role in Pathogenesis. Caister Academic Press. ISBN 978-1-904455-42-4.

- Salyers, A. A. & Whitt, D. D. (2002). Bacterial Pathogenesis: A Molecular Approach, 2nd ed., Washington, D.C.: ASM Press. ISBN 1-55581-171-X

Human Health and Nutrition

This chapter explains in detail the issues caused by the lack of nutrition and it elucidates the importance of nutrition and the issues caused by the lack of it. A detailed analysis of malnutrition, eating disorder, and obesity is dealt with. The aspects elucidated in this chapter are of vital importance, and provide a better understanding of nutrition and health.

Diet (Nutrition)

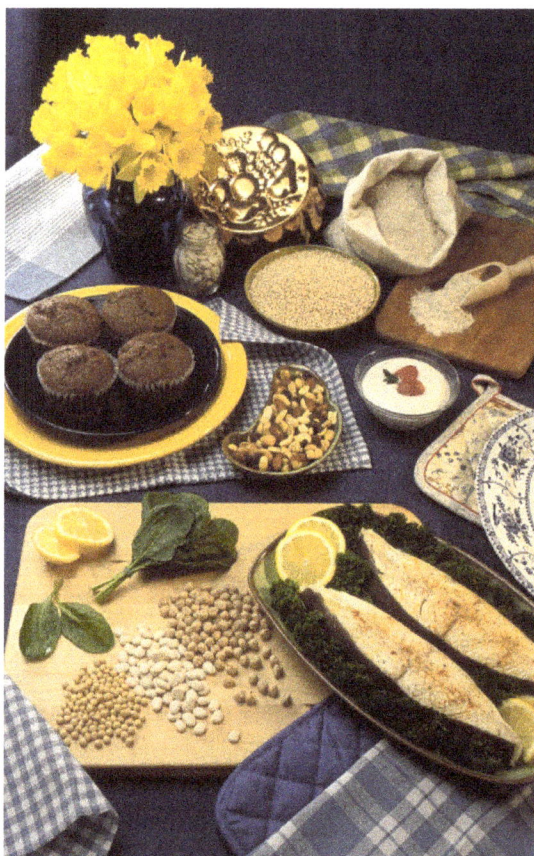

A selection of foods consumed by humans. However, the human diet can vary widely.

In nutrition, diet is the sum of food consumed by a person or other organism. The word diet often implies the use of specific intake of nutrition for health or weight-management reasons (with the two often being related). Although humans are omnivores, each culture and each person holds some food preferences or some food taboos. This may be due to personal tastes or ethical reasons. Individual dietary choices may be more or less healthy.

Complete nutrition requires ingestion and absorption of vitamins, minerals, and food energy in the form of carbohydrates, proteins, and fats. Dietary habits and choices play a significant role in the quality of life, health and longevity.

Religious and Cultural Dietary Choices

Some cultures and religions have restrictions concerning what foods are acceptable in their diet. For example, only Kosher foods are permitted by Judaism, and Halal foods by Islam. Although Buddhists are generally vegetarians, the practice varies and meat-eating may be permitted depending on the sects. In Hinduism, vegetarianism is the ideal. Jains are strictly vegetarian and consumption of roots is not permitted.

Dietary Choices

Many people choose to forgo food from animal sources to varying degrees (e.g. flexitarianism, vegetarianism, veganism, fruitarianism) for health reasons, issues surrounding morality, or to reduce their personal impact on the environment, although some of the public assumptions about which diets have lower impacts are known to be incorrect. Raw foodism is another contemporary trend. These diets may require tuning or supplementation such as vitamins to meet ordinary nutritional needs.

Weight Management

A particular diet may be chosen to seek weight loss or weight gain. Changing a subject's dietary intake, or "going on a diet", can change the energy balance and increase or decrease the amount of fat stored by the body. Some foods are specifically recommended, or even altered, for conformity to the requirements of a particular diet. These diets are often recommended in conjunction with exercise. Specific weight loss programs can be harmful to health, while others may be beneficial (and can thus be coined as healthy diets). The terms "healthy diet" and "diet for weight management" are often related, as the two promote healthy weight management. Having a healthy diet is a way to prevent health problems, and will provide your body with the right balance of vitamins, minerals, and other nutrients.

Eating Disorders

An eating disorder is a mental disorder that interferes with normal food consumption. It is defined by abnormal eating habits that may involve either insufficient or excessive diet.

Health

A healthy diet may improve or maintain optimal health. In developed countries, affluence enables unconstrained caloric intake and possibly inappropriate food choices.

Health agencies recommend that people maintain a normal weight by limiting consumption of energy-dense foods and sugary drinks, eat plant-based food, limit red and processed meat, and limit alcohol.

Diet Classification Table

Food Type	Carnivorous	Ketogenic	Omnivorous	Pescetarian	Vegetarian	Vegan	Raw vegan	Islamic	Hindu	Jewish	Paleolithic	Fruitarian
Fruits and berries	No	No	Yes	Yes	Yes	Yes	Yes	Yes	Yes	Yes	Yes	Yes
Greens	No	No	Yes	Yes	Yes	Yes	Yes	Yes	Yes	Yes	Yes	Yes
Vegetables	No	No	Yes	Yes	Yes	Yes	Yes	Yes	Yes	Yes	Yes	No
Legumes	No	No	Yes	Yes	Yes	Yes	Yes	Yes	Yes	Yes	No	No
Tubers	No	No	Yes	Yes	Yes	Yes	No	Yes	Yes	Yes	Yes	No
Grains	No	No	Yes	Yes	Yes	Yes	No	Yes	Yes	Yes	No	Yes
Poultry	Yes	Yes	Yes	No	No	No	No	Yes	Yes	Yes	Yes	No
Fish (scaled)	Yes	Yes	Yes	Yes	No	No	No	Yes	Yes	Yes	Yes	No
Seafood (non-fish)	Yes	Yes	Yes	Yes	No	No	No	Yes	Yes	No	Yes	No
Beef	Yes	Yes	Yes	No	No	No	No	Yes	No	Yes	Yes	No
Pork	Yes	Yes	Yes	No	No	No	No	No	No	No	Yes	No
Eggs	Yes	Yes	Yes	Yes	Maybe	No	No	Yes	Yes	Yes	Yes	No
Dairy	No	Maybe	Yes	Yes	Maybe	No	No	Yes	Yes	Yes	No	No
Nuts	No	Maybe	Yes	Yes	Yes	Yes	Yes	Yes	Yes	Yes	Yes	Yes
Alcohol	No	Maybe	Yes	Yes	Yes	Yes	No	No	Yes	Yes	No	No

Healthy Diet

A healthy diet is one that helps to maintain or improve overall health.

A healthy diet provides the body with essential nutrition: fluid, adequate essential amino acids from protein, essential fatty acids, vitamins, minerals, and adequate calories. The requirements for a healthy diet can be met from a variety of plant-based and animal-based foods. A healthy diet supports energy needs and provides for human nutrition without exposure to toxicity or excessive weight gain from consuming excessive amounts. Where lack of calories is not an issue, a properly balanced diet (in addition to exercise) is also thought to be important for lowering health risks, such as obesity, heart disease, type 2 diabetes, hypertension and cancer.

Various nutrition guides are published by medical and governmental institutions to educate the public on what they should be eating to promote health. Nutrition facts labels are also mandatory in some countries to allow consumers to choose between foods based on the components relevant to health.

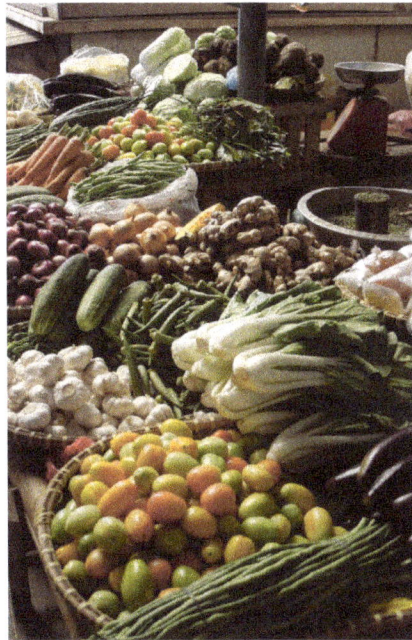

Leafy green, allium, and cruciferous vegetables are key components of a healthy diet

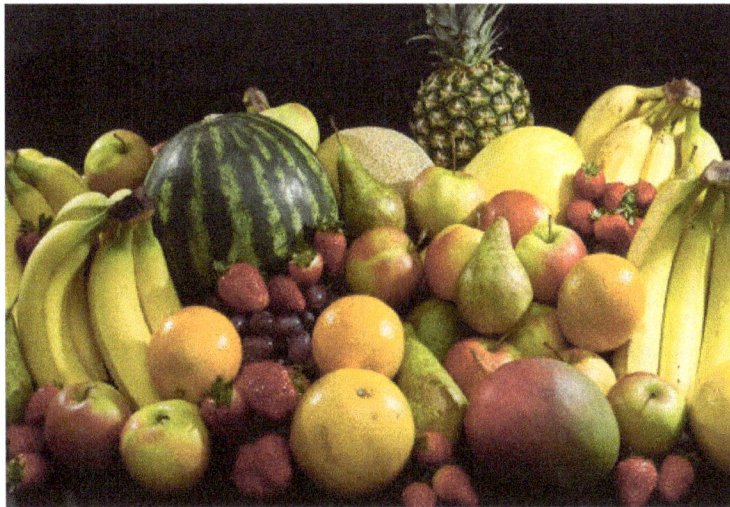

Common colorful culinary fruits. Apples, pears, strawberries, oranges, bananas, grapes, canary melons, watermelon, cantaloupe, pineapple and mango.

The idea of dietary therapy (using dietary choices to maintain health and improve poor health) is quite old and thus has both modern scientific forms (medical nutrition therapy) and prescientific forms (such as dietary therapy in traditional Chinese medicine).

Mainstream Science

Healthy eating is simple, according to Marion Nestle, who expresses the mainstream view among scientists who study nutrition:

The basic principles of good diets are so simple that I can summarize them in just ten words: eat less, move more, eat lots of fruits and vegetables. For additional clarification, a five-word modifier helps: go easy on junk foods. Follow these precepts and you will go a long way toward preventing the major diseases of our overfed society—coronary heart disease, certain cancers, diabetes, stroke, osteoporosis, and a host of others.... These precepts constitute the bottom line of what seem to be the far more complicated dietary recommendations of many health organizations and national and international governments—the forty-one "key recommendations" of the 2005 Dietary Guidelines, for example. ... Although you may feel as though advice about nutrition is constantly changing, the basic ideas behind my four precepts have not changed in half a century. And they leave plenty of room for enjoying the pleasures of food.

David L. Katz, who reviewed the most prevalent popular diets in 2014, noted:

The weight of evidence strongly supports a theme of healthful eating while allowing for variations on that theme. A diet of minimally processed foods close to nature, predominantly plants, is decisively associated with health promotion and disease prevention and is consistent with the salient components of seemingly distinct dietary approaches. Efforts to improve public health through diet are forestalled not for want of knowledge about the optimal feeding of Homo sapiens but for distractions associated with exaggerated claims, and our failure to convert what we reliably know into what we routinely do. Knowledge in this case is not, as of yet, power; would that it were so.

Recommendations

World Health Organization

The World Health Organization (WHO) makes the following 5 recommendations with respect to both populations and individuals:

- Eat roughly the same amount of calories that your body is using. A healthy weight is a balance between energy consumed and energy that is 'burnt off'.

- Limit intake of fats, and prefer unsaturated fats to saturated fats and trans fats.

- Increase consumption of plant foods, particularly fruits, vegetables, legumes, whole grains and nuts.

- Limit the intake of sugar. A 2003 report recommends less than 10% of calorie intake from simple sugars.

- Limit salt / sodium consumption from all sources and ensure that salt is iodized.

Other recommendations include:

- Essential micronutrients such as vitamins and certain minerals.

- Avoiding directly poisonous (e.g. heavy metals) and carcinogenic (e.g. benzene) substances.

- Avoiding foods contaminated by human pathogens (e.g. *E. coli*, tapeworm eggs).

United States Department of Agriculture

The Dietary Guidelines for American by the United States Department of Agriculture (USDA) recommends three healthy patterns of diet, summarized in table below, for a 2000 kcal diet.

It emphasizes both health and environmental sustainability and a flexible approach: the committee that drafted it wrote: "The major findings regarding sustainable diets were that a diet higher in plant-based foods, such as vegetables, fruits, whole grains, legumes, nuts, and seeds, and lower in calories and animal-based foods is more health promoting and is associated with less environmental impact than is the current U.S. diet. This pattern of eating can be achieved through a variety of dietary patterns, including the "Healthy U.S.-style Pattern," the "Healthy Mediterranean-style Pattern," and the "Healthy Vegetarian Pattern". Food group amounts per day, unless noted per week.

Food group/subgroup (units)	Healthy US patterns	Healthy Vegetarian patterns	Healthy Med-style patterns
Fruits (cup eq)	2	2	2.5
Vegetables (cup eq)	2.5	2.5	2.5
Dark green	1.5/wk	1.5/wk	1.5/wk
Red/orange	5.5/wk	5.5/wk	5.5/wk
Starchy	5/wk	5/wk	5/wk
Legumes	1.5/wk	3/wk	1.5/wk
Others	4/wk	4/wk	4/wk
Grains (oz eq)	6	6.5	6
Whole	3	3.5	3
Refined	3	3	3
Dairy (cup eq)	3	3	2
Protein Foods (oz eq)	5.5	3.5	6.5
Meat (red and processed)	12.5/wk	--	12.5/wk
Poultry	10.5/wk	--	10.5/wk
Seafood	8/wk	--	15/wk
Eggs	3/wk	3/wk	3/wk
Nuts/seeds	4/wk	7/wk	4/wk
Processed Soy (including tofu)	0.5/wk	8/wk	0.5/wk
Oils (grams)	27	27	27
Solid fats limit (grams)	18	21	17
Added sugars limit (grams)	30	36	29

American Heart Association / World Cancer Research Fund / American Institute for Cancer Research

The American Heart Association, World Cancer Research Fund, and American Institute for Cancer Research recommends a diet that consists mostly of unprocessed plant foods, with emphasis a wide range of whole grains, legumes, and non-starchy vegetables and fruits. This healthy diet is full of a wide range of various non-starchy vegetables and fruits, that provide different colors including red, green, yellow, white, purple, and orange. They note that tomato cooked with oil, allium vegetables like garlic, and cruciferous vegetables like cauliflower, provide some protection against cancer. This healthy diet is low in energy density, which may protect against weight gain and associated diseases. Finally, limiting consumption of sugary drinks, limiting energy rich foods, including "fast foods" and red meat, and avoiding processed meats improves health and longevity. Overall, researchers and medical policy conclude that this healthy diet can reduce the risk of chronic disease and cancer.

In children less than 25 gms of added sugar (100 calories) is recommended per day. Other recommendations include no extra sugars in those under 2 years old and less than one soft drink per week.

Harvard School of Public Health

The Nutrition Source of Harvard School of Public Health makes the following 10 recommendations for a healthy diet:

- Choose good carbohydrates: whole grains (the less processed the better), vegetables, fruits and beans. Avoid white bread, white rice, and the like as well as pastries, sugared sodas, and other highly processed food.

- Pay attention to the protein package: good choices include fish, poultry, nuts, and beans. Try to avoid red meat.

- Choose foods containing healthy fats. Plant oils, nuts, and fish are the best choices. Limit consumption of saturated fats, and avoid foods with trans fat.

- Choose a fiber-filled diet which includes whole grains, vegetables, and fruits.

- Eat more vegetables and fruits—the more colorful and varied, the better.

- Calcium is important, but milk is not its best or only source. Good sources of calcium are collards, bok choy, fortified soy milk, baked beans, and supplements which contain calcium and vitamin D.

- Water is the best source of liquid. Avoid sugary drinks, and limit intake of juices and milk. Coffee, tea, artificially-sweetened drinks, 100-percent fruit juices, low-fat milk and alcohol can fit into a healthy diet but are best consumed in moderation. Sports drinks are recommended only for people who exercise more than an hour at a stretch to replace substances lost in sweat.

- Limit salt intake. Choose more fresh foods, instead of processed ones.

- Moderate alcohol drinking has health benefits, but is not recommended for everyone.

- Daily multivitamin and extra vitamin D intake has potential health benefits.

Other than nutrition, the guide recommends frequent physical exercise and maintaining a healthy body weight.

For Specific Conditions

In addition to dietary recommendations for the general population, there are many specific diets that have primarily been developed to promote better health in specific population groups, such as people with high blood pressure (as in low sodium diets or the more specific DASH diet), or people who are overweight or obese (in weight control diets). However, some of them may have more or less evidence for beneficial effects in normal people as well.

Hypertension

A low sodium diet is beneficial for people with high blood pressure. A Cochrane review published in 2008 concluded that a long term (more than 4 weeks) low sodium diet has a useful effect to reduce blood pressure, both in people with hypertension and in people with normal blood pressure.

The DASH diet (Dietary Approaches to Stop Hypertension) is a diet promoted by the National Heart, Lung, and Blood Institute (part of the NIH, a United States government organization) to control hypertension. A major feature of the plan is limiting intake of sodium, and it also generally encourages the consumption of nuts, whole grains, fish, poultry, fruits and vegetables while lowering the consumption of red meats, sweets, and sugar. It is also "rich in potassium, magnesium, and calcium, as well as protein". Evidence shows that the Mediterranean diet improves cardiovascular outcomes.

WHO recommends few standards such as an intake of less than 5 grams per person per day so as to prevent one from cardiovascular disease. Unsaturated fatty acids with polyunsaturated vegetable oils, on the other hand plays an essential role in reducing coronary heart disease risk as well as diabetes.

Obesity

Weight control diets aim to maintain a controlled weight. In most cases dieting is used in combination with physical exercise to lose weight in those who are overweight or obese.

Diets to promote weight loss are divided into four categories: low-fat, low-carbohydrate, low-calorie, and very low calorie. A meta-analysis of six randomized controlled trials found no difference between the main diet types (low calorie, low carbohydrate, and low fat), with a 2–4 kilogram weight loss in all studies. At two years, all calorie-reduced diet types cause equal weight loss irrespective of the macronutrients emphasized.

Reduced Disease Risk

There may be a relationship between lifestyle including food consumption and potentially lowering the risk of cancer or other chronic diseases. A diet high in fruits and vegetables appears to decrease the risk of cardiovascular disease and death but not cancer.

A healthy diet may consist mostly of whole plant foods, with limited consumption of energy dense foods, red meat, alcoholic drinks and salt while reducing consumption of sugary drinks, and processed meat. A healthy diet may contain non-starchy vegetables and fruits, including those with red, green, yellow, white, purple or orange pigments. Tomato cooked with oil, allium vegetables like garlic, and cruciferous vegetables like cauliflower "probably" contain compounds which are under research for their possible anti-cancer activity.

A healthy diet is low in energy density, lowering caloric content, thereby possibly inhibiting weight gain and lowering risk against chronic diseases. Chronic Western diseases are associated with pathologically increased IGF-1 levels. Findings in molecular biology and epidemiologic data suggest that milk consumption is a promoter of chronic diseases of Western nations, including atherosclerosis, carcinogenesis and neurodegenerative diseases.

Unhealthy Diets

The Western pattern diet which is typically eaten by Americans and increasingly adapted by people in the developing world as they leave poverty is unhealthy: it is "rich in red meat, dairy products, processed and artificially sweetened foods, and salt, with minimal intake of fruits, vegetables, fish, legumes, and whole grains."

An unhealthy diet is a major risk factor for a number of chronic diseases including: high blood pressure, diabetes, abnormal blood lipids, overweight/obesity, cardiovascular diseases, and cancer.

The WHO estimates that 2.7 million deaths are attributable to a diet low in fruits and vegetables every year. Globally it is estimated to cause about 19% of gastrointestinal cancer, 31% of ischaemic heart disease, and 11% of strokes, thus making it one of the leading preventable causes of death worldwide.

Popular Diets

Popular diets, often referred to as fad diets, make promises of weight loss or other health advantages such as longer life without backing by solid science, and in many cases are characterized by highly restrictive or unusual food choices. Celebrity endorsements (including celebrity doctors) are frequently associated with popular diets, and the individuals who develop and promote these programs often profit handsomely.[-12]

Public Health

Fears of high cholesterol were frequently voiced up until the mid-1990s. However, more recent research has shown that the distinction between high- and low-density lipoprotein ('good' and 'bad' cholesterol, respectively) must be addressed when speaking of the potential ill effects of cholesterol. Different types of dietary fat have different effects on blood levels of cholesterol. For example, polyunsaturated fats tend to decrease both types of cholesterol; monounsaturated fats tend to lower LDL and raise HDL; saturated fats tend to either raise HDL, or raise both HDL and LDL; and trans fat tend to raise LDL and lower HDL.

While dietary cholesterol is only found in animal products such as meat, eggs, and dairy, studies have not found a link between eating cholesterol and blood levels of cholesterol.

Vending machines in particular have come under fire as being avenues of entry into schools for junk food promoters. However, there is little in the way of regulation and it is difficult for most people to properly analyze the real merits of a company referring to itself as "healthy." Recently, the Committee of Advertising Practice in the United Kingdom launched a proposal to limit media advertising for food and soft drink products high in fat, salt or sugar. The British Heart Foundation released its own government-funded advertisements, labeled "Food4Thought", which were targeted at children and adults to discourage unhealthy habits of consuming junk food.

Cultural and Psychological Factors

From a psychological and cultural perspective, a healthier diet may be difficult to achieve for people with poor eating habits. This may be due to tastes acquired in childhood and preferences for sugary, salty and/or fatty foods.

Dietary Supplement

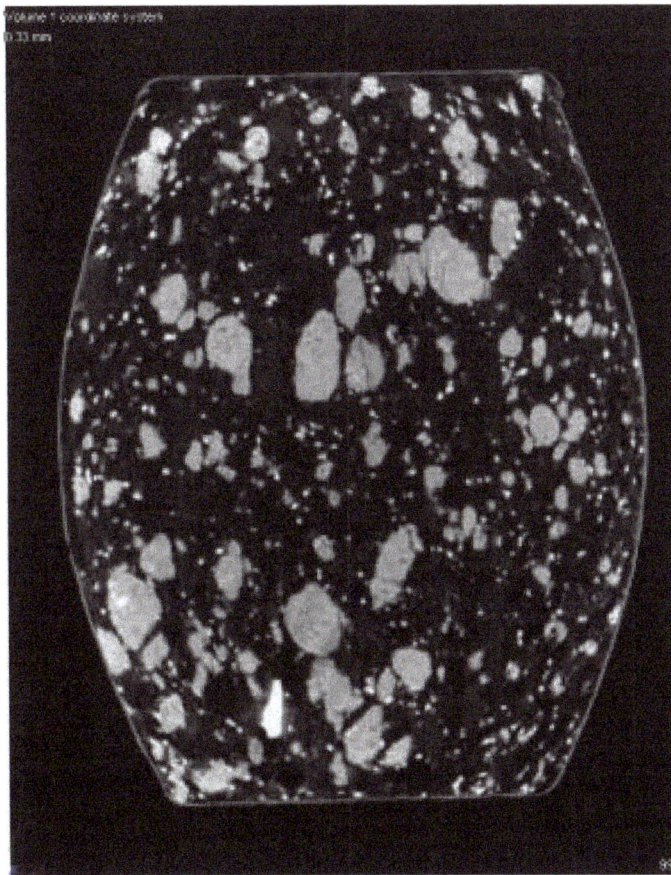

Flight through a CT image stack of a multivitamin tablet "A-Z" by German company Abtei.

A dietary supplement is intended to provide nutrients that may otherwise not be consumed in sufficient quantities.

Supplements as generally understood include vitamins, minerals, fiber, fatty acids, or amino acids, among other substances. U.S. authorities define dietary supplements as foods, while elsewhere they may be classified as drugs or other products.

There are more than 50,000 dietary supplements available. More than half of the U.S. adult population (53% - 55%) consume dietary supplements with most common ones being multivitamins.

These products are not intended to prevent or treat any disease and in some circumstances are dangerous, according to the U.S. National Institutes of Health. For those who fail to consume a balanced diet, the agency says that certain supplements "may have value."

Most supplements should be avoided, and usually people should not eat micronutrients except people with clearly shown deficiency. Those people should first consult a doctor. An exception is vitamin D, which is recommended in Nordic countries due to weak sunlight.

Definition

According to the United States Food and Drug Administration (FDA), dietary supplements are products which are not pharmaceutical drugs, food additives like spices or preservatives, or conventional food, and which also meet any of these criteria:

1. The product is intended to supplement a person's diet, despite it not being usable as a meal replacement.

2. The product is or contains a vitamin, dietary element, herb used for herbalism or botanical used as a medicinal plant, amino acid, any substance which contributes to other food eaten, or any concentrate, metabolite, ingredient, extract, or combination of these things.

3. The product is labeled as a dietary supplement.

In the United States, the FDA has different monitoring procedures for substances depending on whether they are presented as drugs, food additives, food, or dietary supplements. Dietary supplements are eaten or taken by mouth, and are regulated in United States law as a type of food rather than a type of drug. Like food and unlike drugs, no government approval is required to make or sell dietary supplements; the manufacturer checks the safety of dietary supplements but the government does not; and rather than requiring risk–benefit analysis to prove that the product can be sold like a drug, risk–benefit analysis is only used to petition that food or a dietary supplement is unsafe and should be removed from market.

Medical Uses

The intended use of dietary supplements is to ensure that a person gets enough essential nutrients.

Dietary supplements should not be used to treat any disease or as preventive healthcare. An exception to this recommendation is the appropriate use of vitamins.

Dietary supplements are unnecessary if one eats a balanced diet.

Supplements may create harm in several ways, including over-consumption, particularly of minerals and fat-soluble vitamins which can build up in the body. The products may also cause harm related to their rapid absorption in a short period of time, quality issues such as contamination, or by adverse interactions with other foods and medications.

Types

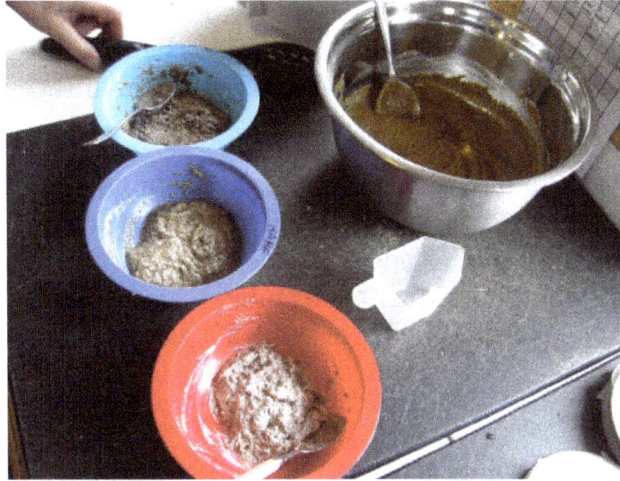

Dietary supplements being mixed into food for pigs.

There are many types of dietary supplements.

Vitamins

Vitamin is an organic compound required by an organism as a vital nutrient in limited amounts. An organic chemical compound (or related set of compounds) is called a vitamin when it cannot be synthesized in sufficient quantities by an organism, and must be obtained from the diet. Thus, the term is conditional both on the circumstances and on the particular organism. For example, ascorbic acid (vitamin C) is a vitamin for humans, but not for most other animals. Supplementation is important for the treatment of certain health problems but there is little evidence of benefit when used by those who are otherwise healthy.

Dietary Element

Dietary elements, commonly called "dietary minerals" or "minerals", are the chemical elements required by living organisms, other than the four elements carbon, hydrogen, nitrogen, and oxygen present in common organic molecules. The term "dietary mineral" is archaic, as the substances it refers are chemical elements rather than actual minerals.

Herbal Medicine

Herbal medicine is the use of plants for medicinal purposes. Plants have been the basis for medical treatments through much of human history, and such traditional medicine is still widely practiced today. Modern medicine recognizes herbalism as a form of alternative medicine, as the practice of herbalism is not strictly based on evidence gathered using the scientific method. Modern medicine, does, however, make use of many plant-derived compounds as the basis for evidence-tested pharmaceutical drugs, and phytotherapy works to apply modern standards of effectiveness testing to herbs and medicines that are derived from natural sources. The scope of herbal medicine is sometimes extended to include fungal and bee products, as well as minerals, shells and certain animal parts.

Amino Acids and Proteins

Amino acids are biologically important organic compounds composed of amine (-NH$_2$) and carboxylic acid (-COOH) functional groups, along with a side-chain specific to each amino acid. The key elements of an amino acid are carbon, hydrogen, oxygen, and nitrogen, though other elements are found in the side-chains of certain amino acids.

Amino acids can be divided into three categories: essential amino acids, non-essential amino acids, and conditional amino acids. Essential amino acids cannot be made by the body, and must be supplied by food. Non-essential amino acids are made by the body from essential amino acids or in the normal breakdown of proteins. Conditional amino acids are usually not essential, except in times of illness, stress, or for someone challenged with a lifelong medical condition.

Essential Fatty Acids

Essential fatty acids, or EFAs, are fatty acids that humans and other animals must ingest because the body requires them for good health but cannot synthesize them. The term "essential fatty acid" refers to fatty acids required for biological processes but does not include the fats that only act as fuel.

Bodybuilding Supplements

Bodybuilding supplements are dietary supplements commonly used by those involved in bodybuilding and athletics. Bodybuilding supplements may be used to replace meals, enhance weight gain, promote weight loss or improve athletic performance. Among the most widely used are vitamin supplements, protein drinks, branched-chain amino acids (BCAA), glutamine, essential fatty acids, meal replacement products, creatine, weight loss products and testosterone boosters. Supplements are sold either as single ingredient preparations or in the form of "stacks" – proprietary blends of various supplements marketed as offering synergistic advantages. While many bodybuilding supplements are also consumed by the general public their salience and frequency of use may differ when used specifically by bodybuilders.

Industry

In 2013, the global market of vitamins, minerals, and nutritional and herbal supplements (VMHS) was valued at $82 billion, with roughly 28 percent of that in the U.S., where sales increased by approximately $6 billion between 2007 and 2012.

The vitamins and dietary supplements sector in the U.S. grew 4% in 2015, to reach US$27.2 billion. The U.S. market was highly competitive in 2015, as no single company accounted for more than a 5% share of value sales.

Controversy

According to University of Helsinki food safety professor Marina Heinonen, more than 90% of dietary supplement health claims are incorrect. In addition, ingredients listed have been found to be different from the contents. For example, Consumer Reports reported unsafe levels of arsenic, cadmium, lead and mercury in several of the protein powders that were tested. Also, the CBC found that protein spiking (the addition of amino acid filler to manipulate analysis) was not uncommon, however many of the companies involved challenged their claim.

Adverse Effects

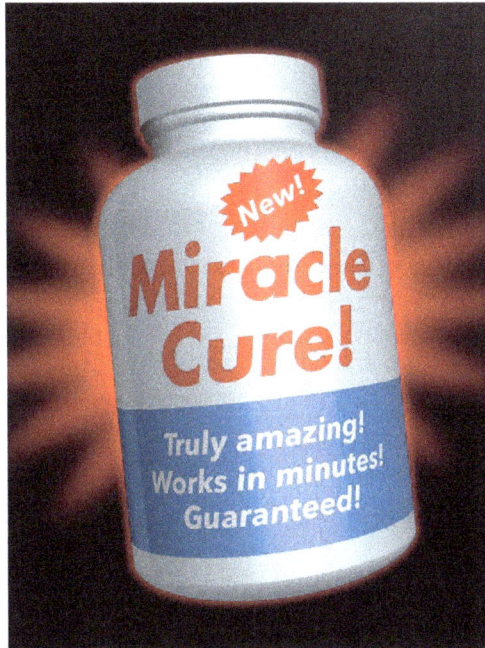

Some products make extraordinary claims and contain active ingredients which may not have been proven effective.

The number of incidents of liver damage from dietary supplements has tripled in a decade. Most of the products causing that effect were bodybuilding supplements. Some of the victims required liver transplants and some died. A third of the supplements involved contained unlisted steroids.

Mild to severe toxicity has occurred on many occasions due to dietary supplements, even when the active ingredients were essential nutrients such as vitamins, minerals or amino acids. This has been a result of adulteration of the product, excessive usage on the part of the consumer, or use by persons at risk for the development of adverse effects. In addition, a number of supplements contain psychoactive drugs, whether of natural or synthetic origin.

Physical and Chemical Properties

Adulteration in North America

BMC Medicine published a study on herbal supplements in 2013. Most of the supplements studied were of low quality, one third did not contain the active ingredient(s) claimed, and one third contained unlisted substances.

An investigation by the New York Attorney General's office analyzed 78 bottles of herbal supplements from Walmart, Target, Walgreens and GNC stores in New York State using DNA barcoding. a method used to detect labeling fraud in the seafood industry. Only about 20% contained the ingredient on the label.

Some supplements were contamined by rodent feces and urine.

Only 0.3% of the 55,000 U.S. market dietary supplements have been studied regarding their common side effects.

Society and Culture

Use as Food Replacement

In early 20th century there were great hopes for supplements, but later research has shown these hopes were unfounded.

"Antioxidant paradox" means the fact that even though fruits and vegetables are related to decreases in mortality, cardiovascular diseases and cancers, antioxidant nutrients do not really seem to help. According to one theory, this is because some other nutrients would be the important ones. Multivitamin pills have neither proved useful but may even increase mortality.

Omega-3 fatty acids and fish oils from food are very healthy, but fish oil supplements are recommended only for those suffering from coronary artery diseases and not eating fish. Latest research has made the benefits of the supplements questionable even for them. Contrary to claims, fish oils do not decrease cholesterol but may even raise the "bad" LDL cholesterol and cause other harms. Also the use of cod liver oil is criticized by scientists.

Alice Lichtenstein, DSc, chairwoman of the American Heart Association (AHA) says that even though omega-3 fatty acids from foods are healthy, the same is not shown in studies on omega-3 supplements. Therefore, one should not eat fish oil supplements unless one suffers from heart diseases.

Legal Regulation

United States

The regulation of food and dietary supplements by the U.S. Food and Drug Administration is governed by various statutes enacted by the United States Congress and interpreted by the U.S. Food and Drug Administration ("FDA"). Pursuant to the Federal Food, Drug, and Cosmetic Act ("the Act") and accompanying legislation, the FDA has authority to oversee the quality of substances sold as food in the United States, and to monitor claims made in the labeling about both the composition and the health benefits of foods.

Substances which the FDA regulates as food are subdivided into various categories, including foods, food additives, added substances (man-made substances which are not intentionally introduced into food, but nevertheless end up in it), and dietary supplements. The specific standards which the FDA exercises differ from one category to the next. Furthermore, the FDA has been granted a variety of means by which it can address violations of the standards for a given category of substances.

Regulation in European Union

The European Union's Food Supplements Directive of 2002 requires that supplements be demonstrated to be safe, both in dosages and in purity. Only those supplements that have been proven to be safe may be sold in the bloc without prescription. As a category of food, food supplements cannot be labeled with drug claims but can bear health claims and nutrition claims.

The dietary supplements industry in the United Kingdom (UK), one of the 28 countries in the bloc, strongly opposed the Directive. In addition, a large number of consumers throughout Europe, including over one million in the UK, and various doctors and scientists, had signed petitions by 2005 against what are viewed by the petitioners as unjustified restrictions of consumer choice.

In 2004, along with two British trade associations, the Alliance for Natural Health (ANH) had a legal challenge to the Food Supplements Directive referred to the European Court of Justice by the High Court in London.

Although the European Court of Justice's Advocate General subsequently said that the bloc's plan to tighten rules on the sale of vitamins and food supplements should be scrapped, he was eventually overruled by the European Court, which decided that the measures in question were necessary and appropriate for the purpose of protecting public health. ANH, however, interpreted the ban as applying only to synthetically produced supplements—and not to vitamins and minerals normally found in or consumed as part of the diet.

Nevertheless, the European judges acknowledged the Advocate General's concerns, stating that there must be clear procedures to allow substances to be added to the permitted list based on scientific evidence. They also said that any refusal to add the product to the list must be open to challenge in the courts.

Research

Effects of most dietary supplements have not been determined in randomized clinical trials and manufacturing is lightly regulated; randomized clinical trials of certain vitamins and antioxidants have found increased mortality rates.

Essential Amino Acid

An essential amino acid or indispensable amino acid is an amino acid that cannot be synthesized de novo *(from scratch)* by the organism, and thus must be supplied in its diet. The nine amino acids humans cannot synthesize are phenylalanine, valine, threonine, tryptophan, methionine, leucine, isoleucine, lysine, and histidine (i.e., F V T W M L I K H).

Six other amino acids are considered conditionally essential in the human diet, meaning their synthesis can be limited under special pathophysiological conditions, such as prematurity in the infant or individuals in severe catabolic distress. These six are arginine, cysteine, glycine, glutamine, proline, and tyrosine (i.e. R C G Q P Y). Five amino acids are dispensable in humans, meaning they can be synthesized in the body. These five are alanine, aspartic acid, asparagine, glutamic acid and serine (i.e., A D N E S).

Essentiality in Humans

Essential	Nonessential **
Histidine	Alanine
Isoleucine	Arginine*
Leucine	Aspartic acid
Lysine	Cysteine*
Methionine	Glutamic acid
Phenylalanine	Glutamine*
Threonine	Glycine*
Tryptophan	Proline*
Valine	Serine*
	Tyrosine*
	Asparagine*
	Selenocysteine

(*) Essential only in certain cases.

(**) Pyrrolysine, sometimes considered "the 22nd amino acid", is not listed here as it is not used by humans.

Eukaryotes can synthesize some of the amino acids from other substrates. Consequently, only a subset of the amino acids used in protein synthesis are essential nutrients.

Minimum Daily Intake

Estimating the daily requirement for the indispensable amino acids has proven to be difficult; these numbers have undergone considerable revision over the last 20 years. The following table lists the WHO recommended daily amounts currently in use for essential amino acids in adult humans, together with their standard one-letter abbreviations. Food sources are identified based on the USDA National Nutrient Database Release.

Amino acid(s)	mg per kg body weight	mg per 70 kg	mg per 100 kg
H Histidine	10	700	1000
I Isoleucine	20	1400	2000
L Leucine	39	2730	3900
K Lysine	30	2100	3000
M Methionine + **C** Cysteine	10.4 + 4.1 (15 total)	1050	1500
F Phenylalanine + **Y** Tyrosine	25 (total)	1750	2500
T Threonine	15	1050	1500

W Tryptophan	4	280	400
V Valine	26	1820	2600

The recommended daily intakes for children aged three years and older is 10% to 20% higher than adult levels and those for infants can be as much as 150% higher in the first year of life. Cysteine (or sulphur-containing amino acids), tyrosine (or aromatic amino acids), and arginine are always required by infants and growing children.

Relative Amino Acid Composition of Protein Sources

Various attempts have been made to express the "quality" or "value" of various kinds of protein. Measures include the biological value, net protein utilization, protein efficiency ratio, protein digestibility-corrected amino acid score and complete proteins concept. These concepts are important in the livestock industry, because the relative lack of one or more of the essential amino acids in animal feeds would have a limiting effect on growth and thus on feed conversion ratio. Thus, various feedstuffs may be fed in combination to increase net protein utilization, or a supplement of an individual amino acid (methionine, lysine, threonine, or tryptophan) can be added to the feed.

Although proteins from plant sources tend to have a relatively lower concentrations of protein by mass in comparison to protein from eggs or milk, they are nevertheless "complete" in that they contain at least trace amounts of all of the amino acids that are essential in human nutrition. Eating various plant foods in combination can provide a protein of higher biological value. Certain native combinations of foods, such as corn and beans, soybeans and rice, or red beans and rice, contain the essential amino acids necessary for humans in adequate amounts.

Additionally, certain types of algae and marine phytoplankton predate the division between animal and plant life on the planet; they have both chlorophyll as do plants, and also all the essential amino acids, as do animal proteins.

Protein Per Calorie

It can be shown that common vegetable sources contain adequate protein, often more protein per Calorie than the standard reference, whole raw egg, while other plant sources, particularly fruits contain less. For example, while 100 g of raw broccoli only provides 28 kcal and 3 g of protein, it has over 100 mg of protein per kcal. An egg contains five times as many calories (143 kcal) but only four times as much protein, roughly 90 mg of protein per kcal. However, a carrot has only 23 mg protein per kcal or twice the minimum recommendation, a banana meets the minimum, and an apple is below recommendation. It is recommended that adult humans obtain 10-35% of their calories as protein, or roughly 11–39 mg of protein per kcal per day (22-78 g for 2000 kcal). The US FDA daily reference value of 50 g protein per 2000 kcal is 25 mg/kcal per day.

Source	protein (g)	Calories (kcal)	protein/Calorie (mg / kcal)	L (mg)	T (mg)	W (mg)	M+C (mg)
Apples, raw (100 g)	0.26	52	5	12	6	1	2

Minimum daily reference	22	2000	**11**				
Bananas, raw (100 g)	1	89	**12**	500	28	9	17
Carrot, raw (100 g)	1	41	**23**	101	191	12	103
US FDA daily / WHO (70 kg)	50	2000	**25**	2730	1050	280	1050
Upper daily reference	78	2000	**39**				
Peanut, valencia, raw (100 g)	48	570	**84**	1,627	859	244	630
Soybeans, dry (100 g)	40	451	**88**	2634	1719	575	1172
Egg, whole, raw (100 g)	13	143	**91**	912	556	167	652
Broccoli, raw (100 g)	3	28	**107**	141	91	29	54
Soy Sauce, typical (100 g)	11	60	**175**	729	403	182	576
Beef, grass-fed, lean (100 g)	23	117	**197**				

Complete Proteins in Non-human Animals

Scientists had known since the early 20th century that rats could not survive on a diet whose only protein source was zein, which comes from maize (corn), but recovered if they were fed casein from cow's milk. This led William Cumming Rose to the discovery of the essential amino acid threonine. Through manipulation of rodent diets, Rose was able to show that ten amino acids are essential for rats: lysine, tryptophan, histidine, phenylalanine, leucine, isoleucine, methionine, valine, and arginine, in addition to threonine. Rose's later work showed that eight amino acids are essential for adult human beings, with histidine also being essential for infants. Longer term studies established histidine as also essential for adult humans.

Interchangeability

The distinction between essential and non-essential amino acids is somewhat unclear, as some amino acids can be produced from others. The sulfur-containing amino acids, methionine and homocysteine, can be converted into each other but neither can be synthesized *de novo* in humans. Likewise, cysteine can be made from homocysteine but cannot be synthesized on its own. So, for convenience, sulfur-containing amino acids are sometimes considered a single pool of nutritionally equivalent amino acids as are the aromatic amino acid pair, phenylalanine and tyrosine. Likewise arginine, ornithine, and citrulline, which are interconvertible by the urea cycle, are considered a single group.

Effects of Deficiency

If one of the nonessential amino acids is less than needed for an individual the utilization of other amino acids will be hindered and thus protein synthesis will be less than what it usually is, even in the presence of adequate total nitrogen intake.

Protein deficiency has been shown to affect all of the body's organs and many of its systems, including the brain and brain function of infants and young children; the immune system, thus elevating risk of infection; gut mucosal function and permeability, which affects absorption and vulnerability to systemic disease; and kidney function. The physical signs of protein deficiency include edema, failure to thrive in infants and children, poor musculature, dull skin, and thin and fragile hair. Biochemical changes reflecting protein deficiency include low serum albumin and low serum transferrin.

The amino acids that are essential in the human diet were established in a series of experiments led by William Cumming Rose. The experiments involved elemental diets to healthy male graduate students. These diets consisted of cornstarch, sucrose, butterfat without protein, corn oil, inorganic salts, the known vitamins, a large brown "candy" made of liver extract flavored with peppermint oil (to supply any unknown vitamins), and mixtures of highly purified individual amino acids. The main outcome measure was nitrogen balance. Rose noted that the symptoms of nervousness, exhaustion, and dizziness were encountered to a greater or lesser extent whenever human subjects were deprived of an essential amino acid.

Essential amino acid deficiency should be distinguished from protein-energy malnutrition, which can manifest as marasmus or kwashiorkor. Kwashiorkor was once attributed to pure protein deficiency in individuals who were consuming enough calories ("sugar baby syndrome"). However, this theory has been challenged by the finding that there is no difference in the diets of children developing marasmus as opposed to kwashiorkor. Still, for instance in Dietary Reference Intakes (DRI) maintained by the USDA, lack of one or more of the essential amino acids is described as protein-energy malnutrition.

Obesity

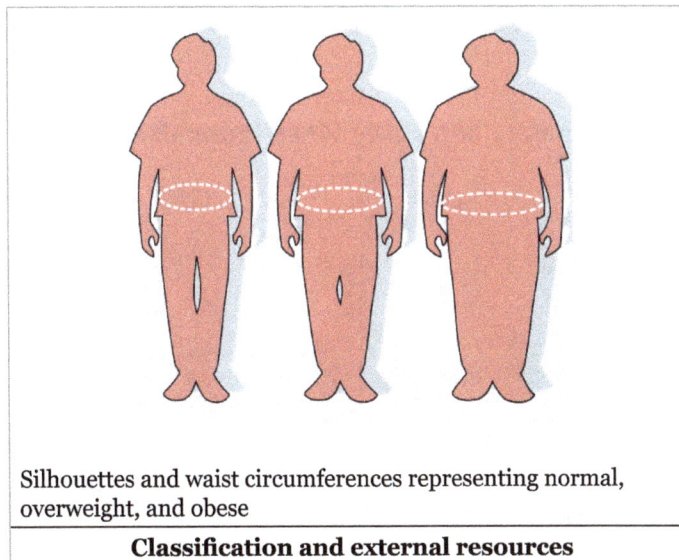

Silhouettes and waist circumferences representing normal, overweight, and obese

Classification and external resources

Obesity is a medical condition in which excess body fat has accumulated to the extent that it may have a negative effect on health. People are generally considered obese when their body mass index (BMI), a measurement obtained by dividing a person's weight by the square of the person's height, is over 30 kg/m^2, with the range 25–30 kg/m^2 defined as overweight. Some

East Asian countries use lower values. Obesity increases the likelihood of various diseases, particularly heart disease, type 2 diabetes, obstructive sleep apnea, certain types of cancer, and osteoarthritis.

Obesity is most commonly caused by a combination of excessive food intake, lack of physical activity, and genetic susceptibility. A few cases are caused primarily by genes, endocrine disorders, medications, or mental illness. Evidence to support the view that obese people eat little yet gain weight due to a slow metabolism is not generally supported. On average, obese people have a greater energy expenditure than their thin counterparts due to the energy required to maintain an increased body mass.

Obesity is mostly preventable through a combination of social changes and personal choices. Changes to diet and exercising are the main treatments. Diet quality can be improved by reducing the consumption of energy-dense foods, such as those high in fat and sugars, and by increasing the intake of dietary fiber. Medications may be taken, along with a suitable diet, to reduce appetite or decrease fat absorption. If diet, exercise, and medication are not effective, a gastric balloon or surgery may be performed to reduce stomach volume or bowel length, leading to feeling full earlier or a reduced ability to absorb nutrients from food.

Obesity is a leading preventable cause of death worldwide, with increasing rates in adults and children. In 2014, 600 million adults (13%) and 42 million children under the age of five were obese. Obesity is more common in women than men. Authorities view it as one of the most serious public health problems of the 21st century. Obesity is stigmatized in much of the modern world (particularly in the Western world), though it was seen as a symbol of wealth and fertility at other times in history and still is in some parts of the world. In 2013, the American Medical Association classified obesity as a disease.

Classification

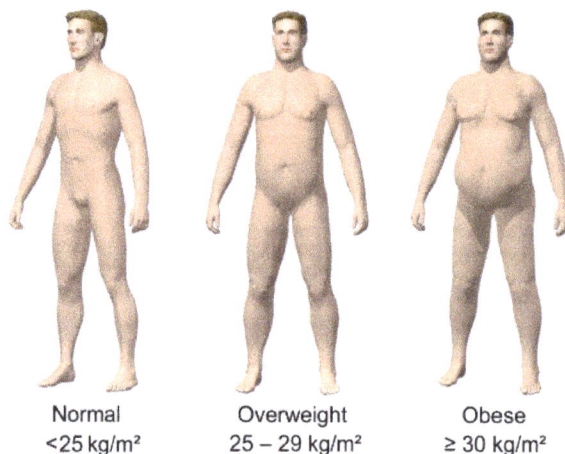

Obesity and Body Mass Index (BMI)

$$BMI = \frac{weight\ (kg)}{height\ (m^2)}$$

Normal	Overweight	Obese
<25 kg/m²	25 – 29 kg/m²	≥ 30 kg/m²

Obesity and BMI

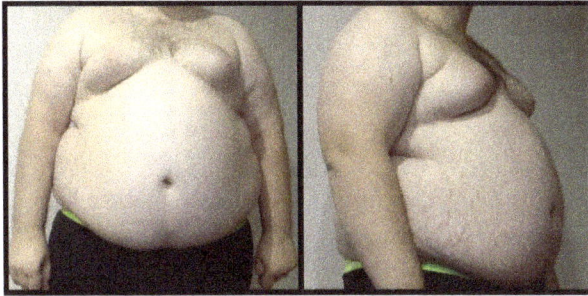

A "super obese" male with a BMI of 53 kg/m²: weight 182 kg (400 lb), height 185 cm (6 ft 1 in)

Obesity is a medical condition in which excess body fat has accumulated to the extent that it may have an adverse effect on health. It is defined by body mass index (BMI) and further evaluated in terms of fat distribution via the waist–hip ratio and total cardiovascular risk factors. BMI is closely related to both percentage body fat and total body fat. In children, a healthy weight varies with age and sex. Obesity in children and adolescents is defined not as an absolute number but in relation to a historical normal group, such that obesity is a BMI greater than the 95th percentile. The reference data on which these percentiles were based date from 1963 to 1994, and thus have not been affected by the recent increases in weight. BMI is defined as the subject's weight divided by the square of their height and is calculated as follows.

$$BMI = \frac{m}{h^2},$$

where m and h are the subject's weight and height respectively.

BMI is usually expressed in kilograms per square metre, resulting when weight is measured in kilograms and height in metres. To convert from pounds per square inch multiply by 703 (kg/m²)/ (lb/sq in).

BMI (kg/m²)		Classification
from	up to	
	18.5	underweight
18.5	25.0	normal weight
25.0	30.0	overweight
30.0	35.0	class I obesity
35.0	40.0	class II obesity
40.0		class III obesity

The most commonly used definitions, established by the World Health Organization (WHO) in 1997 and published in 2000, provide the values listed in the table.

Some modifications to the WHO definitions have been made by particular bodies. The surgical literature breaks down "class III" obesity into further categories whose exact values are still disputed.

- Any BMI ≥ 35 or 40 kg/m² is *severe obesity*.

- A BMI of ≥ 35 kg/m² and experiencing obesity-related health conditions or ≥40–44.9 kg/m² is *morbid obesity.*

- A BMI of ≥ 45 or 50 kg/m² is *super obesity.*

As Asian populations develop negative health consequences at a lower BMI than Caucasians, some nations have redefined obesity; the Japanese have defined obesity as any BMI greater than 25 kg/m² while China uses a BMI of greater than 28 kg/m².

Effects on Health

Excessive body weight is associated with various diseases, particularly cardiovascular diseases, diabetes mellitus type 2, obstructive sleep apnea, certain types of cancer, osteoarthritis and asthma. As a result, obesity has been found to reduce life expectancy.

Mortality

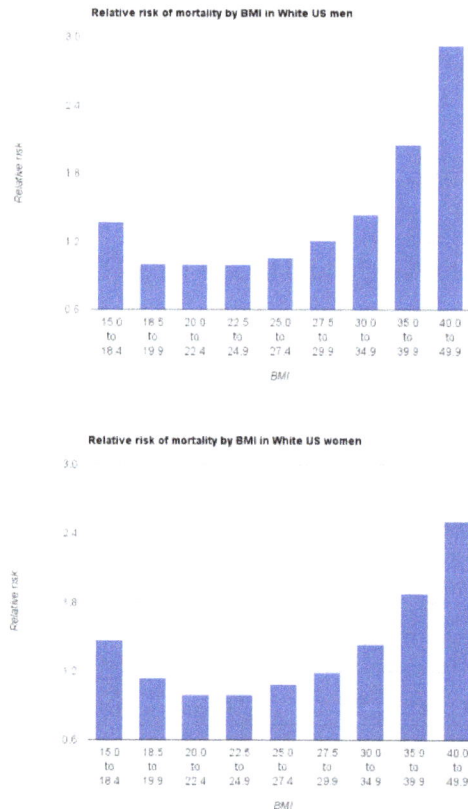

Relative risk of death over 10 years for white men (left) and women (right) who have never smoked in the United States by BMI.

Obesity is one of the leading preventable causes of death worldwide. A number of reviews have found that mortality risk is lowest at a BMI of 20–25 kg/m² in non-smokers and at 24–27 kg/m² in current smokers, with risk increasing along with changes in either direction. This appears to apply in at least four continents. In contrast, a 2013 review found that grade 1 obesity (BMI 30-35) was not associated with higher mortality than normal weight, and that overweight (BMI 25-30) was associated with "lower" mortality than was normal weight (BMI 18.5-25). Other evidence suggests that the association of BMI and waist circumference with mortality is U- or J-shaped, while the association between waist-to-hip ratio and waist-to-height ratio with mortality is more positive. In Asians the risk of negative health effects begins to increase between 22–25 kg/m^2. A BMI above 32 kg/m^2 has been associated with a doubled mortality rate among women over a 16-year period. In the United States obesity is estimated to cause 111,909 to 365,000 deaths per year, while 1 million (7.7%) of deaths in Europe are attributed to excess weight. On average, obesity reduces life expectancy by six to seven years, a BMI of 30–35 kg/m^2 reduces life expectancy by two to four years, while severe obesity (BMI > 40 kg/m^2) reduces life expectancy by ten years.

Morbidity

Obesity increases the risk of many physical and mental conditions. These comorbidities are most commonly shown in metabolic syndrome, a combination of medical disorders which includes: diabetes mellitus type 2, high blood pressure, high blood cholesterol, and high triglyceride levels.

Complications are either directly caused by obesity or indirectly related through mechanisms sharing a common cause such as a poor diet or a sedentary lifestyle. The strength of the link between obesity and specific conditions varies. One of the strongest is the link with type 2 diabetes. Excess body fat underlies 64% of cases of diabetes in men and 77% of cases in women.

Health consequences fall into two broad categories: those attributable to the effects of increased fat mass (such as osteoarthritis, obstructive sleep apnea, social stigmatization) and those due to the increased number of fat cells (diabetes, cancer, cardiovascular disease, non-alcoholic fatty liver disease). Increases in body fat alter the body's response to insulin, potentially leading to insulin resistance. Increased fat also creates a proinflammatory state, and a prothrombotic state.

Medical field	Condition	Medical field	Condition
Cardiology	• coronary heart disease: angina and myocardial infarction • congestive heart failure • high blood pressure • abnormal cholesterol levels • deep vein thrombosis and pulmonary embolism	Dermatology	• stretch marks • acanthosis nigricans • lymphedema • cellulitis • hirsutism • intertrigo
Endocrinology and Reproductive medicine	• diabetes mellitus • polycystic ovarian syndrome • menstrual disorders • infertility • complications during pregnancy • birth defects • intrauterine fetal death	Gastroenterology	• gastroesophageal reflux disease • fatty liver disease • cholelithiasis (gallstones)
Neurology	• stroke • meralgia paresthetica • migraines • carpal tunnel syndrome • dementia • idiopathic intracranial hypertension • multiple sclerosis	Oncology	• esophageal • colorectal • pancreatic • gallbladder, • endometrial • kidney • Leukemia • Hepatocellular carcinoma • malignant melanoma

Psychiatry	• depression in women • social stigmatization	Respirology	• obstructive sleep apnea • obesity hypoventilation syndrome • asthma • increased complications during general anaesthesia
Rheumatology and Orthopedics	• gout • poor mobility • osteoarthritis • low back pain	Urology and Nephrology	• erectile dysfunction • urinary incontinence • chronic renal failure • hypogonadism • buried penis

Survival Paradox

Although the negative health consequences of obesity in the general population are well supported by the available evidence, health outcomes in certain subgroups seem to be improved at an increased BMI, a phenomenon known as the obesity survival paradox. The paradox was first described in 1999 in overweight and obese people undergoing hemodialysis, and has subsequently been found in those with heart failure and peripheral artery disease (PAD).

In people with heart failure, those with a BMI between 30.0 and 34.9 had lower mortality than those with a normal weight. This has been attributed to the fact that people often lose weight as they become progressively more ill. Similar findings have been made in other types of heart disease. People with class I obesity and heart disease do not have greater rates of further heart problems than people of normal weight who also have heart disease. In people with greater degrees of obesity, however, the risk of further cardiovascular events is increased. Even after cardiac bypass surgery, no increase in mortality is seen in the overweight and obese. One study found that the improved survival could be explained by the more aggressive treatment obese people receive after a cardiac event. Another found that if one takes into account chronic obstructive pulmonary disease (COPD) in those with PAD, the benefit of obesity no longer exists.

Causes

At an individual level, a combination of excessive food energy intake and a lack of physical activity is thought to explain most cases of obesity. A limited number of cases are due primarily to genetics, medical reasons, or psychiatric illness. In contrast, increasing rates of obesity at a societal level are felt to be due to an easily accessible and palatable diet, increased reliance on cars, and mechanized manufacturing.

A 2006 review identified ten other possible contributors to the recent increase of obesity: (1) insufficient sleep, (2) endocrine disruptors (environmental pollutants that interfere with lipid metabolism), (3) decreased variability in ambient temperature, (4) decreased rates of smoking, because smoking suppresses appetite, (5) increased use of medications that can cause weight gain (e.g., atypical antipsychotics), (6) proportional increases in ethnic and age groups that tend to be heavier, (7) pregnancy at a later age (which may cause susceptibility to obesity in children), (8) epigenetic risk factors passed on generationally, (9) natural selection for higher BMI, and (10) assortative mating leading to increased concentration of obesity risk factors (this would increase the number of obese people by increasing population variance in weight). While there is substantial evidence supporting the influence of these mechanisms on the increased prevalence of obesity, the evidence is still inconclusive, and the authors state that these are probably less influential than the ones discussed in the previous paragraph.

Diet

1961

2001–03

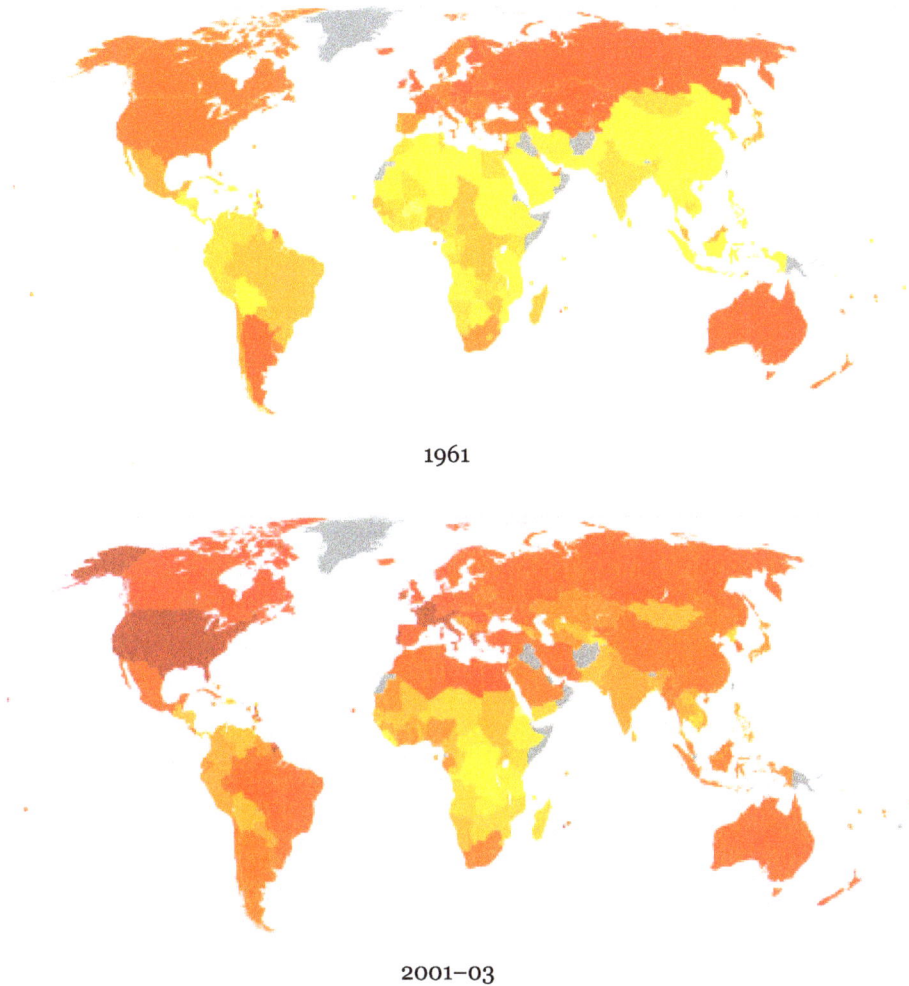

Map of dietary energy availability per person per day in 1961 (left) and 2001–2003 (right)
Calories per person per day (kilojoules per person per day)

no data	2,600–2,800 (10,900–11,700)
<1,600 (<6,700)	2,800–3,000 (11,700–12,600)
1,600–1,800 (6,700–7,500)	3,000–3,200 (12,600–13,400)
1,800–2,000 (7,500–8,400)	3,200–3,400 (13,400–14,200)
2,000–2,200 (8,400–9,200)	3,400–3,600 (14,200–15,100)
2,200–2,400 (9,200–10,000)	>3,600 (>15,100)
2,400–2,600 (10,000–10,900)	

World Food Enegery Consumption

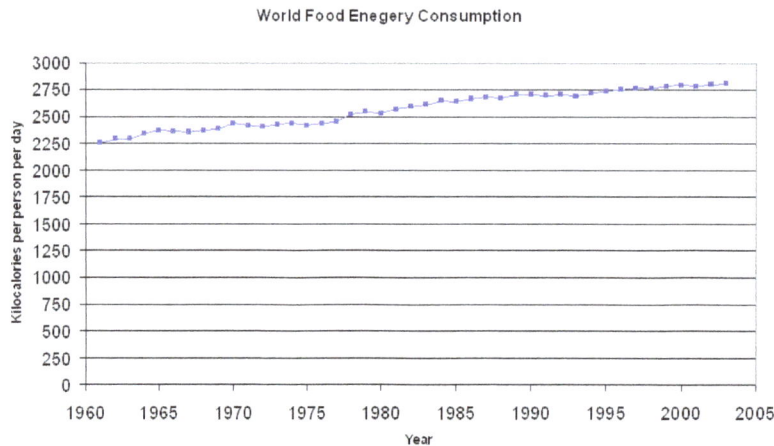

Average per capita energy consumption of the world from 1961 to 2002

Dietary energy supply per capita varies markedly between different regions and countries. It has also changed significantly over time. From the early 1970s to the late 1990s the average food energy available per person per day (the amount of food bought) increased in all parts of the world except Eastern Europe. The United States had the highest availability with 3,654 calories (15,290 kJ) per person in 1996. This increased further in 2003 to 3,754 calories (15,710 kJ). During the late 1990s Europeans had 3,394 calories (14,200 kJ) per person, in the developing areas of Asia there were 2,648 calories (11,080 kJ) per person, and in sub-Saharan Africa people had 2,176 calories (9,100 kJ) per person. Total food energy consumption has been found to be related to obesity.

The widespread availability of nutritional guidelines has done little to address the problems of overeating and poor dietary choice. From 1971 to 2000, obesity rates in the United States increased from 14.5% to 30.9%. During the same period, an increase occurred in the average amount of food energy consumed. For women, the average increase was 335 calories (1,400 kJ) per day (1,542 calories (6,450 kJ) in 1971 and 1,877 calories (7,850 kJ) in 2004), while for men the average increase was 168 calories (700 kJ) per day (2,450 calories (10,300 kJ) in 1971 and 2,618 calories (10,950 kJ) in 2004). Most of this extra food energy came from an increase in carbohydrate consumption rather than fat consumption. The primary sources of these extra carbohydrates are sweetened beverages, which now account for almost 25 percent of daily food energy in young adults in America, and potato chips. Consumption of sweetened drinks such as soft drinks, fruit drinks, iced tea, and energy and vitamin water drinks is believed to be contributing to the rising rates of obesity and to an increased risk of metabolic syndrome and type 2 diabetes.

As societies become increasingly reliant on energy-dense, big-portions, and fast-food meals, the association between fast-food consumption and obesity becomes more concerning. In the United States consumption of fast-food meals tripled and food energy intake from these meals quadrupled between 1977 and 1995.

Agricultural policy and techniques in the United States and Europe have led to lower food prices. In the United States, subsidization of corn, soy, wheat, and rice through the U.S. farm bill has made the main sources of processed food cheap compared to fruits and vegetables. Calorie count laws and nutrition facts labels attempt to steer people toward making healthier food choices, including awareness of how much food energy is being consumed.

Obese people consistently under-report their food consumption as compared to people of normal weight. This is supported both by tests of people carried out in a calorimeter room and by direct observation.

Sedentary Lifestyle

A sedentary lifestyle plays a significant role in obesity. Worldwide there has been a large shift towards less physically demanding work, and currently at least 30% of the world's population gets insufficient exercise. This is primarily due to increasing use of mechanized transportation and a greater prevalence of labor-saving technology in the home. In children, there appear to be declines in levels of physical activity due to less walking and physical education. World trends in active leisure time physical activity are less clear. The World Health Organization indicates people worldwide are taking up less active recreational pursuits, while a study from Finland found an increase and a study from the United States found leisure-time physical activity has not changed significantly.

In both children and adults, there is an association between television viewing time and the risk of obesity. A review found 63 of 73 studies (86%) showed an increased rate of childhood obesity with increased media exposure, with rates increasing proportionally to time spent watching television.

Genetics

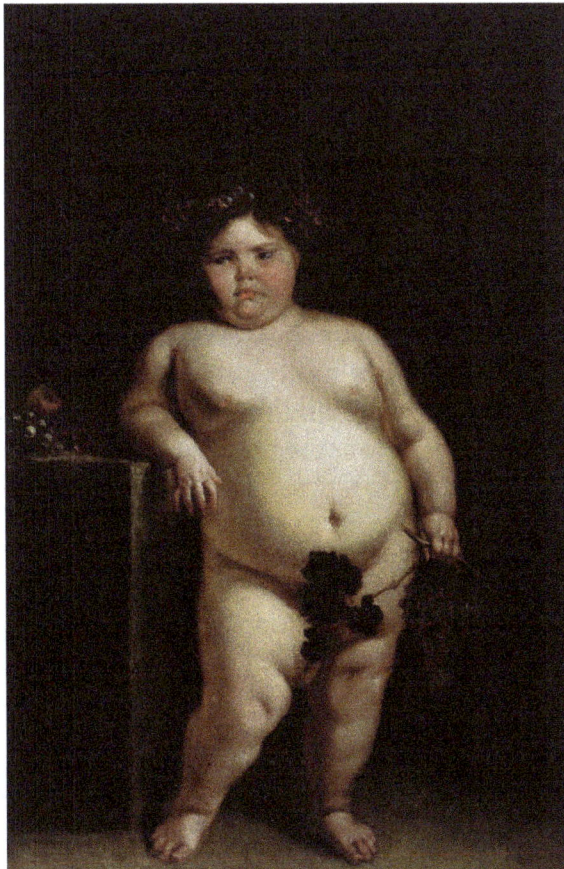

A 1680 painting by Juan Carreno de Miranda of a girl presumed to have Prader–Willi syndrome

Like many other medical conditions, obesity is the result of an interplay between genetic and environmental factors. Polymorphisms in various genes controlling appetite and metabolism predispose to obesity when sufficient food energy is present. As of 2006, more than 41 of these sites on the human genome have been linked to the development of obesity when a favorable environment is present. People with two copies of the FTO gene (fat mass and obesity associated gene) have been found on average to weigh 3–4 kg more and have a 1.67-fold greater risk of obesity compared with those without the risk allele. The differences in BMI between people that are due to genetics varies depending on the population examined from 6% to 85%.

Obesity is a major feature in several syndromes, such as Prader–Willi syndrome, Bardet–Biedl syndrome, Cohen syndrome, and MOMO syndrome. (The term "non-syndromic obesity" is sometimes used to exclude these conditions.) In people with early-onset severe obesity (defined by an onset before 10 years of age and body mass index over three standard deviations above normal), 7% harbor a single point DNA mutation.

Studies that have focused on inheritance patterns rather than on specific genes have found that 80% of the offspring of two obese parents were also obese, in contrast to less than 10% of the offspring of two parents who were of normal weight. Different people exposed to the same environment have different risks of obesity due to their underlying genetics.

The thrifty gene hypothesis postulates that, due to dietary scarcity during human evolution, people are prone to obesity. Their ability to take advantage of rare periods of abundance by storing energy as fat would be advantageous during times of varying food availability, and individuals with greater adipose reserves would be more likely to survive famine. This tendency to store fat, however, would be maladaptive in societies with stable food supplies. This theory has received various criticisms, and other evolutionarily-based theories such as the drifty gene hypothesis and the thrifty phenotype hypothesis have also been proposed.

Other Illnesses

Certain physical and mental illnesses and the pharmaceutical substances used to treat them can increase risk of obesity. Medical illnesses that increase obesity risk include several rare genetic syndromes (listed above) as well as some congenital or acquired conditions: hypothyroidism, Cushing's syndrome, growth hormone deficiency, and the eating disorders: binge eating disorder and night eating syndrome. However, obesity is not regarded as a psychiatric disorder, and therefore is not listed in the DSM-IVR as a psychiatric illness. The risk of overweight and obesity is higher in patients with psychiatric disorders than in persons without psychiatric disorders.

Certain medications may cause weight gain or changes in body composition; these include insulin, sulfonylureas, thiazolidinediones, atypical antipsychotics, antidepressants, steroids, certain anticonvulsants (phenytoin and valproate), pizotifen, and some forms of hormonal contraception.

Social Determinants

While genetic influences are important to understanding obesity, they cannot explain the current dramatic increase seen within specific countries or globally. Though it is accepted that energy consumption in excess of energy expenditure leads to obesity on an individual basis, the cause of the shifts in these two factors on the societal scale is much debated. There are a number of theories as to the cause but most believe it is a combination of various factors.

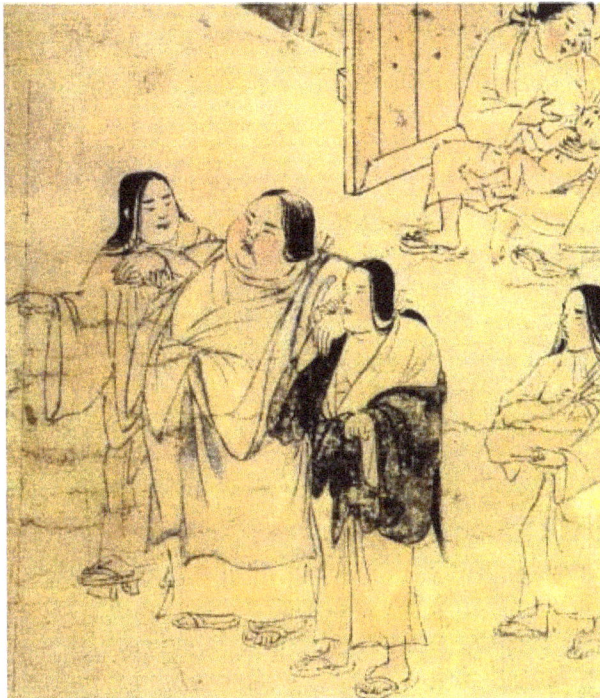

The disease scroll (Yamai no soshi, late 12th century) depicts a woman moneylender with obesity, considered a disease of the rich.

The correlation between social class and BMI varies globally. A review in 1989 found that in developed countries women of a high social class were less likely to be obese. No significant differences were seen among men of different social classes. In the developing world, women, men, and children from high social classes had greater rates of obesity. An update of this review carried out in 2007 found the same relationships, but they were weaker. The decrease in strength of correlation was felt to be due to the effects of globalization. Among developed countries, levels of adult obesity, and percentage of teenage children who are overweight, are correlated with income inequality. A similar relationship is seen among US states: more adults, even in higher social classes, are obese in more unequal states.

Many explanations have been put forth for associations between BMI and social class. It is thought that in developed countries, the wealthy are able to afford more nutritious food, they are under greater social pressure to remain slim, and have more opportunities along with greater expectations for physical fitness. In undeveloped countries the ability to afford food, high energy expenditure with physical labor, and cultural values favoring a larger body size are believed to contribute to the observed patterns. Attitudes toward body weight held by people in one's life may also play a role in obesity. A correlation in BMI changes over time has been found among friends, siblings, and spouses. Stress and perceived low social status appear to increase risk of obesity.

Smoking has a significant effect on an individual's weight. Those who quit smoking gain an average of 4.4 kilograms (9.7 lb) for men and 5.0 kilograms (11.0 lb) for women over ten years. However, changing rates of smoking have had little effect on the overall rates of obesity.

In the United States the number of children a person has is related to their risk of obesity. A woman's risk increases by 7% per child, while a man's risk increases by 4% per child. This could be partly explained by the fact that having dependent children decreases physical activity in Western parents.

In the developing world urbanization is playing a role in increasing rate of obesity. In China overall rates of obesity are below 5%; however, in some cities rates of obesity are greater than 20%.

Malnutrition in early life is believed to play a role in the rising rates of obesity in the developing world. Endocrine changes that occur during periods of malnutrition may promote the storage of fat once more food energy becomes available.

Consistent with cognitive epidemiological data, numerous studies confirm that obesity is associated with cognitive deficits. Whether obesity causes cognitive deficits, or vice versa is unclear at present.

Gut Bacteria

The study of the effect of infectious agents on metabolism is still in its early stages. Gut flora has been shown to differ between lean and obese humans. There is an indication that gut flora in obese and lean individuals can affect the metabolic potential. This apparent alteration of the metabolic potential is believed to confer a greater capacity to harvest energy contributing to obesity. Whether these differences are the direct cause or the result of obesity has yet to be determined unequivocally.

An association between viruses and obesity has been found in humans and several different animal species. The amount that these associations may have contributed to the rising rate of obesity is yet to be determined.

Pathophysiology

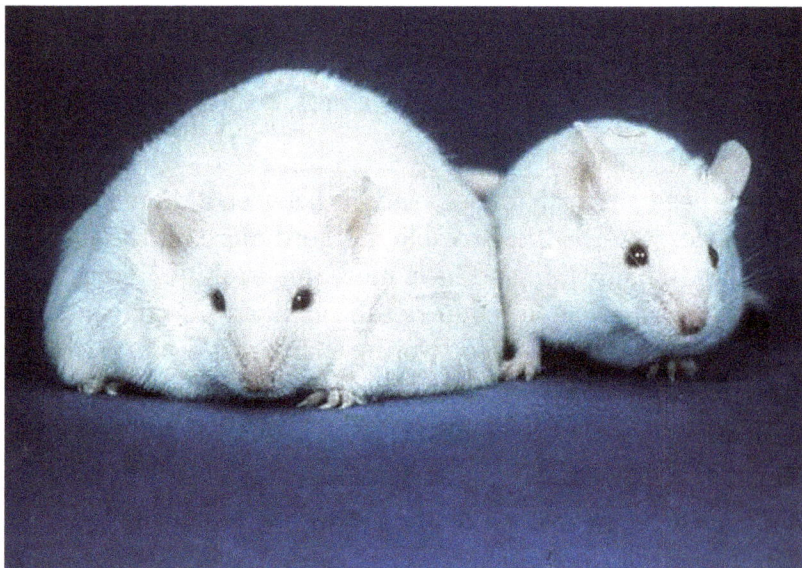

A comparison of a mouse unable to produce leptin thus resulting in obesity (left) and a normal mouse (right)

There are many possible pathophysiological mechanisms involved in the development and maintenance of obesity. This field of research had been almost unapproached until the leptin gene was discovered in 1994 by J. M. Friedman's laboratory. These investigators postulated that leptin was a satiety factor. In the ob/ob mouse, mutations in the leptin gene resulted in the obese phenotype opening the possibility of leptin therapy for human obesity. However, soon thereafter J. F. Caro's laboratory could not detect any mutations in the leptin gene in humans with obesity. On the contrary Leptin expression was increased proposing the possibility of Leptin-resistance in human obesity. Since this discovery, many other hormonal mechanisms have been elucidated that participate in the regulation of appetite and food intake, storage patterns of adipose tissue, and development of insulin resistance. Since leptin's discovery, ghrelin, insulin, orexin, PYY 3-36, cholecystokinin, adiponectin, as well as many other mediators have been studied. The adipokines are mediators produced by adipose tissue; their action is thought to modify many obesity-related diseases.

Leptin and ghrelin are considered to be complementary in their influence on appetite, with ghrelin produced by the stomach modulating short-term appetitive control (i.e. to eat when the stomach is empty and to stop when the stomach is stretched). Leptin is produced by adipose tissue to signal fat storage reserves in the body, and mediates long-term appetitive controls (i.e. to eat more when fat storages are low and less when fat storages are high). Although administration of leptin may be effective in a small subset of obese individuals who are leptin deficient, most obese individuals are thought to be leptin resistant and have been found to have high levels of leptin. This resistance is thought to explain in part why administration of leptin has not been shown to be effective in suppressing appetite in most obese people.

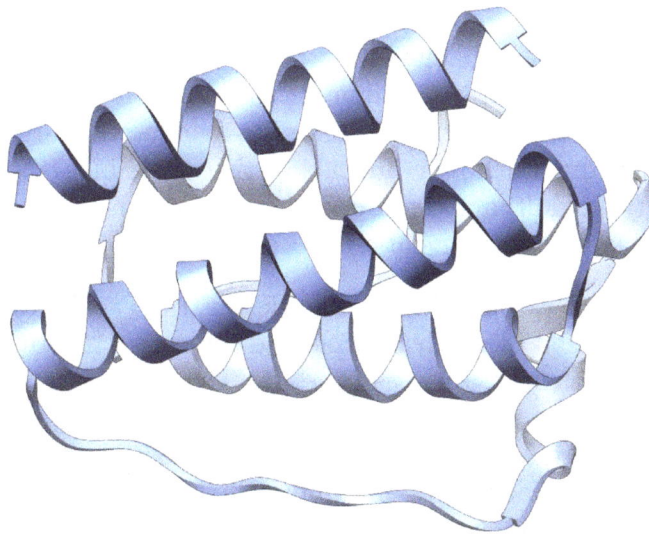

A graphic depiction of a leptin molecule

While leptin and ghrelin are produced peripherally, they control appetite through their actions on the central nervous system. In particular, they and other appetite-related hormones act on the hypothalamus, a region of the brain central to the regulation of food intake and energy expenditure. There are several circuits within the hypothalamus that contribute to its role in integrating appetite, the melanocortin pathway being the most well understood. The circuit begins with an area of the hypothalamus, the arcuate nucleus, that has outputs to the lateral hypothalamus (LH) and ventromedial hypothalamus (VMH), the brain's feeding and satiety centers, respectively.

The arcuate nucleus contains two distinct groups of neurons. The first group coexpresses neuropeptide Y (NPY) and agouti-related peptide (AgRP) and has stimulatory inputs to the LH and inhibitory inputs to the VMH. The second group coexpresses pro-opiomelanocortin (POMC) and cocaine- and amphetamine-regulated transcript (CART) and has stimulatory inputs to the VMH and inhibitory inputs to the LH. Consequently, NPY/AgRP neurons stimulate feeding and inhibit satiety, while POMC/CART neurons stimulate satiety and inhibit feeding. Both groups of arcuate nucleus neurons are regulated in part by leptin. Leptin inhibits the NPY/AgRP group while stimulating the POMC/CART group. Thus a deficiency in leptin signaling, either via leptin deficiency or leptin resistance, leads to overfeeding and may account for some genetic and acquired forms of obesity.

Public Health

The World Health Organization (WHO) predicts that overweight and obesity may soon replace more traditional public health concerns such as undernutrition and infectious diseases as the most significant cause of poor health. Obesity is a public health and policy problem because of its prevalence, costs, and health effects. The United States Preventive Services Task Force recommends screening for all adults followed by behavioral interventions in those who are obese. Public health efforts seek to understand and correct the environmental factors responsible for the increasing prevalence of obesity in the population. Solutions look at changing the factors that cause excess food energy consumption and inhibit physical activity. Efforts include federally reimbursed meal programs in schools, limiting direct junk food marketing to children, and decreasing access to sugar-sweetened beverages in schools. When constructing urban environments, efforts have been made to increase access to parks and to develop pedestrian routes.

Many countries and groups have published reports pertaining to obesity. In 1998, the first US Federal guidelines were published, titled "Clinical Guidelines on the Identification, Evaluation, and Treatment of Overweight and Obesity in Adults: The Evidence Report". In 2006 the Canadian Obesity Network published the "Canadian Clinical Practice Guidelines (CPG) on the Management and Prevention of Obesity in Adults and Children". This is a comprehensive evidence-based guideline to address the management and prevention of overweight and obesity in adults and children.

In 2004, the United Kingdom Royal College of Physicians, the Faculty of Public Health and the Royal College of Paediatrics and Child Health released the report "Storing up Problems", which highlighted the growing problem of obesity in the UK. The same year, the House of Commons Health Select Committee published its "most comprehensive inquiry [...] ever undertaken" into the impact of obesity on health and society in the UK and possible approaches to the problem. In 2006, the National Institute for Health and Clinical Excellence (NICE) issued a guideline on the diagnosis and management of obesity, as well as policy implications for non-healthcare organizations such as local councils. A 2007 report produced by Sir Derek Wanless for the King's Fund warned that unless further action was taken, obesity had the capacity to cripple the National Health Service financially.

Comprehensive approaches are being looked at to address the rising rates of obesity. The Obesity Policy Action (OPA) framework divides measure into 'upstream' policies, 'midstream' policies, 'downstream' policies. 'Upstream' policies look at changing society, 'midstream' policies try to alter individuals' behavior to prevent obesity, and 'downstream' policies try to treat currently afflicted people.

Management

The main treatment for obesity consists of dieting and physical exercise. Diet programs may produce weight loss over the short term, but maintaining this weight loss is frequently difficult and often requires making exercise and a lower food energy diet a permanent part of a person's lifestyle.

In the short-term low carbohydrate diets appear better than low fat diets for weight loss. In the long term; however, all types of low-carbohydrate and low-fat diets appear equally beneficial. A 2014 review found that the heart disease and diabetes risks associated with different diets appear to be similar. Promotion of the Mediterranean diets among the obese may lower the risk of heart disease. Decreased intake of sweet drinks is also related to weight-loss. Success rates of long-term weight loss maintenance with lifestyle changes are low, ranging from 2–20%. Dietary and lifestyle changes are effective in limiting excessive weight gain in pregnancy and improve outcomes for both the mother and the child. Intensive behavioral counseling is recommended in those who are both obese and have other risk factors for heart disease.

Three medications, orlistat, lorcaserin and a combination of phentermine and topiramate are currently available and have evidence for long term use. Weight loss with orlistat is modest, an average of 2.9 kg (6.4 lb) at 1 to 4 years. Its use is associated with high rates of gastrointestinal side effects and concerns have been raised about negative effects on the kidneys. The other two medications are available in the United States but not Europe. Lorcaserin results in an average 3.1 kg weight loss (3% of body weight) greater than placebo over a year; however, it may increase heart valve problems. A combination of phentermine and topiramate is also somewhat effective; however, it may be associated with heart problems. There is no information on how these drugs affect longer-term complications of obesity such as cardiovascular disease or death.

The most effective treatment for obesity is bariatric surgery. Surgery for severe obesity is associated with long-term weight loss, improvement in obesity related conditions, and decreased overall mortality. One study found a weight loss of between 14% and 25% (depending on the type of procedure performed) at 10 years, and a 29% reduction in all cause mortality when compared to standard weight loss measures. Complications occur in about 17% of cases and reoperation is needed in 7% of cases. Due to its cost and risks, researchers are searching for other effective yet less invasive treatments including devices that occupy space in the stomach.

Epidemiology

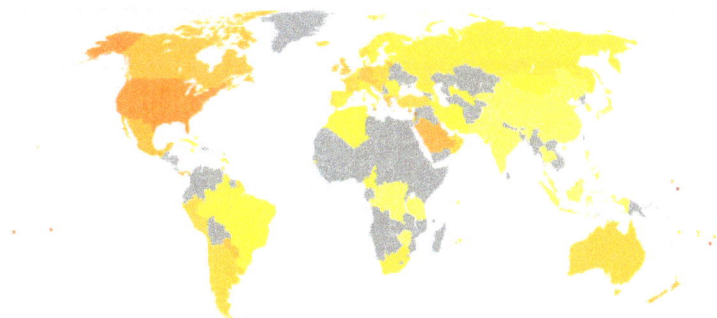

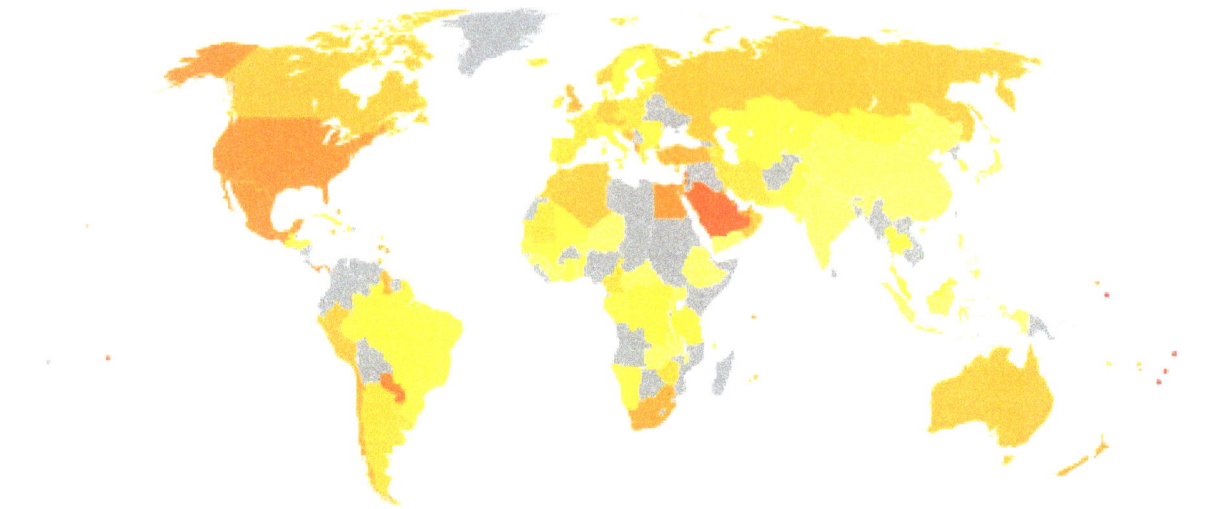

World obesity prevalence among males (left) and females (right).

<5%	15–20%	30–35%	45–50%
5–10%	20–25%	35–40%	50–55%
10–15%	25–30%	40–45%	>55%

In earlier historical periods obesity was rare, and achievable only by a small elite, although already recognised as a problem for health. But as prosperity increased in the Early Modern period, it affected increasingly larger groups of the population. In 1997 the WHO formally recognized obesity as a global epidemic. As of 2008 the WHO estimates that at least 500 million adults (greater than 10%) are obese, with higher rates among women than men. The rate of obesity also increases with age at least up to 50 or 60 years old and severe obesity in the United States, Australia, and Canada is increasing faster than the overall rate of obesity.

Once considered a problem only of high-income countries, obesity rates are rising worldwide and affecting both the developed and developing world. These increases have been felt most dramatically in urban settings. The only remaining region of the world where obesity is not common is sub-Saharan Africa.

Historical Attitudes

Ancient Greek medicine recognizes obesity as a medical disorder, and records that the Ancient Egyptians saw it in the same way. Hippocrates wrote that "Corpulence is not only a disease itself, but the harbinger of others". The Indian surgeon Sushruta (6th century BCE) related obesity to diabetes and heart disorders. He recommended physical work to help cure it and its side effects. For most of human history mankind struggled with food scarcity. Obesity has thus historically been viewed as a sign of wealth and prosperity. It was common among high officials in Europe in the Middle Ages and the Renaissance as well as in Ancient East Asian civilizations. In the 17th century, English medical author Tobias Venner is credited with being one of the first to refer to the term as a societal disease in a published English language book.

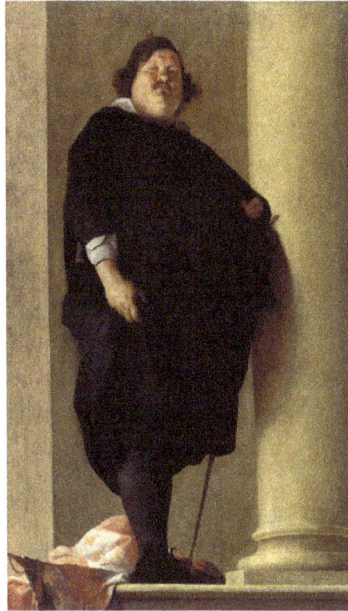

During the Middle Ages and the Renaissance obesity was often seen as a sign of wealth, and was relatively common among the elite: *The Tuscan General Alessandro del Borro*, attributed to Charles Mellin, 1645

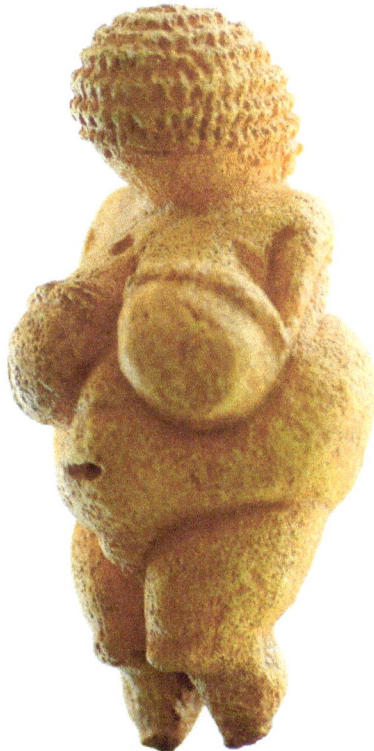

Venus of Willendorf created 24,000–22,000 BC

With the onset of the industrial revolution it was realized that the military and economic might of nations were dependent on both the body size and strength of their soldiers and workers. Increasing the average body mass index from what is now considered underweight to what is now the normal range played a significant role in the development of industrialized societies. Height and weight thus both increased through the 19th century in the developed world. During the 20th century, as populations reached their genetic potential for height, weight began increasing much more than height, resulting in obesity. In the 1950s increasing wealth in the developed world decreased child mortality, but as body weight increased heart and kidney disease became more common. During this time period insurance companies realized the connection between weight and life expectancy and increased premiums for the obese.

Many cultures throughout history have viewed obesity as the result of a character flaw. The *obesus* or fat character in Greek comedy was a glutton and figure of mockery. During Christian times food was viewed as a gateway to the sins of sloth and lust. In modern Western culture, excess weight is often regarded as unattractive, and obesity is commonly associated with various negative stereotypes. People of all ages can face social stigmatization, and may be targeted by bullies or shunned by their peers.

Public perceptions in Western society regarding healthy body weight differ from those regarding the weight that is considered ideal – and both have changed since the beginning of the 20th century. The weight that is viewed as an ideal has become lower since the 1920s. This is illustrated by the fact that the average height of Miss America pageant winners increased by 2% from 1922 to 1999, while their average weight decreased by 12%. On the other hand, people's views concerning healthy weight have changed in the opposite direction. In Britain the weight at which people considered themselves to be overweight was significantly higher in 2007 than in 1999. These changes are believed to be due to increasing rates of adiposity leading to increased acceptance of extra body fat as being normal.

Obesity is still seen as a sign of wealth and well-being in many parts of Africa. This has become particularly common since the HIV epidemic began.

The Arts

The first sculptural representations of the human body 20,000–35,000 years ago depict obese females. Some attribute the Venus figurines to the tendency to emphasize fertility while others feel they represent "fatness" in the people of the time. Corpulence is, however, absent in both Greek and Roman art, probably in keeping with their ideals regarding moderation. This continued through much of Christian European history, with only those of low socioeconomic status being depicted as obese.

During the Renaissance some of the upper class began flaunting their large size, as can be seen in portraits of Henry VIII of England and Alessandro del Borro. Rubens (1577–1640) regularly depicted full-bodied women in his pictures, from which derives the term Rubenesque. These women, however, still maintained the "hourglass" shape with its relationship to fertility. During the 19th century, views on obesity changed in the Western world. After centuries of obesity being synonymous with wealth and social status, slimness began to be seen as the desirable standard.

Society and Culture

Economic Impact

In addition to its health impacts, obesity leads to many problems including disadvantages in employment and increased business costs. These effects are felt by all levels of society from individuals, to corporations, to governments.

In 2005, the medical costs attributable to obesity in the US were an estimated $190.2 billion or 20.6% of all medical expenditures, while the cost of obesity in Canada was estimated at CA$2 billion in 1997 (2.4% of total health costs). The total annual direct cost of overweight and obesity in Australia in 2005 was A$21 billion. Overweight and obese Australians also received A$35.6 billion in government subsidies. The estimate range for annual expenditures on diet products is $40 billion to $100 billion in the US alone.

Obesity prevention programs have been found to reduce the cost of treating obesity-related disease. However, the longer people live, the more medical costs they incur. Researchers therefore conclude that reducing obesity may improve the public's health, but it is unlikely to reduce overall health spending.

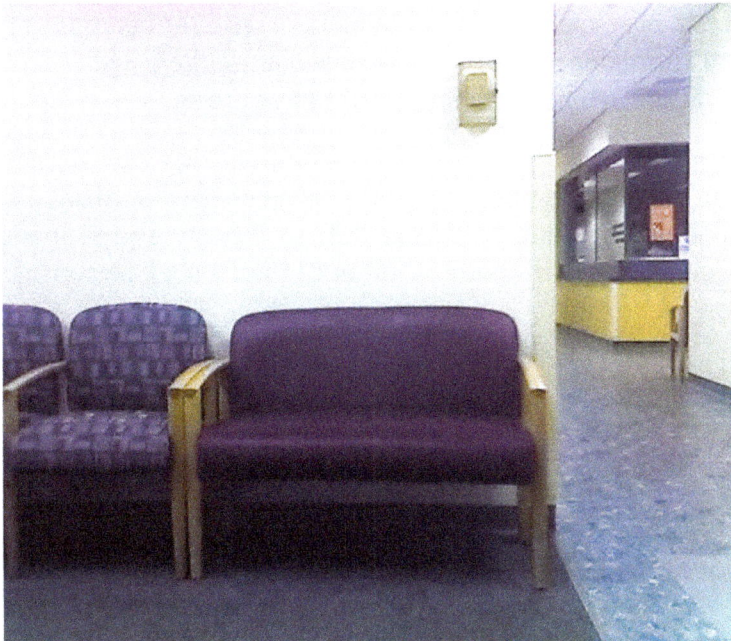

Services must accommodate obese people with specialist equipment such as much wider chairs.

Obesity can lead to social stigmatization and disadvantages in employment. When compared to their normal weight counterparts, obese workers on average have higher rates of absenteeism from work and take more disability leave, thus increasing costs for employers and decreasing productivity. A study examining Duke University employees found that people with a BMI over 40 kg/m² filed twice as many workers' compensation claims as those whose BMI was 18.5–24.9 kg/m². They also had more than 12 times as many lost work days. The most common injuries in this group were due to falls and lifting, thus affecting the lower extremities, wrists or hands, and backs. The Alabama State Employees' Insurance Board approved a controversial plan to charge obese workers $25 a month for health insurance that would otherwise be free unless they take steps to lose weight and improve their health. These measures started in January 2010 and apply to those state workers whose BMI exceeds 35 kg/m² and who fail to make improvements in their health after one year.

Some research shows that obese people are less likely to be hired for a job and are less likely to be promoted. Obese people are also paid less than their non-obese counterparts for an equivalent job; obese women on average make 6% less and obese men make 3% less.

Specific industries, such as the airline, healthcare and food industries, have special concerns. Due to rising rates of obesity, airlines face higher fuel costs and pressures to increase seating width. In 2000, the extra weight of obese passengers cost airlines US$275 million. The healthcare industry has had to invest in special facilities for handling severely obese patients, including special lifting equipment and bariatric ambulances. Costs for restaurants are increased by litigation accusing them of causing obesity. In 2005 the US Congress discussed legislation to prevent civil lawsuits against the food industry in relation to obesity; however, it did not become law.

With the American Medical Association's 2013 classification of obesity as a chronic disease, it is thought that health insurance companies will more likely pay for obesity treatment, counseling and surgery, and the cost of research and development of fat treatment pills or gene therapy treatments should be more affordable if insurers help to subsidize their cost. The AMA classification is not legally binding, however, so health insurers still have the right to reject coverage for a treatment or procedure.

In 2014, The European Court of Justice ruled that morbid obesity is a disability. The Court argued that if an employee's obesity prevents him from "full and effective participation of that person in professional life on an equal basis with other workers", then it shall be considered a disability and that firing someone on such grounds is discriminatory.

Size Acceptance

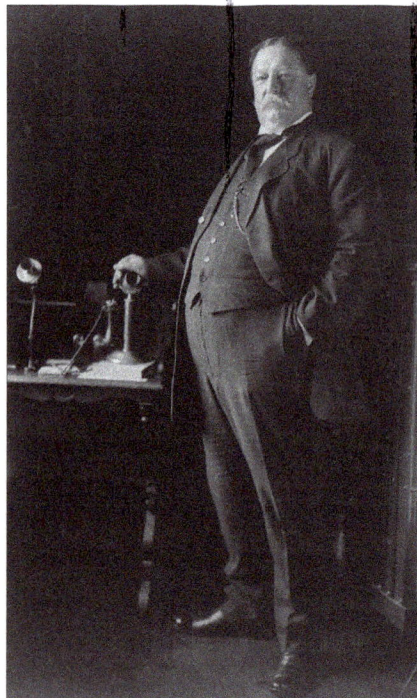

United States President William Howard Taft was often ridiculed for being overweight

The principal goal of the fat acceptance movement is to decrease discrimination against people who are overweight and obese. However, some in the movement are also attempting to challenge the established relationship between obesity and negative health outcomes.

A number of organizations exist that promote the acceptance of obesity. They have increased in prominence in the latter half of the 20th century. The US-based National Association to Advance Fat Acceptance (NAAFA) was formed in 1969 and describes itself as a civil rights organization dedicated to ending size discrimination.

The International Size Acceptance Association (ISAA) is a non-governmental organization (NGO) which was founded in 1997. It has more of a global orientation and describes its mission as promoting size acceptance and helping to end weight-based discrimination. These groups often argue for the recognition of obesity as a disability under the US Americans With Disabilities Act (ADA). The American legal system, however, has decided that the potential public health costs exceed the benefits of extending this anti-discrimination law to cover obesity.

Childhood Obesity

The healthy BMI range varies with the age and sex of the child. Obesity in children and adolescents is defined as a BMI greater than the 95th percentile. The reference data that these percentiles are based on is from 1963 to 1994 and thus has not been affected by the recent increases in rates of obesity. Childhood obesity has reached epidemic proportions in the 21st century, with rising rates in both the developed and developing world. Rates of obesity in Canadian boys have increased from 11% in the 1980s to over 30% in the 1990s, while during this same time period rates increased from 4 to 14% in Brazilian children.

As with obesity in adults, many factors contribute to the rising rates of childhood obesity. Changing diet and decreasing physical activity are believed to be the two most important causes for the recent increase in the incidence of child obesity. Because childhood obesity often persists into adulthood and is associated with numerous chronic illnesses, children who are obese are often tested for hypertension, diabetes, hyperlipidemia, and fatty liver. Treatments used in children are primarily lifestyle interventions and behavioral techniques, although efforts to increase activity in children have had little success. In the United States, medications are not FDA approved for use in this age group.

Other Animals

Obesity in pets is common in many countries. In the United States, 23–41% of dogs are overweight, and about 5.1% are obese. The rate of obesity in cats was slightly higher at 6.4%. In Australia the rate of obesity among dogs in a veterinary setting has been found to be 7.6%. The risk of obesity in dogs is related to whether or not their owners are obese; however, there is no similar correlation between cats and their owners.

Malnutrition

Malnutrition or malnourishment is a condition that results from eating a diet in which nutrients are either not enough or are too much such that the diet causes health problems. It may involve calories, protein, carbohydrates, vitamins or minerals. Not enough nutrients is called undernutrition or undernourishment while too much is called overnutrition. Malnutrition is often used specifically to refer to undernutrition where there is not enough calories, protein, or micronutrients. If undernutrition occurs during pregnancy, or before two years of age, it may result in permanent problems with physical and mental development. Extreme undernourishment, known as starvation, may have symptoms that include: a short height, thin body, very poor energy levels, and swollen legs and abdomen. People also often get infections and are frequently cold. The symptoms of micronutrient deficiencies depend on the micronutrient that is lacking.

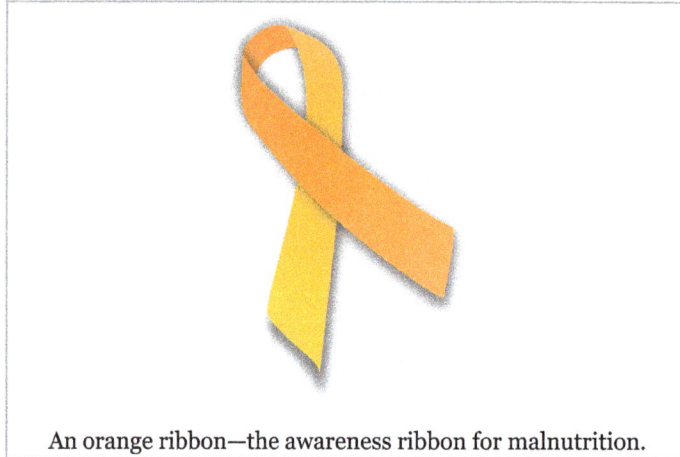

An orange ribbon—the awareness ribbon for malnutrition.

Undernourishment is most often due to not enough high-quality food being available to eat. This is often related to high food prices and poverty. A lack of breastfeeding may contribute, as may a number of infectious diseases such as: gastroenteritis, pneumonia, malaria, and measles, which increase nutrient requirements. There are two main types of undernutrition: protein-energy malnutrition and dietary deficiencies. Protein-energy malnutrition has two severe forms: marasmus (a lack of protein and calories) and kwashiorkor (a lack of just protein). Common micronutrient deficiencies include: a lack of iron, iodine, and vitamin A. During pregnancy, due to the body's increased need, deficiencies may become more common. In some developing countries, overnutrition in the form of obesity is beginning to present within the same communities as undernutrition. Other causes of malnutrition include anorexia nervosa and bariatric surgery.

Efforts to improve nutrition are some of the most effective forms of development aid. Breastfeeding can reduce rates of malnutrition and death in children, and efforts to promote the practice increase the rates of breastfeeding. In young children, providing food (in addition to breastmilk) between six months and two years of age improves outcomes. There is also good evidence supporting the supplementation of a number of micronutrients to women during pregnancy and among young children in the developing world. To get food to people who need it most, both delivering food and providing money so people can buy food within local markets are effective. Simply feeding students at school is insufficient. Management of severe malnutrition within the person's home with ready-to-use therapeutic foods is possible much of the time. In those who have severe malnutrition complicated by other health problems, treatment in a hospital setting is recommended. This often involves managing low blood sugar and body temperature, addressing dehydration, and gradual feeding. Routine antibiotics are usually recommended due to the high risk of infection. Longer-term measures include: improving agricultural practices, reducing poverty, improving sanitation, and the empowerment of women.

There were 793 million undernourished people in the world in 2015 (13% of the total population). This is a reduction of 216 million people since 1990 when 23% were undernourished. In 2012 it was estimated that another billion people had a lack of vitamins and minerals. In 2013, protein-energy malnutrition was estimated to have resulted in 469,000 deaths—down from 510,000 deaths in 1990. Other nutritional deficiencies, which include iodine deficiency and iron deficiency anemia, result in another 84,000 deaths. In 2010, malnutrition was the cause of 1.4% of all disability adjusted life years. About a third of deaths in children are believed to be due to undernutrition, although the deaths are rarely labelled as such. In 2010, it was estimated to have contributed to about 1.5 million deaths in women and children, though some estimate the number may be greater than 3 million. An additional 165 million children were estimated to have stunted growth from malnutrition in 2013. Undernutrition is more common in developing countries. Certain groups have higher rates of undernutrition, including women—in particular while pregnant or breastfeeding—children under five years of age, and the elderly. In the elderly, undernutrition becomes more common due to physical, psychological, and social factors.

Definitions

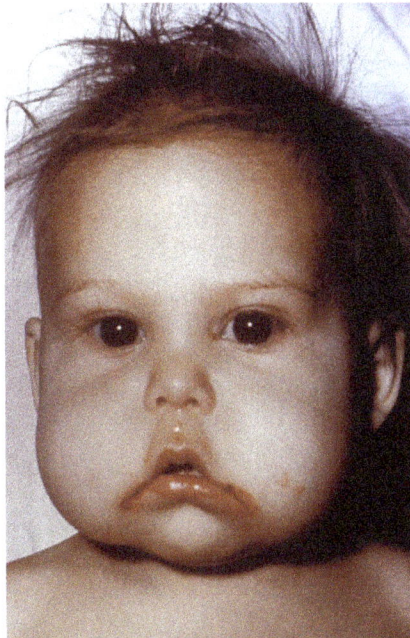

Child in the United States with signs of Kwashiorkor, a dietary protein deficiency.

Unless specifically mentioned otherwise, the term malnutrition refers to undernutrition for the remainder of this article. Malnutrition can divided in two different types, SAM and MAM. SAM is refers to children with severe acute malnutrition. MAM refers to moderate acute malnutrition.

Undernutrition and Overnutrition

Malnutrition is caused by eating a diet in which nutrients are *not enough* or are *too much* such that it causes health problems. It is a category of diseases that includes undernutrition and overnutrition. Overnutrition can result in obesity and being overweight. In some developing countries, overnutrition in the form of obesity is beginning to present within the same communities as undernutrition.

However, the term malnutrition is commonly used to refer to undernutrition only. This applies particularly to the context of development cooperation. Therefore, "malnutrition" in documents by the World Health Organization, UNICEF, Save the Children or other international non-governmental organizations (NGOs) usually is equated to undernutrition.

Protein-energy Malnutrition

Undernutrition is sometimes used as a synonym of protein–energy malnutrition (PEM). While other include both micronutrient deficiencies and protein energy malnutrition in its definition. It differs from calorie restriction in that calorie restriction may not result in negative health effects. The term hypoalimentation means underfeeding.

The term "severe malnutrition" or "severe undernutrition" is often used to refer specifically to PEM. PEM is often associated with micronutrient deficiency. Two forms of PEM are kwashiorkor and marasmus, and they commonly coexist.

Kwashiorkor

Kwashiorkor ('displaced child') is mainly caused by inadequate protein intake resulting in a low concentration of amino acids. The main symptoms are edema, wasting, liver enlargement, hypoalbuminaemia, steatosis, and possibly depigmentation of skin and hair. Kwashiorkor is identified by swelling of the extremities and belly, which is deceiving of actual nutritional status.

Marasmus

Marasmus ('to waste away') is caused by an inadequate intake of protein and energy. The main symptoms are severe wasting, leaving little or no edema, minimal subcutaneous fat, severe muscle wasting, and non-normal serum albumin levels. Marasmus can result from a sustained diet of inadequate energy and protein, and the metabolism adapts to prolong survival. It is traditionally seen in famine, significant food restriction, or more severe cases of anorexia. Conditions are characterized by extreme wasting of the muscles and a gaunt expression.

Undernutrition, Hunger

Undernutrition encompasses stunted growth (stunting), wasting, and deficiencies of essential vitamins and minerals (collectively referred to as micronutrients). The term hunger, which describes a feeling of discomfort from not eating, has been used to describe undernutrition, especially in reference to food insecurity.

Definition by Gomez

In 1956, Gómez and Galvan studied factors associated with death in a group of malnourished (undernourished) children in a hospital in Mexico City, Mexico and defined categories of malnutrition: first, second, and third degree. The degrees were based on weight below a specified percentage of median weight for age. The risk of death increases with increasing degree of malnutrition. An adaptation of Gomez's original classification is still used today. While it provides a way to compare malnutrition within and between populations, the classification has been criticized for being "arbitrary" and for not considering overweight as a form of malnutrition. Also, height alone may not be the best indicator of malnutrition; children who are born prematurely may be considered short for their age even if they have good nutrition.

Degree of PEM	% of desired body weight for age and sex
Normal	90%-100%
Mild: Grade I (1st degree)	75%-89%
Moderate: Grade II (2nd degree)	60%-74%
Severe: Grade III (3rd degree)	<60%
SOURCE:"Serum Total Protein and Albumin Levels in Different Grades of Protein Energy Malnutrition"	

Definition by Waterlow

John Conrad Waterlow established a new classification for malnutrition. Instead of using just weight for age measurements, the classification established by Waterlow combines weight-for-height (indicating acute episodes of malnutrition) with height-for-age to show the stunting that results from chronic malnutrition. One advantage of the Waterlow classification over the Gomez classification is that weight for height can be examined even if ages are not known.

Degree of PEM	Stunting (%) Height for age	Wasting (%) Weight for height
Normal: Grade 0	>95%	>90%
Mild: Grade I	87.5-95%	80-90%
Moderate: Grade II	80-87.5%	70-80%
Severe: Grade III	<80%	<70%
SOURCE: "Classification and definition of protein-calorie malnutrition." by Waterlow, 1972		

These classifications of malnutrition are commonly used with some modifications by WHO.

Effects

Malnutrition increases the risk of infection and infectious disease, and moderate malnutrition weakens every part of the immune system. For example, it is a major risk factor in the onset of active tuberculosis. Protein and energy malnutrition and deficiencies of specific micronutrients (including iron, zinc, and vitamins) increase susceptibility to infection. Malnutrition affects HIV transmission by increasing the risk of transmission from mother to child and also increasing replication of the virus. In communities or areas that lack access to safe drinking water, these additional health risks present a critical problem. Lower energy and impaired function of the brain also represent the downward spiral of malnutrition as victims are less able to perform the tasks they need to in order to acquire food, earn an income, or gain an education.

Vitamin-deficiency-related diseases (such as scurvy and rickets).

Hypoglycemia (low blood sugar) can result from a child not eating for 4 to 6 hours. Hypoglycemia should be considered if there is lethargy, limpness, convulsion, or loss of consciousness. If blood sugar can be measured immediately and quickly, perform a finger or heel stick.

Signs

In those with malnutrition some of the signs of dehydration differ. Children; however, may still be interested in drinking, have decreased interactions with the world around them, have decreased urine output, and may be cool to touch.

Site	Sign
Face	Moon face (kwashiorkor), simian facies (marasmus)
Eye	Dry eyes, pale conjunctiva, Bitot's spots (vitamin A), periorbital edema
Mouth	Angular stomatitis, cheilitis, glossitis, spongy bleeding gums (vitamin C), parotid enlargement
Teeth	Enamel mottling, delayed eruption
Hair	Dull, sparse, brittle hair, hypopigmentation, flag sign (alternating bands of light and normal color), broomstick eyelashes, alopecia
Skin	Loose and wrinkled (marasmus), shiny and edematous (kwashiorkor), dry, follicular hyperkeratosis, patchy hyper- and hypopigmentation, erosions, poor wound healing
Nail	Koilonychia, thin and soft nail plates, fissures or ridges
Musculature	Muscles wasting, particularly in the buttocks and thighs
Skeletal	Deformities usually a result of calcium, vitamin D, or vitamin C deficiencies
Abdomen	Distended - hepatomegaly with fatty liver, ascites may be present
Cardiovascular	Bradycardia, hypotension, reduced cardiac output, small vessel vasculopathy
Neurologic	Global development delay, loss of knee and ankle reflexes, poor memory
Hematological	Pallor, petechiae, bleeding diathesis
Behavior	Lethargic, apathetic
Source: "Protein Energy Malnutrition"	

Cognitive Development

Protein-calorie malnutrition can cause cognitive impairments. For humans, "critical period varies from the final third of gestation to the first 2 years of life". Iron deficiency anemia in children under two years of age likely affects brain function acutely and probably also chronically. Folate deficiency has been linked to neural tube defects.

Malnutrition in the form of iodine deficiency is "the most common preventable cause of mental impairment worldwide." "Even moderate deficiency, especially in pregnant women and infants, lowers intelligence by 10 to 15 I.Q. points, shaving incalculable potential off a nation's development. The most visible and severe effects — disabling goiters, cretinism and dwarfism — affect a tiny minority, usually in mountain villages. But 16 percent of the world's people have at least mild goiter, a swollen thyroid gland in the neck."

Causes

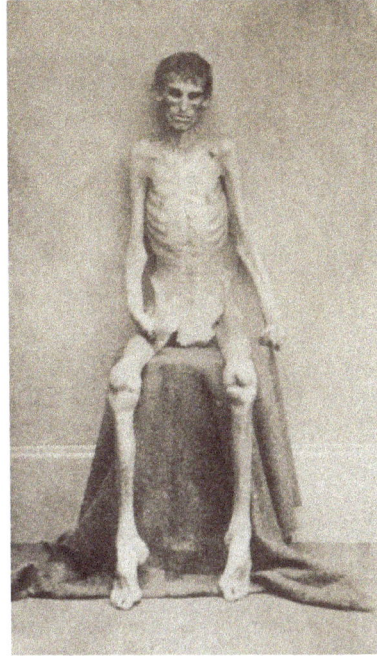

Union Army soldier on his release from Andersonville prison, 1865

Major causes of malnutrition include poverty and food prices, dietary practices and agricultural productivity, with many individual cases being a mixture of several factors. Clinical malnutrition, such as in cachexia, is a major burden also in developed countries. Various scales of analysis also have to be considered in order to determine the sociopolitical causes of malnutrition. For example, the population of a community may be at risk if the area lacks health-related services, but on a smaller scale certain households or individuals may be at even higher risk due to differences in income levels, access to land, or levels of education.

Diseases

Malnutrition can be a consequence of health issues such as gastroenteritis or chronic illness, especially the HIV/AIDS pandemic. Diarrhea and other infections can cause malnutrition through decreased nutrient absorption, decreased intake of food, increased metabolic requirements, and direct nutrient loss. Parasite infections, in particular intestinal worm infections (helminthiasis), can also lead to malnutrition. A leading cause of diarrhea and intestinal worm infections in children in developing countries is lack of sanitation and hygiene.

People may become malnourished due to abnormal nutrient loss (due to diarrhea or chronic illness) or increased energy expenditure (secondary malnutrition).

Dietary Practices

Undernutrition

A lack of adequate breastfeeding leads to malnutrition in infants and children, associated with the deaths of an estimated one million children annually. Illegal advertising of breast milk substitutes continues three decades after its 1981 prohibition under the *WHO International Code of Marketing Breast Milk Substitutes.*

Deriving too much of one's diet from a single source, such as eating almost exclusively corn or rice, can cause malnutrition. This may either be from a lack of education about proper nutrition, or from only having access to a single food source.

It is not just the total amount of calories that matters but specific nutritional deficiencies such as vitamin A deficiency, iron deficiency or zinc deficiency can also increase risk of death.

Overnutrition

Overnutrition caused by overeating is also a form of malnutrition. In the United States, more than half of all adults are now overweight — a condition that, like hunger, increases susceptibility to disease and disability, reduces worker productivity, and lowers life expectancy. Overeating is much more common in the United States, where for the majority of people, access to food is not an issue. Many parts of the world have access to a surplus of non-nutritious food, in addition to increased sedentary lifestyles. Yale psychologist Kelly Brownell calls this a "toxic food environment" where fat and sugar laden foods have taken precedence over healthy nutritious foods.

The issue in these developed countries is choosing the right kind of food. More fast food is consumed per capita in the United States than in any other country. The reason for this mass consumption of fast food is its affordability and accessibility. Often fast food, low in cost and nutrition, is high in calories and heavily promoted. When these eating habits are combined with increasingly urbanized, automated, and more sedentary lifestyles, it becomes clear why weight gain is difficult to avoid.

Not only does obesity occur in developed countries, problems are also occurring in developing countries in areas where income is on the rise. Overeating is also a problem in countries where hunger and poverty persist. In China, consumption of high-fat foods has increased while consumption of rice and other goods has decreased.

Overeating leads to many diseases, such as heart disease and diabetes, that may result in death.

Poverty and Food Prices

In Bangladesh, poor socioeconomic position was associated with chronic malnutrition since it inhibits purchase of nutritious foods such as milk, meat, poultry, and fruits. As much as food shortages may be a contributing factor to malnutrition in countries with lack of technology, the FAO (Food and Agriculture Organization) has estimated that eighty percent of malnourished children living in the developing world live in countries that produce food surpluses. The economist Amartya Sen observed that, in recent decades, famine has always been a problem of food distribution and/or poverty, as there has been sufficient food to feed the whole population of the world. He states that malnutrition and famine were more related to problems of food distribution and purchasing power.

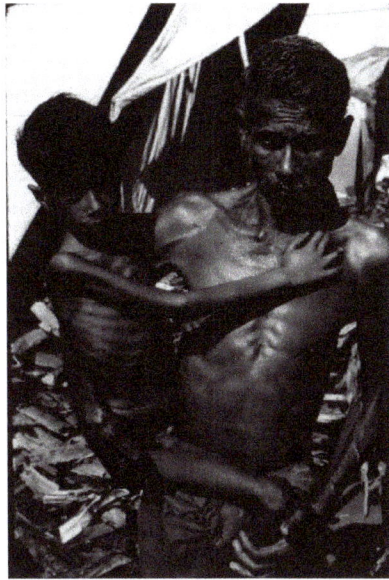

A child with extreme malnutrition

It is argued that commodity speculators are increasing the cost of food. As the real estate bubble in the United States was collapsing, it is said that trillions of dollars moved to invest in food and primary commodities, causing the 2007–2008 food price crisis.

The use of biofuels as a replacement for traditional fuels and raises the price of food. The United Nations special rapporteur on the right to food, Jean Ziegler proposes that agricultural waste, such as corn cobs and banana leaves, rather than crops themselves be used as fuel.

Agricultural Productivity

Local food shortages can be caused by a lack of arable land, adverse weather, lower farming skills such as crop rotation, or by a lack of technology or resources needed for the higher yields found in modern agriculture, such as fertilizers, pesticides, irrigation, machinery and storage facilities. As a result of widespread poverty, farmers cannot afford or governments cannot provide the resources necessary to improve local yields. The World Bank and some wealthy donor countries also press nations that depend on aid to cut or eliminate subsidized agricultural inputs such as fertilizer, in the name of free market policies even as the United States and Europe extensively subsidized their own farmers. Many, if not most, farmers cannot afford fertilizer at market prices, leading to low agricultural production and wages and high, unaffordable food prices. Reasons for the unavailability of fertilizer include moves to stop supplying fertilizer on environmental grounds, cited as the obstacle to feeding Africa by the Green Revolution pioneers Norman Borlaug and Keith Rosenberg.

Future Threats

There are a number of potential disruptions to global food supply that could cause widespread malnutrition.

Climate change is of importance to food security, with 95 percent of all malnourished peoples living in the relatively stable climate region of the sub-tropics and tropics. According to the latest IPCC reports, temperature increases in these regions are "very likely." Even small changes in temperatures can lead to increased frequency of extreme weather conditions. Many of these have great impact on agricultural production and hence nutrition. For example, the 1998–2001 central Asian drought brought about an 80 percent livestock loss and 50 percent reduction in wheat and barley crops in Iran. Similar figures were present in other nations. An increase in extreme weather such as drought in regions such as Sub-Saharan Africa would have even greater consequences in terms of malnutrition. Even without an increase of extreme weather events, a simple increase in temperature reduces the productivity of many crop species, also decreasing food security in these regions.

Colony collapse disorder is a phenomenon where bees die in large numbers. Since many agricultural crops worldwide are pollinated by bees, this represents a threat to the supply of food.

An epidemic of wheat stem rust caused by race Ug99 is currently spreading across Africa and into Asia and, it is feared, could wipe out more than 80 percent of the world's wheat crops.

Prevention

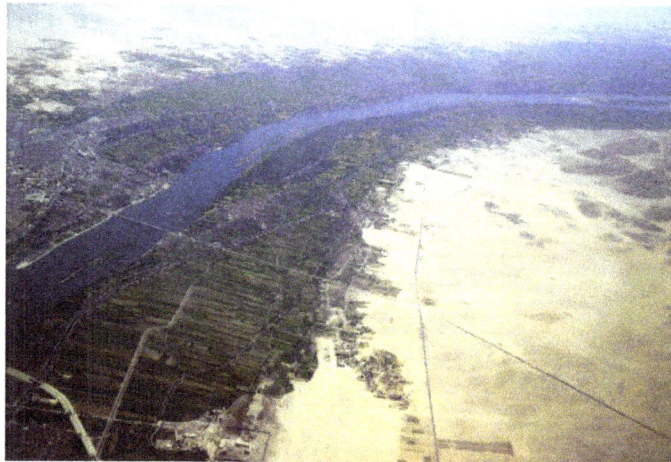

Irrigation canals have opened dry desert areas of Egypt to agriculture.

Food Security

The effort to bring modern agricultural techniques found in the West, such as nitrogen fertilizers and pesticides, to Asia, called the Green Revolution, resulted in decreases in malnutrition similar to those seen earlier in Western nations. This was possible because of existing infrastructure and institutions that are in short supply in Africa, such as a system of roads or public seed companies that made seeds available. Investments in agriculture, such as subsidized fertilizers and seeds, increases food harvest and reduces food prices. For example, in the case of Malawi, almost five million of its 13 million people used to need emergency food aid. However, after the government changed policy and subsidies for fertilizer and seed were introduced against World Bank strictures, farmers produced record-breaking corn harvests as production leaped to 3.4 million in 2007 from 1.2 million in 2005, making Malawi a major food exporter. This lowered food prices and increased wages for farm workers. Such investments in agriculture are still needed in other

African countries like the Democratic Republic of the Congo. The country has one of the highest prevalence of malnutrition even though it is blessed with great agricultural potential John Ulimwengu explains in his article for D+C. Proponents for investing in agriculture include Jeffrey Sachs, who has championed the idea that wealthy countries should invest in fertilizer and seed for Africa's farmers.

New technology in agricultural production also has great potential to combat undernutrition. By improving agricultural yields, farmers could reduce poverty by increasing income as well as open up area for diversification of crops for household use. The World Bank itself claims to be part of the solution to malnutrition, asserting that the best way for countries to succeed in breaking the cycle of poverty and malnutrition is to build export-led economies that will give them the financial means to buy foodstuffs on the world market.

Breastfeeding

As of 2016 is estimated that about 821,000 deaths of children less than five years old could be prevented globally per year through more widespread breastfeeding.

Fortified Foods

Manufacturers are trying to fortify everyday foods with micronutrients that can be sold to consumers such as wheat flour for Beladi bread in Egypt or fish sauce in Vietnam and the iodization of salt.

For example, flour has been fortified with iron, zinc, folic acid and other B vitamins such as thiamine, riboflavin,niacin and vitamin B12.

World Population

Restricting population size is a proposed solution. Thomas Malthus argued that population growth could be controlled by natural disasters and voluntary limits through "moral restraint." Robert Chapman suggests that an intervention through government policies is a necessary ingredient of curtailing global population growth. However, there are many who believe that the world has more than enough resources to sustain its population. Instead, these theorists point to unequal distribution of resources and under- or unutilized arable land as the cause for malnutrition problems. For example, Amartya Sen advocates that, "no matter how a famine is caused, methods of breaking it call for a large supply of food in the public distribution system. This applies not only to organizing rationing and control, but also to undertaking work programmes and other methods of increasing purchasing power for those hit by shifts in exchange entitlements in a general inflationary situation."

Food Sovereignty

One suggested policy framework to resolve access issues is termed food sovereignty—the right of peoples to define their own food, agriculture, livestock, and fisheries systems, in contrast to having food largely subjected to international market forces. Food First is one of the primary think tanks working to build support for food sovereignty. Neoliberals advocate for an increasing role of the free market.

Health Facilities

Another possible long term solution would be to increase access to health facilities to rural parts of the world. These facilities could monitor undernourished children, act as supplemental food distribution centers, and provide education on dietary needs. These types of facilities have already proven very successful in countries such as Peru and Ghana.

Global Initiatives

In April 2012, the Food Assistance Convention was signed, the world's first legally binding international agreement on food aid. The May 2012 Copenhagen Consensus recommended that efforts to combat hunger and malnutrition should be the first priority for politicians and private sector philanthropists looking to maximize the effectiveness of aid spending. They put this ahead of other priorities, like the fight against malaria and AIDS.

The main global policy to reduce hunger and poverty are the Sustainable Development Goals. In particular Goal 2: Zero hunger sets globally agreed targets to end hunger, achieve food security and improved nutrition and promote sustainable agriculture. The partnership Compact2025, led by IFPRI with the involvement of UN organisations, NGOs and private foundations develops and disseminates evidence-based advice to politicians and other decision-makers aimed at ending hunger and undernutrition in the coming 10 years, by 2025.

The EndingHunger campaign is an online communication campaign aimed at raising awareness of the hunger problem. It has many worked through viral videos depicting celebrities voicing their anger about the large number of hungry people in the world. Another initiative focused on improving the hunger situation by improving nutrition is the Scaling up Nutrition movement (SUN). Started in 2010 this movement of people from governments, civil society, the United Nations, donors, businesses and researchers, publishes a yearly progress report on the changes in their 55 partner countries.

Management

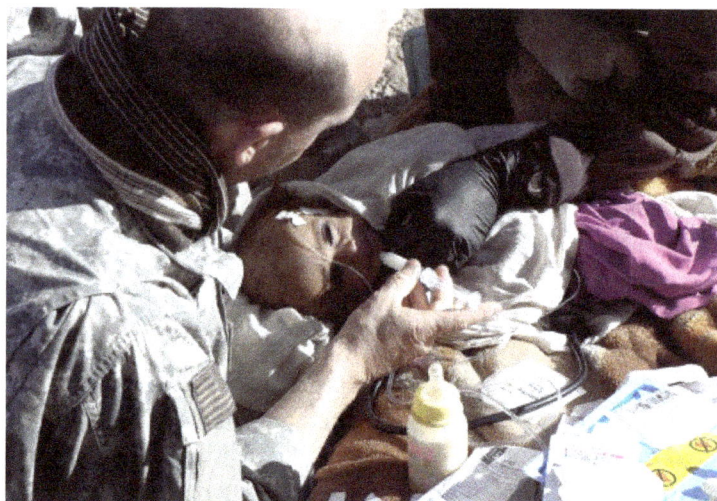

A malnourished Afghan child being treated by a medical team.

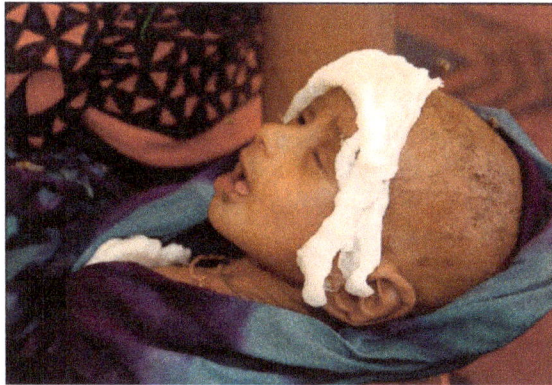

A Somali boy receiving treatment for malnourishment at a health facility.

In response to child malnutrition, the Bangladeshi government recommends ten steps for treating severe malnutrition. They are to prevent or treat dehydration, low blood sugar, low body temperature, infection, correct electrolyte imbalances and micronutrient deficiencies, start feeding cautiously, achieve catch-up growth, provide psychological support, and prepare for discharge and follow-up after recovery.

Among those patients who are hospitalized, nutritional support improves protein, colorie intake and weight.

Food

The evidence for benefit of supplementary feeding is poor. This is due to the small amount of research done on this treatment.

Specially formulated foods do however appear useful in those from the developing world with moderate acute malnutrition. In young children with severe acute malnutrition it is unclear if ready-to-use therapeutic food differs from a normal diet. They may have some benefits in humanitarian emergencies as they can be eaten directly from the packet, do not require refrigeration or mixing with clean water, and can be stored for years.

In those who are severely malnourished, feeding too much too quickly can result in refeeding syndrome. This can result regardless of route of feeding and can present itself a couple of days after eating with heart failure, dysrhythmias and confusion that can result in death.

Micronutrients

Treating malnutrition, mostly through fortifying foods with micronutrients (vitamins and minerals), improves lives at a lower cost and shorter time than other forms of aid, according to the World Bank. The Copenhagen Consensus, which look at a variety of development proposals, ranked micronutrient supplements as number one.

In those with diarrhea, once an initial four-hour rehydration period is completed, zinc supplementation is recommended. Daily zinc increases the chances of reducing the severity and duration of the diarrhea, and continuing with daily zinc for ten to fourteen days makes diarrhea less likely recur in the next two to three months.

In addition, malnourished children need both potassium and magnesium. This can be obtained by following the above recommendations for the dehydrated child to continue eating within two to three hours of starting rehydration, and including foods rich in potassium as above. Low blood potassium is worsened when base (as in Ringer's/Hartmann's) is given to treat acidosis without simultaneously providing potassium. As above, available home products such as salted and unsalted cereal water, salted and unsalted vegetable broth can be given early during the course of a child's diarrhea along with continued eating. Vitamin A, potassium, magnesium, and zinc should be added with other vitamins and minerals if available.

For a malnourished child with diarrhea from any cause, this should include foods rich in potassium such as bananas, green coconut water, and unsweetened fresh fruit juice.

Diarrhea

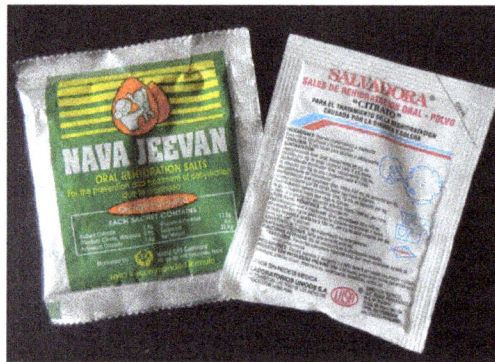

Examples of commercially available oral rehydration salts (Nepal on left, Peru on right).

The World Health Organization (WHO) recommends rehydrating a severely undernourished child who has diarrhea relatively slowly. The preferred method is with fluids by mouth using a drink called oral rehydration solution (ORS). The oral rehydration solution is both slightly sweet and slightly salty and the one recommended in those with severe undernutrition should have half the usual sodium and greater potassium. Fluids by nasogastric tube may be use in those who do not drink. Intravenous fluids are recommended only in those who have significant dehydration due to their potential complications. These complications include congestive heart failure. Over time, ORS developed into ORT, or oral rehydration therapy, which focused on increasing fluids by supplying salts, carbohydrates, and water. This switch from type of fluid to amount of fluid was crucial in order to prevent dehydration from diarrhea.

Breast feeding and eating should resume as soon as possible. Drinks such as soft drinks, fruit juices, or sweetened teas are not recommended as they contain too much sugar and may worsen diarrhea. Broad spectrum antibiotics are recommended in all severely undernourished children with diarrhea requiring admission to hospital.

To prevent dehydration readily available fluids, preferably with a modest amount of sugars and salt such as vegetable broth or salted rice water, may be used. The drinking of additional clean water is also recommended. Once dehydration develops oral rehydration solutions are preferred. As much of these drinks as the person wants can be given, unless there are signs of swelling. If vomiting occurs, fluids can be paused for 5–10 minutes and then restarting more slowly. Vomiting rarely prevents rehydration as fluid are still absorbed and the vomiting rarely last long. A severely malnourished child with what appears to be dehydration but who has not had diarrhea should be treated as if they have an infection.

For babies a dropper or syringe without the needle can be used to put small amounts of fluid into the mouth; for children under 2, a teaspoon every one to two minutes; and for older children and adults, frequent sips directly from a cup. After the first two hours, rehydration should be continued at the same or slower rate, determined by how much fluid the child wants and any ongoing diarrheal loses. After the first two hours of rehydration it is recommended that to alternate between rehydration and food.

In 2003, WHO and UNICEF recommended a reduced-osmolarity ORS which still treats dehydration but also reduced stool volume and vomiting. Reduced-osmolarity ORS is the current standard ORS with reasonably wide availability. For general use, one packet of ORS (glucose sugar, salt, potassium chloride, and trisodium citrate) is added to one liter of water; however, for malnourished children it's recommended that one packet of ORS be added to two liters of water along with an extra 50 grams of sucrose sugar and some stock potassium solution.

Malnourished children have an excess of body sodium. Recommendations for home remedies agree with one liter of water (34 oz.) and 6 teaspoons sugar and disagree regarding whether it's then one teaspoon of salt added or only 1/2, with perhaps most sources recommending 1/2 teaspoon of added salt to one liter water.

Low Blood Sugar

Hypoglycemia, whether known or suspected, can be treated with a mixture of sugar and water. If the child is conscious, the initial dose of sugar and water can be given by mouth. If the child is unconscious, give glucose by intravenous or nasogastric tube. If seizures occur after despite glucose, rectal diazepam is recommended. Blood sugar levels should be re-checked on two hour intervals.

Hypothermia

Hypothermia can occur. To prevent or treat this, the child can be kept warm with covering including of the head or by direct skin-to-skin contact with the mother or father and then covering both parent and child. Prolonged bathing or prolonged medical exams should be avoided. Warming methods are usually most important at night.

Economics

There is a growing realization among aid groups that giving cash or cash vouchers instead of food is a cheaper, faster, and more efficient way to deliver help to the hungry, particularly in areas where food is available but unaffordable. The UN's World Food Program, the biggest non-governmental distributor of food, announced that it will begin distributing cash and vouchers instead of food in some areas, which Josette Sheeran, the WFP's executive director, described as a "revolution" in food aid. The aid agency Concern Worldwide is piloting a method through a mobile phone operator, Safaricom, which runs a money transfer program that allows cash to be sent from one part of the country to another.

However, for people in a drought living a long way from and with limited access to markets, delivering food may be the most appropriate way to help. Fred Cuny stated that "the chances of saving lives at the outset of a relief operation are greatly reduced when food is imported. By the time it arrives in the country and gets to people, many will have died." U.S. law, which requires buying food at home rather than where the hungry live, is inefficient because approximately half of what is spent goes for transport. Cuny further pointed out "studies of every recent famine have shown that food was available in-country — though not always in the immediate food deficit area" and "even though by local standards the prices are too high for the poor to purchase it, it would usually be cheaper for a donor to buy the hoarded food at the inflated price than to import it from abroad."

Ethiopia has been pioneering a program that has now become part of the World Bank's prescribed method for coping with a food crisis and had been seen by aid organizations as a model of how to best help hungry nations. Through the country's main food assistance program, the Productive Safety Net Program, Ethiopia has been giving rural residents who are chronically short of food, a chance to work for food or cash. Foreign aid organizations like the World Food Program were then able to buy food locally from surplus areas to distribute in areas with a shortage of food. Ethiopia been pioneering a program, and Brazil has established a recycling program for organic waste that benefits farmers, urban poor, and the city in general. City residents separate organic waste from their garbage, bag it, and then exchange it for fresh fruit and vegetables from local farmers. As a result, the country's waste is reduced and the urban poor get a steady supply of nutritious food.

Epidemiology

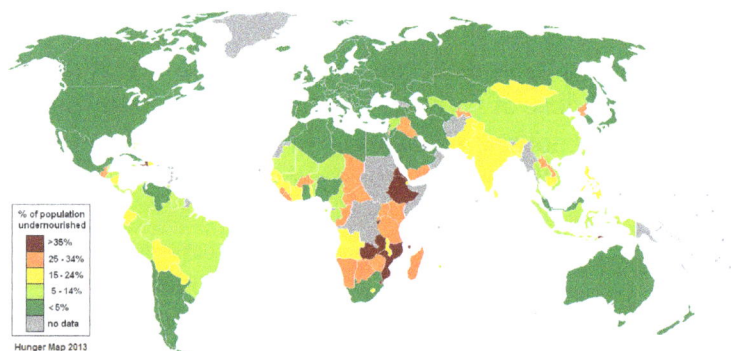

Percentage of population affected by undernutrition by country

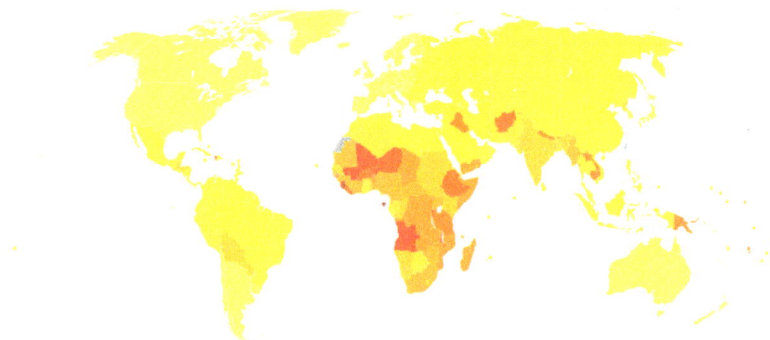

Disability-adjusted life year for nutritional deficiencies per 100,000 inhabitants in 2004. Nutritional deficiencies included: protein-energy malnutrition, iodine deficiency, vitamin A deficiency, and iron deficiency anaemia.

no data	1200-1400
<200	1400-1600
200-400	1600-1800
400-600	1800-2000
600-800	2000-2200
800-1000	2200
1000-1200	

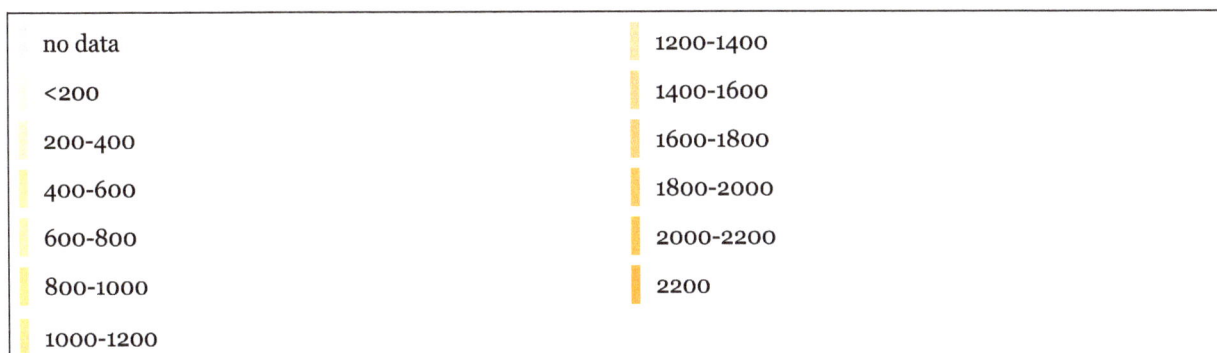

The figures provided in this section on epidemiology all refer to *undernutrition* even if the term malnutrition is used which, by definition, could also apply to too much nutrition.

People Affected

There were 793 million undernourished people in the world in 2015. This was 216 million fewer people than in 1990 when it was 991 million undernourished people. This is despite the world's farmers producing enough food to feed around 12 billion people - almost double the current world population.

Malnutrition, as of 2010, was the cause of 1.4% of all disability adjusted life years.

Number of undernourished globally							
Year	**1970**	**1980**	**1990**	**1995**	**2005**	**2007/08**	**2014/16**
Number in millions			843	788	848	923	793
Percentage in the developing world	37%	28%	20%		16%	17%	13.5%

Mortality

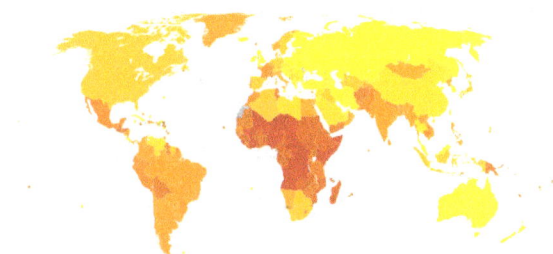

Deaths from nutritional deficiencies per million persons in 2012

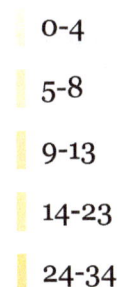

	0-4
	5-8
	9-13
	14-23
	24-34

- 35-56
- 57-91
- 92-220
- 221-365
- 366-1,207

Mortality due to malnutrition accounted for 58 percent of the total mortality in 2006: "In the world, approximately 62 million people, all causes of death combined, die each year. One in twelve people worldwide is malnourished and according to the Save the Children 2012 report, one in four of the world's children are chronically malnourished. In 2006, more than 36 million died of hunger or diseases due to deficiencies in micronutrients".

In 2010 protein-energy malnutrition resulted in 600,000 deaths down from 883,000 deaths in 1990. Other nutritional deficiencies, which include iodine deficiency and iron deficiency anemia, result in another 84,000 deaths. In 2010 malnutrition caused about 1.5 million deaths in women and children.

According to the World Health Organization, malnutrition is the biggest contributor to child mortality, present in half of all cases. Six million children die of hunger every year. Underweight births and intrauterine growth restrictions cause 2.2 million child deaths a year. Poor or non-existent breastfeeding causes another 1.4 million. Other deficiencies, such as lack of vitamin A or zinc, for example, account for 1 million. Malnutrition in the first two years is irreversible. Malnourished children grow up with worse health and lower education achievement. Their own children tend to be smaller. Malnutrition was previously seen as something that exacerbates the problems of diseases as measles, pneumonia and diarrhea. But malnutrition actually causes diseases and can be fatal in its own right.

Society and Culture

Roughly $300 million of aid goes to basic nutrition each year, less than $2 for each child below two in the 20 worst affected countries. In contrast, HIV/AIDS, which causes fewer deaths than child malnutrition, received $2.2 billion—$67 per person with HIV in all countries.

The International Crops Research Institute for the Semi-Arid Tropics (ICRISAT), a member of the CGIAR consortium, partners with farmers, governments, researchers and NGOs to help farmers grow nutritious crops, such as chickpea, groundnut, pigeonpea, millet and sorghum. This helps their communities have more balanced diets and become more resilient to pests and drought. The Harnessing Opportunities for Productivity Enhancement of Sorghum and Millets in Sub-Saharan Africa and South Asia (HOPE) project, for example, is increasing yields of finger millet in Tanzania by encouraging farmers to grow improved varieties. Finger millet is very high in calcium, rich in iron and fiber, and has a better energy content than other cereals. These characteristics make it ideal for feeding to infants and the elderly.

Some organizations have begun working with teachers, policymakers, and managed food service contractors to mandate improved nutritional content and increased nutritional resources in school cafeterias from primary to university-level institutions. Health and nutrition have been proven to have close links with overall educational success.

The verb form is "malnourish"; "malnourishment" is sometimes used instead of "malnutrition."

Special Populations

Undernutrition is an important determinant of maternal and child health, accounting for more than a third of child deaths and more than 10 percent of the total global disease burden according to 2008 studies.

Children

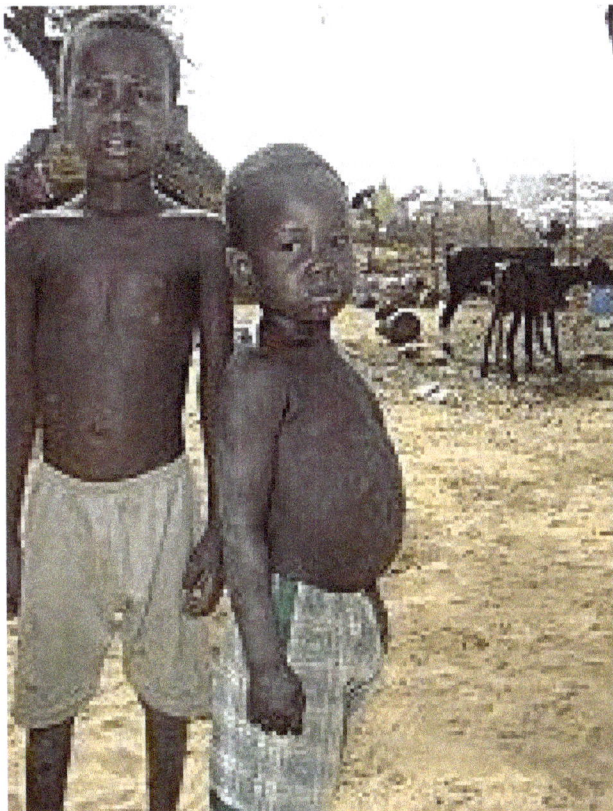

Malnourished children in Niger, during the 2005 famine.

The World Health Organization estimates that malnutrition accounts for 54 percent of child mortality worldwide, about 1 million children. Another estimate also by WHO states that childhood underweight is the cause for about 35% of all deaths of children under the age of five years worldwide.

As underweight children are more vulnerable to almost all infectious diseases, the *indirect* disease burden of malnutrition is estimated to be an order of magnitude higher than the disease burden of the *direct* effects of malnutrition. The combination of direct and indirect deaths from malnutrition caused by unsafe water, sanitation and hygiene (WASH) practices is estimated to lead to 860,000 deaths per year in children under five years of age.

Women

Gender

Researchers from the Centre for World Food Studies in 2003 found that the gap between levels of undernutrition in men and women is generally small, but that the gap varies from region to region and from country to country. These small-scale studies showed that female undernutrition prevalence rates exceeded male undernutrition prevalence rates in South/Southeast Asia and Latin America and were lower in Sub-Saharan Africa. Datasets for Ethiopia and Zimbabwe reported undernutrition rates between 1.5 and 2 times higher in men than in women; however, in India and Pakistan, datasets rates of undernutrition were 1.5-2 times higher in women than in men. Intra-country variation also occurs, with frequent high gaps between regional undernutrition rates. Gender inequality in nutrition in some countries such as India is present in all stages of life.

Studies on nutrition concerning gender bias within households look at patterns of food allocation, and one study from 2003 suggested that women often receive a lower share of food requirements than men. Gender discrimination, gender roles, and social norms affecting women can lead to early marriage and childbearing, close birth spacing, and undernutrition, all of which contribute to malnourished mothers.

Within the household, there may be differences in levels of malnutrition between men and women, and these differences have been shown to vary significantly from one region to another, with problem areas showing relative deprivation of women. Samples of 1000 women in India in 2008 demonstrated that malnutrition in women is associated with poverty, lack of development and awareness, and illiteracy. The same study showed that gender discrimination in households can prevent a woman's access to sufficient food and healthcare. How socialization affects the health of women in Bangladesh, Najma Rivzi explains in an article about a research program on this topic. In some cases, such as in parts of Kenya in 2006, rates of malnutrition in pregnant women were even higher than rates in children.

Women in some societies are traditionally given less food than men since men are perceived to have heavier workloads. Household chores and agricultural tasks can in fact be very arduous and require additional energy and nutrients; however, physical activity, which largely determines energy requirements, is difficult to estimate.

Physiology

Women have unique nutritional requirements, and in some cases need more nutrients than men; for example, women need twice as much calcium as men.

Pregnancy and Breastfeeding

During pregnancy and breastfeeding, women must ingest enough nutrients for themselves and their child, so they need significantly more protein and calories during these periods, as well as more vitamins and minerals (especially iron, iodine, calcium, folic acid, and vitamins A, C, and K). In 2001 the FAO of the UN reported that iron deficiency afflicted 43 percent of women in developing countries and increased the risk of death during childbirth. A 2008 review of interventions estimated that universal supplementation with calcium, iron, and folic acid during pregnancy could prevent 105,000 maternal deaths (23.6 percent of all maternal deaths).

Frequent pregnancies with short intervals between them and long periods of breastfeeding add an additional nutritional burden.

Educating Children

According to the FAO, women are often responsible for preparing food and have the chance to educate their children about beneficial food and health habits, giving mothers another chance to improve the nutrition of their children.

Elderly

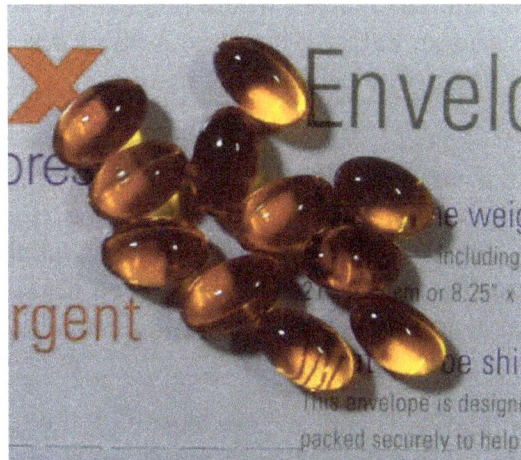

Essential nutrients are one of the main requirements of elderly care.

Malnutrition and being underweight are more common in the elderly than in adults of other ages. If elderly people are healthy and active, the aging process alone does not usually cause malnutrition. However, changes in body composition, organ functions, adequate energy intake and ability to eat or access food are associated with aging, and may contribute to malnutrition. Sadness or depression can play a role, causing changes in appetite, digestion, energy level, weight, and well-being. A study on the relationship between malnutrition and other conditions in the elderly found that Malnutrition in the elderly can result from gastrointestinal and endocrine system disorders, loss of taste and smell, decreased appetite and inadequate dietary intake. Poor dental health, ill-fitting dentures, or chewing and swallowing problems can make eating difficult. As a result of these factors, malnutrition is seen to develop more easily in the elderly.

Rates of malnutrition tend to increase with age with less than 10 percent of the "young" elderly (up to age 75) malnourished, while 30 to 65 percent of the elderly in home care, long-term care facilities, or acute hospitals are malnourished. Many elderly people require assistance in eating, which may contribute to malnutrition. Because of this, one of the main requirements of elderly care is to provide an adequate diet and all essential nutrients.

In Australia malnutrition or risk of malnutrition occurs in 80 percent of elderly people presented to hospitals for admission. Malnutrition and weight loss can contribute to sarcopenia with loss of lean body mass and muscle function. Abdominal obesity or weight loss coupled with sarcopenia lead to immobility, skeletal disorders, insulin resistance, hypertension, atherosclerosis, and metabolic disorders.

Eating Disorder

Eating disorders are mental disorders defined by abnormal eating habits that negatively affect a person's physical or mental health. They include binge eating disorder where people eat a large amount in a short period of time, anorexia nervosa where people eat very little and thus have a low body weight, bulimia nervosa where people eat a lot and then try to rid themselves of the food, pica where people eat non-food items, rumination disorder where people regurgitate food, avoidant/restrictive food intake disorder where people have a lack of interest in food, and a group of other specified feeding or eating disorders. Anxiety disorders, depression, and substance abuse are common among people with eating disorders. These disorders do not include obesity.

The cause of eating disorders is not clear. Both biological and environmental factors appear to play a role. Cultural idealization of thinness is believed to contribute. Eating disorders affect about 12 percent of dancers. Those who have experienced sexual abuse are also more likely to develop eating disorders. Some disorders such as pica and rumination disorder occur more often in people with intellectual disabilities. Only one eating disorder can be diagnosed at a given time.

Treatment can be effective for many eating disorders. This typically involves counselling, a proper diet, a normal amount of exercise, and the reduction of efforts to eliminate food. Hospitalization is occasionally needed. Medications may be used to help with some of the associated symptoms. At five years about 70% of people with anorexia and 50% of people with bulimia recover. Recovery from binge eating disorder is less clear and estimated at 20% to 60%. Both anorexia and bulimia increase the risk of death.

In the developed world binge eating disorder affects about 1.6% of women and 0.8% of men in a given year. Anorexia affects about 0.4% and bulimia affects about 1.3% of young women in a given year. During the entire life up to 4% of women have anorexia, 2% have bulimia, and 2% have binge eating disorder. Anorexia and bulimia occur nearly ten times more often in females than males. Typically they begin in late childhood or early adulthood. Rates of other eating disorders are not clear. Rates of eating disorders appear to be lower in less developed countries.

Classification

Bulimia nervosa is a disorder characterized by binge eating and purging, as well as excessive evaluation of one's self-worth in terms of body weight or shape. Purging can include self-induced vomiting, over-exercising, and the use of diuretics, enemas, and laxatives. Anorexia nervosa is characterized by extreme food restriction and excessive weight loss, accompanied by the fear of being fat. The extreme weight loss often causes women and girls who have begun menstruating to stop having menstrual periods, a condition known as amenorrhea. Although amenorrhea was once a required criterion for the disorder, it is no longer required to meet criteria for anorexia nervosa due to its exclusive nature for sufferers who are male, post-menopause, or who do not menstruate for other reasons. The DSM-5 specifies two subtypes of anorexia nervosa—the restricting type and the binge/purge type. Those who suffer from the restricting type of anorexia nervosa restrict food intake and do not engage in binge eating, whereas those suffering from the binge/purge type lose control over their eating at least occasionally and may compensate for these binge episodes. The most notable difference between anorexia nervosa binge/purge type and bulimia nervosa is the body weight of the person. Those diagnosed with anorexia nervosa binge/purge type are under-weight, while those with bulimia nervosa may have a body weight that falls within the range from normal to obese.

ICD and DSM

These eating disorders are specified as mental disorders in standard medical manuals, such as in the ICD-10, the DSM-5, or both.

- Anorexia nervosa (AN), characterized by lack of maintenance of a healthy body weight, an obsessive fear of gaining weight or refusal to do so, and an unrealistic perception, or non-recognition of the seriousness, of current low body weight. Anorexia can cause menstrua-tion to stop, and often leads to bone loss, loss of skin integrity, etc. It greatly stresses the heart, increasing the risk of heart attacks and related heart problems. The risk of death is greatly increased in individuals with this disease. The most underlining factor researchers are starting to take notice of is that it may not just be a vanity, social, or media issue, but it could also be related to biological and or genetic components. The DSM-5 contains many changes that better represent patients with these conditions. The DSM-IV required amen-orrhea (the absence of the menstrual cycle) to be present in order to diagnose a patient with anorexia. This is no longer a requirement in the DSM-5.

- Bulimia nervosa (BN), characterized by recurrent binge eating followed by compensatory behaviors such as purging (self-induced vomiting, eating to the point of vomiting, excessive use of laxatives/diuretics, or excessive exercise). Fasting and over-exercising may also be used as a method of purging following a binge.

- Muscle dysmorphia is characterized by appearance preoccupation that one's own body is too small, too skinny, insufficiently muscular, or insufficiently lean. Muscle dysmorphia affects mostly males.

- Binge Eating Disorder (BED), characterized by recurring binge eating at least once a week for over a period of 3 months while experiencing lack of control and guilt after overeating. The disorder can develop within individuals of a wide range of ages and socioeconomic classes.

- Other Specified Feeding or Eating Disorder (OSFED) is an eating or feeding disorder that does not meet full DSM-5 criteria for AN, BN, or BED. Examples of otherwise-specified eating disorders include individuals with atypical anorexia nervosa, who meet all criteria for AN except being underweight, despite substantial weight loss; atypical bulimia nervosa, who meet all criteria for BN except that bulimic behaviors are less frequent or have not been ongoing for long enough; purging disorder; and night eating syndrome.

Other

- Compulsive overeating, (COE), in which individuals habitually graze on large quantities of food rather than binging, as would be typical of binge eating disorder.

- Prader-Willi syndrome

- Diabulimia, characterized by the deliberate manipulation of insulin levels by diabetics in an effort to control their weight.

- Food maintenance, characterized by a set of aberrant eating behaviors of children in foster care.

- Orthorexia nervosa, a term used by Steven Bratman to characterize an obsession with a "pure" diet, in which people develop an obsession with avoiding unhealthy foods to the point where it interferes with a person's life.

- Selective eating disorder, also called picky eating, is an extreme sensitivity to how something tastes. A person with SED may or may not be a supertaster.

- Drunkorexia, commonly characterized by purposely restricting food intake in order to reserve food calories for alcoholic calories, exercising excessively in order to burn calories consumed from drinking, and over-drinking alcohols in order to purge previously consumed food.

- Pregorexia, characterized by extreme dieting and over-exercising in order to control pregnancy weight gain. Under-nutrition during pregnancy is associated with low birth weight, coronary heart disease, type 2 diabetes, stroke, hypertension, cardiovascular disease risk, and depression.

- Gourmand syndrome, a rare condition occurring after damage to the frontal lobe, resulting in an obsessive focus on fine foods.

Signs and Symptoms

Symptoms and complications vary according to the nature and severity of the eating disorder:

Possible Symptoms and Complications of Eating Disorders			
acne	xerosis	amenorrhoea	tooth loss, cavities
constipation	diarrhea	water retention and/or edema	lanugo
telogen effluvium	cardiac arrest	hypokalemia	death
osteoporosis	electrolyte imbalance	hyponatremia	brain atrophy
pellagra	scurvy	kidney failure	suicide

Some physical symptoms of eating disorders are weakness, fatigue, sensitivity to cold, reduced beard growth in men, reduction in waking erections, reduced libido, weight loss and failure of growth. Unexplained hoarseness may be a symptom of an underlying eating disorder, as the result of acid reflux, or entry of acidic gastric material into the laryngoesophageal tract. Patients who induce vomiting, such as those with anorexia nervosa, binge eating-purging type or those with purging-type bulimia nervosa are at risk for acid reflux. Polycystic ovary syndrome (PCOS) is the most common endocrine disorder to affect women. Though often associated with obesity it can occur in normal weight individuals. PCOS has been associated with binge eating and bulimic behavior.

Pro-Ana Subculture

Several websites promote eating disorders, and can provide a means for individuals to communicate in order to maintain eating disorders. Members of these websites typically feel that their eating disorder is the only aspect of a chaotic life that they can control. These websites are often interactive and have discussion boards where individuals can share strategies, ideas, and experiences, such as diet and exercise plans that achieve extremely low weights. A study comparing the personal web-blogs that were pro-eating disorder with those focused on recovery found that the pro-eating disorder blogs contained language reflecting lower cognitive processing, used a more closed-minded writing style, contained less emotional expression and fewer social references, and focused more on eating-related contents than did the recovery blogs.

Psychopathology

The psychopathology of eating disorders centers around body image disturbance, such as concerns with weight and shape; self-worth being too dependent on weight and shape; fear of gaining weight even when underweight; denial of how severe the symptoms are and a distortion in the way the body is experienced.

Causes

The cause of eating disorder is not clear.

Many people with eating disorders suffer also from body dysmorphic disorder, altering the way a person sees himself or herself. Studies have found that a high proportion of individuals diagnosed with body dysmorphic disorder also had some type of eating disorder, with 15% of individuals having either anorexia nervosa or bulimia nervosa. This link between body dysmorphic disorder and anorexia stems from the fact that both BDD and anorexia nervosa are characterized by a preoccupation with physical appearance and a distortion of body image. There are also many other possibilities such as environmental, social and interpersonal issues that could promote and sustain these illnesses.} Also, the media are oftentimes blamed for the rise in the incidence of eating disorders due to the fact that media images of idealized slim physical shape of people such as models and celebrities motivate or even force people to attempt to achieve slimness themselves. The media are accused of distorting reality, in the sense that people portrayed in the media are either naturally thin and thus unrepresentative of normality or unnaturally thin by forcing their bodies to look like the ideal image by putting excessive pressure on themselves to look a certain way. While past findings have described the causes of eating disorders as primarily psychological, environmental, and sociocultural, new studies have uncovered evidence that there is a prevalent genetic/heritable aspect of the causes of eating disorders.

Genetics

- Genetic: Numerous studies have been undertaken that show a possible genetic predisposition toward eating disorders as a result of Mendelian inheritance. It has also been shown that eating disorders can be heritable. Recent twin studies have found slight instances of genetic variance when considering the different criterion of both anorexia nervosa and bulimia nervosa as endophenotypes contributing to the disorders as a whole. In another recent study, twin and family studies led researchers to discover a genetic link on chromosome 1 that can be found in multiple family members of an individual with anorexia nervosa, indicating an inheritance pattern found between family members of others that have been previously diagnosed with an eating disorder. A study found that an individual who is a first degree relative of someone who has suffered or currently suffers from an eating disorder is seven to twelve times more likely to suffer from an eating disorder themselves. Twin studies also have shown that at least a portion of the vulnerability to develop eating disorders can be inherited, and there has been sufficient evidence to show that there is a genetic locus that shows susceptibility for developing anorexia nervosa.

- Epigenetics: Epigenetic mechanisms are means by which environmental effects alter gene expression via methods such as DNA methylation; these are independent of and do not alter the underlying DNA sequence. They are heritable, but also may occur throughout the lifespan, and are potentially reversible. Dysregulation of dopaminergic neurotransmission due to epigenetic mechanisms has been implicated in various eating disorders. One study has found that "epigenetic mechanisms may contribute to the known alterations of ANP homeostasis in women with eating disorders." Other candidate genes for epigenetic studies in eating disorders include leptin, pro-opiomelanocortin (POMC) and brain-derived neurotrophic factor (BDNF).

Psychological

Eating disorders are classified as Axis I disorders in the Diagnostic and Statistical Manual of Mental Health Disorders (DSM-IV) published by the American Psychiatric Association. There are various other psychological issues that may factor into eating disorders, some fulfill the criteria for a separate Axis I diagnosis or a personality disorder which is coded Axis II and thus are considered comorbid to the diagnosed eating disorder. Axis II disorders are subtyped into 3 "clusters": A, B and C. The causality between personality disorders and eating disorders has yet to be fully established. Some people have a previous disorder which may increase their vulnerability to developing an eating disorder. Some develop them afterwards. The severity and type of eating disorder symptoms have been shown to affect comorbidity. The DSM-IV should not be used by laypersons to diagnose themselves, even when used by professionals there has been considerable controversy over the diagnostic criteria used for various diagnoses, including eating disorders. There has been controversy over various editions of the DSM including the latest edition, DSM-V, due in May 2013.

Cognitive Attentional Bias Issues

Attentional bias may have an effect on eating disorders. Many studies have been performed to test this theory.

Comorbid Disorders	
Axis I	**Axis II**
depression	obsessive compulsive personality disorder
substance abuse, alcoholism	borderline personality disorder
anxiety disorders	narcissistic personality disorder
obsessive compulsive disorder	histrionic personality disorder
Attention-deficit hyperactivity disorder	avoidant personality disorder

Personality Traits

There are various childhood personality traits associated with the development of eating disorders. During adolescence these traits may become intensified due to a variety of physiological and cultural influences such as the hormonal changes associated with puberty, stress related to the approaching demands of maturity and socio-cultural influences and perceived expectations, especially in areas that concern body image. Eating disorders have been associated with a fragile sense of self and with disordered mentalization. Many personality traits have a genetic component and are highly heritable. Maladaptive levels of certain traits may be acquired as a result of anoxic or traumatic brain injury, neurodegenerative diseases such as Parkinson's disease, neurotoxicity such as lead exposure, bacterial infection such as Lyme disease or viral infection such as Toxoplasma gondii as well as hormonal influences. While studies are still continuing via the use of various imaging techniques such as fMRI; these traits have been shown to originate in various regions of the brain such as the amygdala and the prefrontal cortex. Disorders in the prefrontal cortex and the executive functioning system have been shown to affect eating behavior.

Celiac Disease

People with gastrointestinal disorders may be more risk of developing disorders eating practices than the general population, principally restrictive eating disturbances. An association of anorexia nervosa with celiac disease has been found. The role that gastrointestinal symptoms play in the development of eating disorders seems rather complex. Some authors report that unresolved symptoms prior to gastrointestinal disease diagnosis may create a food aversion in these persons, causing alterations to their eating patterns. Other authors report that greater symptoms throughout their diagnosis led to greater risk. It has been documented that some people with celiac disease, irritable bowel syndrome or inflammatory bowel disease who are not conscious about the importance of strictly following their diet, choose to consume their trigger foods to promote weight loss. On the other hand, individuals with good dietary management may develop anxiety, food aversion and eating disorders because of concerns around cross contamination of their foods. Some authors suggest that medical professionals should evaluate the presence of an unrecognized celiac disease in all people with eating disorder, especially if they present any gastrointestinal symptom (such as decreased appetite, abdominal pain, bloating, distension, vomiting, diarrhea or constipation), weight loss, or growth failure; and also routinely ask celiac patients about weight or body shape concerns, dieting or vomiting for weight control, to evaluate the possible presence of eating disorders, specially in women.

Environmental Influences

Child Maltreatment

Child abuse which encompasses physical, psychological and sexual abuse, as well as neglect has been shown by innumerable studies to be a precipitating factor in a wide variety of psychiatric disorders, including eating disorders. Children who are subjected to abuse may develop eating disorders in an effort to gain some sense of control or for a sense of comfort, or they may be in an environment where the diet is unhealthy or insufficient. Child abuse and neglect can cause profound changes in both the physiological structure and the neurochemistry of the developing brain. Children who, as wards of the state, were placed in orphanages or foster homes are especially susceptible to developing a disordered eating pattern. In a study done in New Zealand 25% of the study subjects in foster care exhibited an eating disorder (Tarren-Sweeney M. 2006). An unstable home environment is detrimental to the emotional well-being of children, even in the absence of blatant abuse or neglect the stress of an unstable home can contribute to the development of an eating disorder.

Social Isolation

Social isolation has been shown to have a deleterious effect on an individual's physical and emotional well-being. Those that are socially isolated have a higher mortality rate in general as compared to individuals that have established social relationships. This effect on mortality is markedly increased in those with pre-existing medical or psychiatric conditions, and has been especially noted in cases of coronary heart disease. "The magnitude of risk associated with social isolation is comparable with that of cigarette smoking and other major biomedical and psychosocial risk factors." (Brummett *et al.*)

Social isolation can be inherently stressful, depressing and anxiety-provoking. In an attempt to ameliorate these distressful feelings an individual may engage in emotional eating in which food serves as a source of comfort. The loneliness of social isolation and the inherent stressors thus associated have been implicated as triggering factors in binge eating as well.

Waller, Kennerley and Ohanian (2007) argued that both bingeing–vomiting and restriction are emotion suppression strategies, but they are just utilized at different times. For example, restriction is used to pre-empt any emotion activation, while bingeing–vomiting is used after an emotion has been activated.

Parental Influence

Parental influence has been shown to be an intrinsic component in the development of eating behaviors of children. This influence is manifested and shaped by a variety of diverse factors such as familial genetic predisposition, dietary choices as dictated by cultural or ethnic preferences, the parents' own body shape and eating patterns, the degree of involvement and expectations of their children's eating behavior as well as the interpersonal relationship of parent and child. This is in addition to the general psychosocial climate of the home and the presence or absence of a nurturing stable environment. It has been shown that maladaptive parental behavior has an important role in the development of eating disorders. As to the more subtle aspects of parental influence, it has been shown that eating patterns are established in early childhood and that children should be allowed to decide when their appetite is satisfied as early as the age of two. A direct link has been shown between obesity and parental pressure to eat more.

Coercive tactics in regard to diet have not been proven to be efficacious in controlling a child's eating behavior. Affection and attention have been shown to affect the degree of a child's finickiness and their acceptance of a more varied diet.

Hilde Bruch, a pioneer in the field of studying eating disorders, asserts that anorexia nervosa often occurs in girls who are high achievers, obedient, and always trying to please their parents. Their parents have a tendency to be over-controlling and fail to encourage the expression of emotions, inhibiting daughters from accepting their own feelings and desires. Adolescent females in these overbearing families lack the ability to be independent from their families, yet realize the need to, often resulting in rebellion. Controlling their food intake may make them feel better, as it provides them with a sense of control.

Peer Pressure

In various studies such as one conducted by The McKnight Investigators, peer pressure was shown to be a significant contributor to body image concerns and attitudes toward eating among subjects in their teens and early twenties.

Eleanor Mackey and co-author, Annette M. La Greca of the University of Miami, studied 236 teen girls from public high schools in southeast Florida. "Teen girls' concerns about their own weight, about how they appear to others and their perceptions that their peers want them to be thin are significantly related to weight-control behavior", says psychologist Eleanor Mackey of the Children's National Medical Center in Washington and lead author of the study. "Those are really important."

According to one study, 40% of 9- and 10-year-old girls are already trying to lose weight. Such dieting is reported to be influenced by peer behavior, with many of those individuals on a diet reporting that their friends also were dieting. The number of friends dieting and the number of friends who pressured them to diet also played a significant role in their own choices.

Elite athletes have a significantly higher rate in eating disorders. Female athletes in sports such as gymnastics, ballet, diving, etc. are found to be at the highest risk among all athletes. Women are more likely than men to acquire an eating disorder between the ages of 13–30. 0–15% of those with bulimia and anorexia are men.

Cultural Pressure

There is a cultural emphasis on thinness which is especially pervasive in western society. There is an unrealistic stereotype of what constitutes beauty and the ideal body type as portrayed by the media, fashion and entertainment industries. "The cultural pressure on men and women to be 'perfect' is an important predisposing factor for the development of eating disorders". Further, when women of all races base their evaluation of their self upon what is considered the culturally ideal body, the incidence of eating disorders increases. Eating disorders are becoming more prevalent in non-Western countries where thinness is not seen as the ideal, showing that social and cultural pressures are not the only causes of eating disorders. For example, observations of anorexia in all of the non-Western regions of the world point to the disorder not being "culture-bound" as once thought. However, studies on rates of bulimia suggest that it might be culturally bound. In non-Western countries, bulimia is less prevalent than anorexia, but these non-Western countries where it is observed can be said to have probably or definitely been influenced or exposed to Western culture and ideology.

Socioeconomic status (SES) has been viewed as a risk factor for eating disorders, presuming that possessing more resources allows for an individual to actively choose to diet and reduce body weight. Some studies have also shown a relationship between increasing body dissatisfaction with increasing SES. However, once high socioeconomic status has been achieved, this relationship weakens and, in some cases, no longer exists.

The media plays a major role in the way in which people view themselves. Countless magazine ads and commercials depict thin celebrities like Lindsay Lohan, Nicole Richie, Victoria Beckham and Mary Kate Olsen, who appear to gain nothing but attention from their looks. Society has taught people that being accepted by others is necessary at all costs. Unfortunately this has led to the belief that in order to fit in one must look a certain way. Televised beauty competitions such as the Miss America Competition contribute to the idea of what it means to be beautiful because competitors are evaluated on the basis of their opinion.

In addition to socioeconomic status being considered a cultural risk factor so is the world of sports. Athletes and eating disorders tend to go hand in hand, especially the sports where weight is a competitive factor. Gymnastics, horse back riding, wrestling, body building, and dancing are just a few that fall into this category of weight dependent sports. Eating disorders among individuals that participate in competitive activities, especially women, often lead to having physical and biological changes related to their weight that often mimic prepubescent stages. Oftentimes as women's bodies change they lose their competitive edge which leads them to taking extreme measures to maintain their younger body shape. Men often struggle with binge eating followed by excessive exercise while focusing on building muscle rather than losing fat, but this goal of gaining muscle is just as much an eating disorder as obsessing over thinness. The following statistics taken from Susan Nolen-Hoeksema's book, *(ab)normal psychology*, shows the estimated percentage of athletes that struggle with eating disorders based on the category of sport.

- Aesthetic sports (dance, figure skating, gymnastics) – 35%

- Weight dependent sports (judo, wrestling) – 29%

- Endurance sports (cycling, swimming, running) – 20%

- Technical sports (golf, high jumping) – 14%

- Ball game sports (volleyball, soccer) – 12%

Although most of these athletes develop eating disorders to keep their competitive edge, others use exercise as a way to maintain their weight and figure. This is just as serious as regulating food intake for competition. Even though there is mixed evidence showing at what point athletes are challenged with eating disorders, studies show that regardless of competition level all athletes are at higher risk for developing eating disorders that non-athletes, especially those that participate in sports where thinness is a factor.

Pressure from society is also seen within the homosexual community. Homosexual men are at greater risk of eating disorder symptoms than heterosexual men. Within the gay culture, muscularity gives the advantages of both social and sexual desirability and also power. These pressures and ideas that another homosexual male may desire a mate who is thinner or muscular can possibly lead to eating disorders. The higher eating disorder symptom score reported, the more concern about how others perceive them and the more frequent and excessive exercise sessions occur. High levels of body dissatisfaction are also linked to external motivation to working out and old age; however, having a thin and muscular body occurs within younger homosexual males than older.

It is important to realize some of the limitations and challenges of many studies that try to examine the roles of culture, ethnicity, and SES. For starters, most of the cross-cultural studies use definitions from the DSM-IV-TR, which has been criticized as reflecting a Western cultural bias. Thus, assessments and questionnaires may not be constructed to detect some of the cultural differences associated with different disorders. Also, when looking at individuals in areas potentially influenced by Western culture, few studies have attempted to measure how much an individual has adopted the mainstream culture or retained the traditional cultural values of the area. Lastly, the majority of the cross-cultural studies on eating disorders and body image disturbances occurred in Western nations and not in the countries or regions being examined.

While there are many influences to how an individual processes their body image, the media does play a major role. Along with the media, parental influence, peer influence, and self-efficacy beliefs also play a large role in an individual's view of themselves. The way the media presents images can have a lasting effect on an individual's perception of their body image. Eating disorders are a worldwide issue and while women are more likely to be affected by an eating disorder it still affects both genders (Schwitzer 2012). The media influences eating disorders whether shown in a positive or negative light, it then has a responsibility to use caution when promoting images that projects an ideal that many turn to eating disorders to attain.

To combat unhealthy body image in the fashion world, in 2015, France passed a law requiring models to be declared healthy by a doctor to participate in fashion shows. It also requires retouched images to be marked as such in magazines.

Mechanisms

- Biochemical: Eating behavior is a complex process controlled by the neuroendocrine system, of which the Hypothalamus-pituitary-adrenal-axis (HPA axis) is a major component. Dysregulation of the HPA axis has been associated with eating disorders, such as irregularities in the manufacture, amount or transmission of certain neurotransmitters, hormones or neuropeptides and amino acids such as homocysteine, elevated levels of which are found in AN and BN as well as depression.

  o Serotonin: a neurotransmitter involved in depression also has an inhibitory effect on eating behavior.

  o Norepinephrine is both a neurotransmitter and a hormone; abnormalities in either capacity may affect eating behavior.

o Dopamine: which in addition to being a precursor of norepinephrine and epinephrine is also a neurotransmitter which regulates the rewarding property of food.

o Neuropeptide Y also known as NPY is a hormone that encourages eating and decreases metabolic rate. Blood levels of NPY are elevated in patients with anorexia nervosa, and studies have shown that injection of this hormone into the brain of rats with restricted food intake increases their time spent running on a wheel. Normally the hormone stimulates eating in healthy patients, but under conditions of starvation it increases their activity rate, probably to increase the chance of finding food. The increased levels of NPY in the blood of patients with eating disorders can in some ways explain the instances of extreme over-exercising found in most anorexia nervosa patients.

- Leptin and ghrelin: leptin is a hormone produced primarily by the fat cells in the body; it has an inhibitory effect on appetite by inducing a feeling of satiety. Ghrelin is an appetite inducing hormone produced in the stomach and the upper portion of the small intestine. Circulating levels of both hormones are an important factor in weight control. While often associated with obesity, both hormones and their respective effects have been implicated in the pathophysiology of anorexia nervosa and bulimia nervosa. Leptin can also be used to distinguish between constitutional thinness found in a healthy person with a low BMI and an individual with anorexia nervosa.

- Gut bacteria and immune system: studies have shown that a majority of patients with anorexia and bulimia nervosa have elevated levels of autoantibodies that affect hormones and neuropeptides that regulate appetite control and the stress response. There may be a direct correlation between autoantibody levels and associated psychological traits. Later study revealed that autoantibodies reactive with alpha-MSH are, in fact, generated against ClpB, a protein produced by certain gut bacteria e.g. Escherichia coli. ClpB protein was identified as a conformational antigen-mimetic of alpha-MSH. In patients with eating disorders plasma levels of anti-ClpB IgG and IgM correalated with patients' psychological traits

- Infection: PANDAS, is an abbreviation for Pediatric Autoimmune Neuropsychiatric Disorders Associated with Streptococcal Infections. Children with PANDAS "have obsessive-compulsive disorder (OCD) and/or tic disorders such as Tourette syndrome, and in whom symptoms worsen following infections such as "strep throat" and scarlet fever". (NIMH) There is a possibility that PANDAS may be a precipitating factor in the development of anorexia nervosa in some cases, (PANDAS AN).

- Lesions: studies have shown that lesions to the right frontal lobe or temporal lobe can cause the pathological symptoms of an eating disorder.

- Tumors: tumors in various regions of the brain have been implicated in the development of abnormal eating patterns.

- Brain calcification: a study highlights a case in which prior calcification of the right thalamus may have contributed to development of anorexia nervosa.

- somatosensory homunculus: is the representation of the body located in the somatosensory cortex, first described by renowned neurosurgeon Wilder Penfield. The illustration was originally termed "Penfield's Homunculus", homunculus meaning little man. "In normal development this representation should adapt as the body goes through its pubertal growth spurt. However, in AN it is hypothesized that there is a lack of plasticity in this area, which may result in impairments of sensory processing and distortion of body image". (Bryan Lask, also proposed by VS Ramachandran)

- Obstetric complications: There have been studies done which show maternal smoking, obstetric and perinatal complications such as maternal anemia, very pre-term birth (less than 32 weeks), being born small for gestational age, neonatal cardiac problems, preeclampsia, placental infarction and sustaining a cephalhematoma at birth increase the risk factor for developing either anorexia nervosa or bulimia nervosa. Some of this developmental risk as in the case of placental infarction, maternal anemia and cardiac problems may cause intra-uterine hypoxia, umbilical cord occlusion or cord prolapse may cause ischemia, resulting in cerebral injury, the prefrontal cortex in the fetus and neonate is highly susceptible to damage as a result of oxygen deprivation which has been shown to contribute to executive dysfunction, ADHD, and may affect personality traits associated with both eating disorders and comorbid disorders such as impulsivity, mental rigidity and obsessionality. The problem of perinatal brain injury, in terms of the costs to society and to the affected individuals and their families, is extraordinary. (Yafeng Dong, PhD)

- Symptom of starvation: Evidence suggests that the symptoms of eating disorders are actually symptoms of the starvation itself, not of a mental disorder. In a study involving thirty-six healthy young men that were subjected to semi-starvation, the men soon began displaying symptoms commonly found in patients with eating disorders. In this study, the healthy men ate approximately half of what they had become accustomed to eating and soon began developing symptoms and thought patterns (preoccupation with food and eating, ritualistic eating, impaired cognitive ability, other physiological changes such as decreased body temperature) that are characteristic symptoms of anorexia nervosa. The men used in the study also developed hoarding and obsessive collecting behaviors, even though they had no use for the items, which revealed a possible connection between eating disorders and obsessive compulsive disorder.

Diagnosis

The initial diagnosis should be made by a competent medical professional. "The medical history is the most powerful tool for diagnosing eating disorders"(American Family Physician). There are many medical disorders that mimic eating disorders and comorbid psychiatric disorders. All organic causes should be ruled out prior to a diagnosis of an eating disorder or any other psychiatric disorder. In the past 30 years eating disorders have become increasingly conspicuous and it is uncertain whether the changes in presentation reflect a true increase. Anorexia nervosa and bulimia nervosa are the most clearly defined subgroups of a wider range of eating disorders. Many patients present with subthreshold expressions of the two main diagnoses: others with different patterns and symptoms.

Medical

The diagnostic workup typically includes complete medical and psychosocial history and follows a rational and formulaic approach to the diagnosis. Neuroimaging using fMRI, MRI, PET and

SPECT scans have been used to detect cases in which a lesion, tumor or other organic condition has been either the sole causative or contributory factor in an eating disorder. "Right frontal intracerebral lesions with their close relationship to the limbic system could be causative for eating disorders, we therefore recommend performing a cranial MRI in all patients with suspected eating disorders" (Trummer M *et al.* 2002), "intracranial pathology should also be considered however certain is the diagnosis of early-onset anorexia nervosa. Second, neuroimaging plays an important part in diagnosing early-onset anorexia nervosa, both from a clinical and a research prospective". (O'Brien *et al.* 2001).

Psychological

Eating Disorder Specific Psychometric Tests	
Eating Attitudes Test	SCOFF questionnaire
Body Attitudes Test	Body Attitudes Questionnaire
Eating Disorder Inventory	Eating Disorder Examination Interview

After ruling out organic causes and the initial diagnosis of an eating disorder being made by a medical professional, a trained mental health professional aids in the assessment and treatment of the underlying psychological components of the eating disorder and any comorbid psychological conditions. The clinician conducts a clinical interview and may employ various psychometric tests. Some are general in nature while others were devised specifically for use in the assessment of eating disorders. Some of the general tests that may be used are the Hamilton Depression Rating Scale and the Beck Depression Inventory. longitudinal research showed that there is an increase in chance that a young adult female would develop bulimia due to their current psychological pressure and as the person ages and matures, their emotional problems change or are resolved and then the symptoms decline.

Differential Diagnoses

There are multiple medical conditions which may be misdiagnosed as a primary psychiatric disorder, complicating or delaying treatment. These may have a synergistic effect on conditions which mimic an eating disorder or on a properly diagnosed eating disorder.

- Lyme disease which is known as the "great imitator", as it may present as a variety of psychiatric or neurological disorders including anorexia nervosa.

- Gastrointestinal diseases, such as celiac disease, Crohn's disease, peptic ulcer, eosinophilic esophagitis or non-celiac gluten sensitivity, among others. Celiac disease is also known as the "great imitator", because it may involve several organs and cause an extensive variety of non-gastrointestinal symptoms, such as psychiatric and neurological disorders, including anorexia nervosa.

- Addison's Disease is a disorder of the adrenal cortex which results in decreased hormonal production. Addison's disease, even in subclinical form may mimic many of the symptoms of anorexia nervosa.

- Gastric adenocarcinoma is one of the most common forms of cancer in the world. Complications due to this condition have been misdiagnosed as an eating disorder.

- Hypothyroidism, hyperthyroidism, hypoparathyroidism and hyperparathyroidism may mimic some of the symptoms of, can occur concurrently with, be masked by or exacerbate an eating disorder.

- Toxoplasma seropositivity: even in the absence of symptomatic toxoplasmosis, toxoplasma gondii exposure has been linked to changes in human behavior and psychiatric disorders including those comorbid with eating disorders such as depression. In reported case studies the response to antidepressant treatment improved only after adequate treatment for toxoplasma.

- Neurosyphilis: It is estimated that there may be up to one million cases of untreated syphilis in the US alone. "The disease can present with psychiatric symptoms alone, psychiatric symptoms that can mimic any other psychiatric illness". Many of the manifestations may appear atypical. Up to 1.3% of short term psychiatric admissions may be attributable to neurosyphilis, with a much higher rate in the general psychiatric population. (Ritchie, M Perdigao J,)

- Dysautonomia: a wide variety of autonomic nervous system (ANS) disorders may cause a wide variety of psychiatric symptoms including anxiety, panic attacks and depression. Dysautonomia usually involves failure of sympathetic or parasympathetic components of the ANS system but may also include excessive ANS activity. Dysautonomia can occur in conditions such as diabetes and alcoholism.

Psychological disorders which may be confused with an eating disorder, or be co-morbid with one:

- Emetophobia is an anxiety disorder characterized by an intense fear of vomiting. A person so afflicted may develop rigorous standards of food hygiene, such as not touching food with their hands. They may become socially withdrawn to avoid situations which in their perception may make them vomit. Many who suffer from emetophobia are diagnosed with anorexia or self-starvation. In severe cases of emetophobia they may drastically reduce their food intake.

- Phagophobia is an anxiety disorder characterized by a fear of eating, it is usually initiated by an adverse experience while eating such as choking or vomiting. Persons with this disorder may present with complaints of pain while swallowing.

- Body dysmorphic disorder (BDD) is listed as a somatoform disorder that affects up to 2% of the population. BDD is characterized by excessive rumination over an actual or perceived physical flaw. BDD has been diagnosed equally among men and women. While BDD has been misdiagnosed as anorexia nervosa, it also occurs comorbidly in 39% of eating disorder cases. BDD is a chronic and debilitating condition which may lead to social isolation, major depression and suicidal ideation and attempts. Neuroimaging studies to measure response to facial recognition have shown activity predominately in the left hemisphere in the left lateral prefrontal cortex, lateral temporal lobe and left parietal lobe showing hemispheric imbalance in information processing. There is a reported case of the development of BDD in a 21-year-old male following an inflammatory brain process. Neuroimaging showed the presence of a new atrophy in the frontotemporal region.

Prevention

Prevention aims to promote a healthy development before the occurrence of eating disorders. It also intends early identification of an eating disorder before it is too late to treat. Children as young as ages 5–7 are aware of the cultural messages regarding body image and dieting. Prevention comes in bringing these issues to the light. The following topics can be discussed with young children (as well as teens and young adults).

- Emotional Bites: a simple way to discuss emotional eating is to ask children about why they might eat besides being hungry. Talk about more effective ways to cope with emotions, emphasizing the value of sharing feelings with a trusted adult.

- Say No to Teasing: another concept is to emphasize that it is wrong to say hurtful things about other people's body sizes.

- Body Talk: emphasize the importance of listening to one's body. That is, eating when you are hungry (not starving) and stopping when you are satisfied (not stuffed). Children intuitively grasp these concepts.

- Fitness Comes in All Sizes: educate children about the genetics of body size and the normal changes occurring in the body. Discuss their fears and hopes about growing bigger. Focus on fitness and a balanced diet.

Internet and modern technologies provide new opportunities for prevention. On-line programs have the potential to increase the use of prevention programs. The development and practice of prevention programs via on-line sources make it possible to reach a wide range of people at minimal cost. Such an approach can also make prevention programs to be sustainable.

Treatment

Treatment varies according to type and severity of eating disorder, and usually more than one treatment option is utilized. There is no well-established treatment for eating disorders, meaning that current views about treatment are based mainly on clinical experience. Family doctors play an important role in early treatment of people with eating disorders by encouraging those who are also reluctant to see a psychiatrist. Treatment can take place in a variety of different settings such as community programs, hospitals, day programs, and groups. That said, some treatment methods are:

- Cognitive behavioral therapy (CBT), which postulates that an individual's feelings and behaviors are caused by their own thoughts instead of external stimuli such as other people, situations or events; the idea is to change how a person thinks and reacts to a situation even if the situation itself does not change.

  o Acceptance and commitment therapy: a type of CBT

  o Cognitive Remediation Therapy (CRT), a set of cognitive drills or compensatory interventions designed to enhance cognitive functioning.

- Dialectical behavior therapy

- Family therapy including "conjoint family therapy" (CFT), "separated family therapy" (SFT) and Maudsley Family Therapy.

- Behavioral therapy: focuses on gaining control and changing unwanted behaviors.

- Interpersonal psychotherapy (IPT)

- Cognitive Emotional Behaviour Therapy (CEBT)

- Music Therapy

- Recreation Therapy

- Art therapy

- Nutrition counseling and Medical nutrition therapy

- Medication: Orlistat is used in obesity treatment. Olanzapine seems to promote weight gain as well as the ability to ameliorate obsessional behaviors concerning weight gain. zinc supplements have been shown to be helpful, and cortisol is also being investigated.

- Self-help and guided self-help have been shown to be helpful in AN, BN and BED; this includes support groups and self-help groups such as Eating Disorders Anonymous and Overeaters Anonymous.

- Psychoanalysis

- Inpatient care

There are few studies on the cost-effectiveness of the various treatments. Treatment can be expensive; due to limitations in health care coverage, people hospitalized with anorexia nervosa may be discharged while still underweight, resulting in relapse and rehospitalization.

For children with anorexia, the only well-established treatment is the family treatment-behavior. For other eating disorders in children, however, there is no well-established treatments, though family treatment-behavior has been used in treating bulimia.

Outcomes

Outcome estimates are complicated by non-uniform criteria used by various studies, but for anorexia nervosa, bulimia nervosa, and binge eating disorder, there seems to be general agreement that full recovery rates are in the 50% to 85% range, with larger proportions of people experiencing at least partial remission. The outcomes of eating disorders (ED) vary among the cases. For many, it can be a lifelong struggle or it can be overcome within months. In the United States, twenty million women and ten million men have an eating disorders at least once in their lifetime. Depending on the type of eating disorder, the age that it began, previous psychiatric disorders, etc., the severity of the outcomes differ.

- Miscarriages: Pregnant women with a Binge Eating Disorder have shown to have a greater chance of having a miscarriage compared to pregnant women with any other eating disorders. According to a study done, out of a group of pregnant women being evaluated, 46.7% of the pregnancies ended with a miscarriage in women that were diagnosed with BED, with 23.0% in the control. In the same study, 21.4% of women diagnosed with Bulimia Nervosa had their pregnancies end with miscarriages and only 17.7% of the controls.

- Relapse: An individual who is in remission from BN and EDNOS (Eating Disorder Not Otherwise Specified) is at a high risk of falling back into the habit of self-harming themselves. Factors such as high stress regarding their job, pressures from society, as well as other occurrences that inflict stress on a person, can push a person back to what they feel will ease the pain. A study tracked a group of selected people that were either diagnosed with BN or EDNOS for 60 months. After the 60 months were complete, the researchers recorded whether or not the patients were suffering from a relapse. The results found that the probability of a person previously diagnosed with EDNOS had a 41% chance of relapsing; a person with BN had a 47% chance.

- Attachment insecurity: People who are showing signs of attachment anxiety will most likely have trouble communicating their emotional status as well as having trouble seeking effective social support. Signs that a person has adopted this symptom include not showing recognition to their caregiver or when he/she is feeling pain. In a clinical sample, it is clear that at the pretreatment step of a patient's recovery, more severe eating disorder symptoms directly corresponds to higher attachment anxiety. The more this symptom increases, the more difficult it is to achieve eating disorder reduction prior to treatment.

Anorexia Nervosa symptoms include the increasing chance of getting osteoporosis. This disease causes the bones of an individual to become brittle, weak, and low in density. Thinning of the hair as well as dry hair and skin is also very common. The muscles of the heart will also start to change if no treatment is inflicted on the patient. This causes the heart to have an abnormally slow heart rate along with low blood pressure. Heart failure becomes a major consideration when this begins to occur. Muscles throughout the body begin to lose their strength. This will cause the individual to begin feeling faint, drowsy, and weak. Along with these symptoms, the body will begin to grow a layer of hair called lanugo. The human body does this in response to the lack of heat and insulation due to the low percentage of body fat.

Bulimia nervosa symptoms include heart problems like an irregular heartbeat that can lead to heart failure and death may occur. This occurs because of the electrolyte imbalance that is a result of the constant binge and purge process. The probability of a gastric rupture increases. A gastric rupture is when there is a sudden rupture of the stomach lining that can be fatal. The acids that are contained in the vomit can cause a rupture in the esophagus as well as tooth decay. As a result, to laxative abuse, irregular bowel movements may occur along with constipation. Sores along the lining of the stomach called peptic ulcers begin to appear and the chance of developing pancreatitis increases.

Binge eating symptoms include high blood pressure, which can cause heart disease if it is not treated. Many patients recognize an increase in the levels of cholesterol. The chance of being diagnosed with gallbladder disease increases, which affects an individual's digestive tract.

Epidemiology

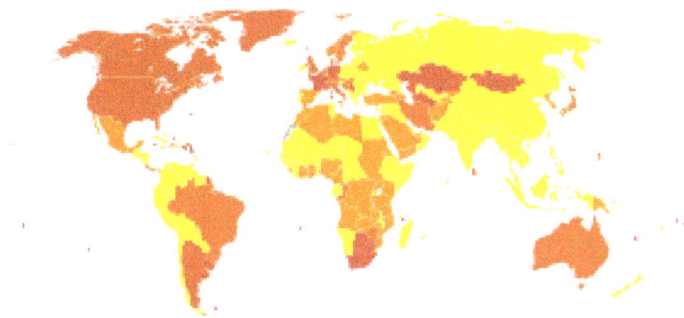

Deaths due to eating disorders per million persons in 2012

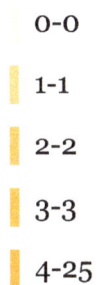

0-0

1-1

2-2

3-3

4-25

Eating disorders result in about 7,000 deaths a year as of 2010, making them the mental illnesses with the highest mortality rate.

One study in the United States found a higher rate in college students who are transgender.

Economics

Total costs in USA for hospital stays involving eating disorders rose from $165 million in 1999–2000 to $277 million in 2008–2009; this was a 68% increase. The mean cost per discharge of a person with an eating disorder rose by 29% over the decade, from $7,300 to $9,400.

Over the decade, hospitalizations involving eating disorders increased among all age groups. The greatest increases occurred among those 45 to 65 years of age (an 88% increase), followed by hospitalizations among people younger than 12 years of age (a 72% increase).

The majority of eating disorder inpatients were female. During 2008–2009, 88% of cases involved females, and 12% were males. The report also showed a 53% increase in hospitalizations for males with a principal diagnosis of an eating disorder, from 10% to 12% over the decade.

References

- Robert S. Goodhart; Maurice E. Shils (1980). Modern Nutrition in Health and Disease (6th ed.). Philadelphia: Lea and Febinger. pp. 134–138. ISBN 0-8121-0645-8.

- Kushner, Robert (2007). Treatment of the Obese Patient (Contemporary Endocrinology). Totowa, NJ: Humana Press. p. 158. ISBN 1-59745-400-1. Retrieved April 5, 2009.

- Woodhouse R (2008). "Obesity in art: A brief overview". Front Horm Res. Frontiers of Hormone Research. 36: 271–86. doi:10.1159/000115370. ISBN 978-3-8055-8429-6. PMID 18230908.

- Kolata,Gina (2007). Rethinking thin: The new science of weight loss – and the myths and realities of dieting. Picador. p. 122. ISBN 0-312-42785-9.

- Wilkinson, Richard; Pickett, Kate (2009). The Spirit Level: Why More Equal Societies Almost Always Do Better. London: Allen Lane. pp. 91–101. ISBN 978-1-84614-039-6.

- Boulpaep, Emile L.; Boron, Walter F. (2003). Medical physiology: A cellular and molecular approach. Philadelphia: Saunders. p. 1227. ISBN 0-7216-3256-4.

- Loscalzo, Joseph; Fauci, Anthony S.; Braunwald, Eugene; Dennis L. Kasper; Hauser, Stephen L; Longo, Dan L. (2008). Harrison's principles of internal medicine. McGraw-Hill Medical. ISBN 0-07-146633-9.

- Satcher D (2001). The Surgeon General's Call to Action to Prevent and Decrease Overweight and Obesity. U.S. Dept. of Health and Human Services, Public Health Service, Office of Surgeon General. ISBN 978-0-16-051005-2.

- Great Britain Parliament House of Commons Health Committee (May 2004). Obesity – Volume 1 – HCP 23-I, Third Report of session 2003–04. Report, together with formal minutes. London, UK: TSO (The Stationery Office). ISBN 978-0-215-01737-6. Retrieved 2007-12-17.

- Wanless, Sir Derek; Appleby, John; Harrison, Anthony; Patel, Darshan (2007). Our Future Health Secured? A review of NHS funding and performance. London, UK: The King's Fund. ISBN 1-85717-562-X.

- Theodore Mazzone; Giamila Fantuzzi (2006). Adipose Tissue And Adipokines in Health And Disease (Nutrition and Health). Totowa, NJ: Humana Press. p. 222. ISBN 1-58829-721-7.

- Fumento, Michael (1997). The Fat of the Land: Our Health Crisis and How Overweight Americans Can Help Themselves. Penguin (Non-Classics). p. 126. ISBN 0-14-026144-3.

- Prentice, editor-in-chief, Benjamin Caballero ; editors, Lindsay Allen, Andrew (2005). Encyclopedia of human nutrition (2nd ed.). Amsterdam: Elsevier/Academic Press. p. 68. ISBN 9780080454283.

- Ann Ashworth (2003). Guidelines for the inpatient treatment of severely malnourished children. Geneva: World Health Organization. ISBN 9241546093.

- editors, Ronnie A. Rosenthal, Michael E. Zenilman, Mark R. Katlic, (2011). Principles and practice of geriatric surgery (2nd ed.). Berlin: Springer. p. 78. ISBN 9781441969996.

- Walker, [edited by] Christopher Duggan, John B. Watkins, W. Allan (2008). Nutrition in pediatrics: basic science, clinical application. Hamilton: BC Decker. pp. 127–141. ISBN 978-1-55009-361-2.

- Management of diarrhoea with severe malnutrition". The Treatment of diarrhoea : a manual for physicians and other senior health workers. (PDF) (4 ed.). Geneva: World Health Organization. 2005. pp. 22–24. ISBN 924159318 0.

Processes Vital for Nutrition and Metabolism

The following chapter elucidates the various processes that are related to nutrition and metabolism. The major categories that this chapter explains are processes like metabolic pathway, ketogenesis, fatty acid metabolism, fermentation and oxidative phosphorylation. The aspects elucidated are of vital importance, and provide a better understanding on the topic.

Metabolic Pathway

In biochemistry, a metabolic pathway is a linked series of chemical reactions occurring within a cell. The reactants, products, and intermediates of an enzymatic reaction are known as metabolites, which are modified by a sequence of chemical reactions catalyzed by enzymes. In a metabolic pathway, the product of one enzyme acts as the substrate for the next. These enzymes often require dietary minerals, vitamins, and other cofactors to function.

Different metabolic pathways function based on the position within a eukaryotic cell and the significance of the pathway in the given compartment of the cell. For instance, the citric acid cycle, electron transport chain, and oxidative phosphorylation all take place in the mitochondrial membrane. In contrast, glycolysis, pentose phosphate pathway, and fatty acid biosynthesis all occur in the cytosol of a cell.

There are two types of metabolic pathways that are characterized by their ability to either synthesize molecules with the utilization of energy (anabolic pathway) or break down of complex molecules by releasing energy in the process (catabolic pathway). The two pathways compliment each other in that the energy released from one is used up by the other. The degradative process of a catabolic pathway provides the energy required to conduct a biosynthesis of an anabolic pathway. In addition to the two distinct metabolic pathways is the amphibolic pathway, which can be either catabolic or anabolic based on the need for or the availability of energy.

Pathways are required for the maintenance of homeostasis within an organism and the flux of metabolites through a pathway is regulated depending on the needs of the cell and the availability of the substrate. The end product of a pathway may be used immediately, initiate another metabolic pathway or be stored for later use. The metabolism of a cell consists of an elaborate network of interconnected pathways that enable the synthesis and breakdown of molecules (anabolism and catabolism)

Overview

Each metabolic pathway consists of a series of biochemical reactions that are connected by their intermediates: the products of one reaction are the substrates for subsequent reactions, and so on. Metabolic pathways are often considered to flow in one direction. Although all chemical reactions are technically reversible, conditions in the cell are often such that it is thermodynamically more favorable for flux to flow in one direction of a reaction. For example, one pathway may be responsible for the synthesis of a particular amino acid, but the breakdown of that amino acid may occur via a separate and distinct pathway. One example of an exception to this "rule" is the metabolism of glucose. Glycolysis results in the breakdown of glucose, but several reactions in the glycolysis pathway are reversible and participate in the re-synthesis of glucose (gluconeogenesis).

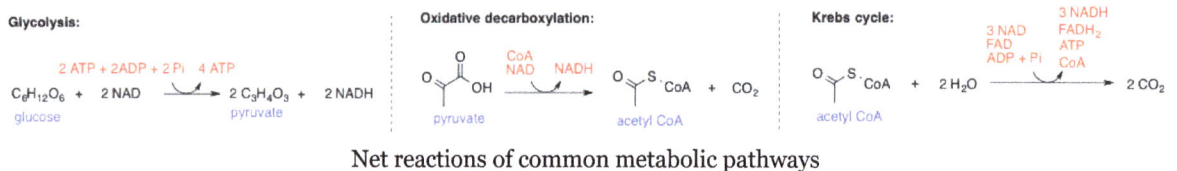

Net reactions of common metabolic pathways

- Glycolysis was the first metabolic pathway discovered:

1. As glucose enters a cell, it is immediately phosphorylated by ATP to glucose 6-phosphate in the irreversible first step.

2. In times of excess lipid or protein energy sources, certain reactions in the glycolysis pathway may run in reverse in order to produce glucose 6-phosphate which is then used for storage as glycogen or starch.

- Metabolic pathways are often regulated by feedback inhibition.

- Some metabolic pathways flow in a 'cycle' wherein each component of the cycle is a sub-strate for the subsequent reaction in the cycle, such as in the Krebs Cycle.

- Anabolic and catabolic pathways in eukaryotes often occur independently of each other, separated either physically by compartmentalization within organelles or separated biochemically by the requirement of different enzymes and co-factors.

Major Metabolic Pathways

Catabolic Pathway (Catabolism)

A catabolic pathway is a series of reactions that bring about a net release of energy in the form of a high energy phosphate bond formed with the energy carriers Adenosine Diphosphate (ADP) and Guanosine Diphosphate (GDP) to produce Adenosine Triphosphate (ATP) and Guanosine Triphosphate (GTP), respectively. The net reaction is, therefore, thermodynamically favorable, for it results in a lower free energy for the final products. A catabolic pathway is an exergonic system that produces chemical energy in the form of ATP, GTP, NADH, NADPH, FADH2, etc. from energy containing sources such as carbohydrates, fats, and proteins. The end products are often carbon dioxide, water, and ammonia. Coupled with an endergonic reaction of anabolism, the cell can synthesize new macromolecules using the original precursors of the anabolic pathway. An example of a coupled reaction is the phosphorylation of fructose-6-phosphate to form the intermediate fructose-1,6-bisphosphate by the enzyme phsophofructokinase accompanied by the hydrolysis of ATP in the pathway of glycolysis. The resulting chemical reaction within the metabolic pathway is highly thermodynamically favorable and, as a result, irreversible in the cell.

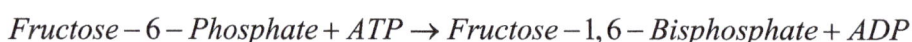

$$Fructose-6-Phosphate+ATP \rightarrow Fructose-1,6-Bisphosphate+ADP$$

Cellular Respiration

A core set of energy-producing catabolic pathways occur within all living organisms in some form. These pathways transfer the energy released by breakdown of nutrients into ATP and other small molecules used for energy (e.g. GTP, NADPH, FADH). All cells can perform anaerobic respiration by glycolysis. Additionally, most organisms can perform more efficient aerobic respiration through the citric acid cycle and oxidative phosphorylation. Additionally plants, algae and cyanobacteria are able to use sunlight to anabolically synthesize compounds from non-living matter by photosynthesis.

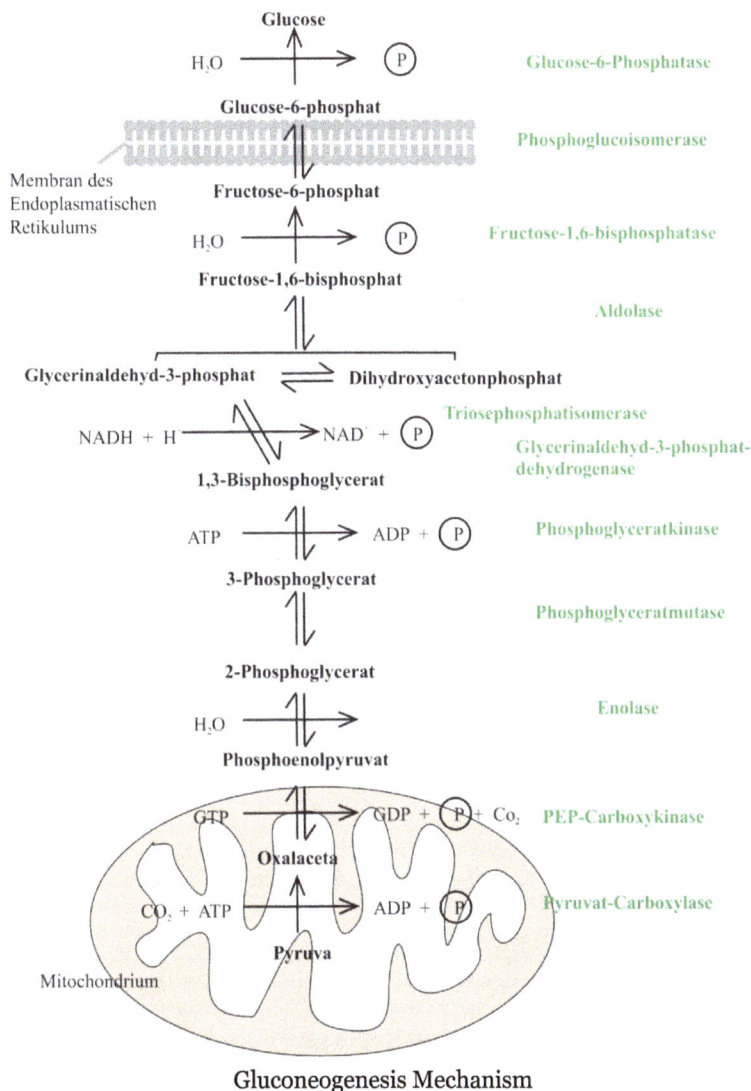

Gluconeogenesis Mechanism

Anabolic Pathway (Anabolism)

In contrast to the catabolic pathways, are the anabolic pathways that require an input of energy in order to conduct the construction of macromolecules such as polypeptides, nucleic acids, proteins, polysaccharides, and lipids. The isolated reaction of anabolism is unfavorable in a cell due to a positive Gibbs Free Energy ($+\Delta G$); thus, an input of chemical energy through a coupling with an exergonic reaction is necessary. The coupled reaction of the catabolic pathway affects the thermodynamics of the reaction by lowering the overall activation energy of an anabolic pathway and allowing the reaction to take place. Otherwise, an endergonic reaction is non-spontaneous.

An anabolic pathway is a biosynthetic pathway, meaning that it combines smaller molecules to form larger and more complex ones. An example is the reversed pathway of glycolysis, otherwise known as gluconeogenesis, which occurs in the liver and sometimes in the kidney in order to maintain proper glucose concentration in the blood and to be able to supply the brain and muscle tissues with adequate amount of glucose. Although gluconeogenesis is similar to the reverse pathway of glycolysis, it contains three distinct enzymes from glycolysis that allow the pathway to occur spontaneously. An example of the pathway for gluconeogenesis is illustrated in the image titled "Gluconeogenesis Mechanism".

Amphibolic Pathway

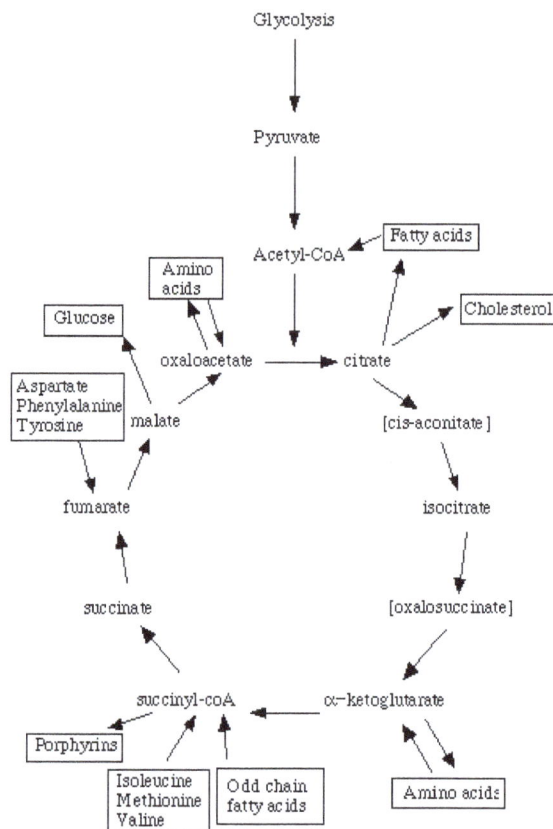

Amphibolic Properties of the Citric Acid Cycle

An amphibolic pathway is one that can be either catabolic or anabolic based on the availability of or the need for energy. The currency of energy in a biological cell is adenosine triphosphate (ATP), which stores its energy in the phosphoanhydride bonds. The energy is utilized to conduct biosynthesis, facilitate movement, and regulate active transport inside of the cell. Examples of amphibolic pathways are the citric acid cycle and the glyoxylate cycle. These sets of chemical reactions contain both energy producing and utilizing pathways. To the right is an illustration of the amphibolic properties of the TCA cycle.

The glyoxylate shunt pathway is an alternative to the tricarboxylic acid (TCA) cycle, for it redirects the pathway of TCA to prevent full oxidation of carbon compounds, and to preserve high energy carbon sources as future energy sources. This pathway occurs only in plants and bacteria and transpires in the absence of glucose molecules.

Regulation

The flux of the entire pathway is regulated by the rate-determining steps. These are the slowest steps in a network of reactions. The rate-limiting step occurs near the beginning of the pathway and is regulated by feedback inhibition, which ultimately controls the overall rate of the pathway. The metabolic pathway in the cell is regulated by covalent or non-covalent modifications. A covalent modification involves an addition or removal of a chemical bond, whereas a non-covalent modification (also known as allosteric regulation) is the binding of the regulator to the enzyme via hydrogen bonds, electrostatic interactions, and Van Der Waals forces.

The rate of turnover in a metabolic pathway, otherwise known as the metabolic flux, is regulated based on the stoichiometric reaction model, the utilization rate of metabolites, and the translocation pace of molecules across the lipid bilayer. The regulation methods are based on experiments involving 13C-labeling, which is then analyzed by Nuclear Magnetic Resonance (NMR) or gas chromatography-mass spectrometry (GC-MS)-derived mass compositions. The aforementioned techniques synthesize a statistical interpretation of mass distribution in proteinogenic amino acids to the catalytic activities of enzymes in a cell.

Ketogenesis

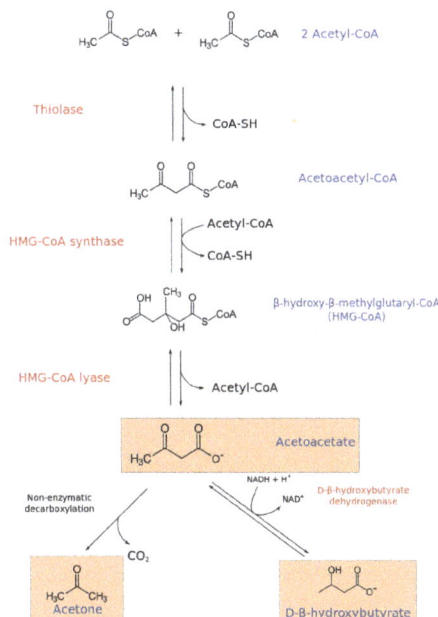

Ketogenesis pathway. The three ketone bodies (acetoacetate, acetone, and beta-hydroxy-butyrate) are marked within an orange box

Ketogenesis is the biochemical process by which organisms produce a group of substances collectively known as ketone bodies by the breakdown of fatty acids and ketogenic amino acids. This process supplies energy to certain organs (particularly the brain) under circumstances such as fasting, but insufficient ketogenesis can cause hypoglycemia and excessive production of ketone bodies leads to a dangerous state known as ketoacidosis.

Production

Ketone bodies are produced mainly in the mitochondria of liver cells, and synthesis can occur in response to an unavailability of blood glucose, such as during fasting.

Ketogenesis takes place in the setting of low glucose levels in the blood, after exhaustion of other cellular carbohydrate stores, such as glycogen. It can also take place when there is insufficient insulin (e.g. in diabetes), particularly during periods of "ketogenic stress" such as intercurrent illness.

The production of ketone bodies is then initiated to make available energy that is stored as fatty acids. Fatty acids are enzymatically broken down in β-oxidation to form acetyl-CoA. Under normal conditions, acetyl-CoA is further oxidized by the citric acid cycle (TCA/Krebs cycle) and then by the mitochondrial electron transport chain to release energy. However, if the amounts of acetyl-CoA generated in fatty-acid β-oxidation challenge the processing capacity of the TCA cycle; i.e. if activity in TCA cycle is low due to low amounts of intermediates such as oxaloacetate, acetyl-CoA is then used instead in biosynthesis of ketone bodies via acetoacyl-CoA and β-hydroxy-β-methylglutaryl-CoA (HMG-CoA). Deaminated amino acids that are ketogenic, such as leucine, also feed TCA cycle, forming acetoacetate & ACoA and thereby produce ketones. Besides its role in the synthesis of ketone bodies, HMG-CoA is also an intermediate in the synthesis of cholesterol, but the steps are compartmentalised. Ketogenesis occurs in the mitochondria, whereas cholesterol synthesis occurs in the cytosol, hence both the processes are independently regulated.

Ketone Bodies

The three ketone bodies, each synthesized from acetyl-CoA molecules, are:

- Acetoacetate, which can be converted by the liver into β-hydroxybutyrate, or spontaneously turn into acetone

- Acetone, which is generated through the decarboxylation of acetoacetate, either spontaneously or through the enzyme acetoacetate decarboxylase. It can then be further metabolized either by CYP2E1 into hydroxyacetone (acetol) and then via propylene glycol to pyruvate, lactate and acetate (usable for energy) and propionaldehyde, or via methylglyoxal to pyruvate and lactate.

- β-hydroxybutyrate (not technically a ketone according to IUPAC nomenclature) is generated through the action of the enzyme D-β-hydroxybutyrate dehydrogenase on acetoacetate.

Regulation

Ketogenesis may or may not occur, depending on levels of available carbohydrates in the cell or body. This is closely related to the paths of acetyl-CoA:

- When the body has ample carbohydrates available as energy source, glucose is completely oxidized to CO_2; acetyl-CoA is formed as an intermediate in this process, first entering the citric acid cycle followed by complete conversion of its chemical energy to ATP in oxidative phosphorylation.

- When the body has excess carbohydrates available, some glucose is fully metabolized, and some of it is stored in the form of glycogen or, upon citrate excess, as fatty acids. (CoA is also recycled here.)

- When the body has no free carbohydrates available, fat must be broken down into acetyl-CoA in order to get energy. Acetyl-CoA is not being recycled through the citric acid cycle because the citric acid cycle intermediates (mainly oxaloacetate) have been depleted to feed the gluconeogenesis pathway, and the resulting accumulation of acetyl-CoA activates ketogenesis.

Pathology

Both acetoacetate and beta-hydroxybutyrate are acidic, and, if levels of these ketone bodies are too high, the pH of the blood drops, resulting in ketoacidosis. Ketoacidosis is known to occur in untreated type I diabetes and in alcoholics after prolonged binge-drinking without intake of sufficient carbohydrates.

Ketogenesis can be ineffective in people with beta oxidation defects.

Fatty Acid Metabolism

Fatty acids are a family of molecules classified within the lipid macronutrient class. One role of fatty acids within animal metabolism is energy production, captured in the form of adenosine triphosphate (ATP). When compared to other macronutrient classes (carbohydrates and protein), fatty acids yield the most ATP on an energy per gram basis, when they are completely oxidized to CO_2 and water by β-oxidation and the citric acid cycle. Fatty acids (mainly in the form of triglycerides) are therefore the foremost storage form of fuel in most animals, and to a lesser extent in plants. In addition, fatty acids are important components of the phospholipids that form the phospholipid bilayers out of which all the membranes of the cell are constructed (the cell wall, and the membranes that enclose all the organelles within the cells, such as the nucleus, the mitochondria, endoplasmic reticulum, and the Golgi apparatus). Fatty acids can also be cleaved, or partially cleaved, from their chemical attachments in the cell membrane to form second messengers within the cell, and local hormones in the immediate vicinity of the cell. The prostaglandins made from arachidonic acid stored in the cell wall, are probably the most well known group of these local hormones. Fatty acid metabolism consists of catabolic processes that generate energy, and anabolic processes that create biologically important molecules (triglycerides, phospholipids, second messengers, local hormones and ketone bodies).

Fatty Acid Catabolism

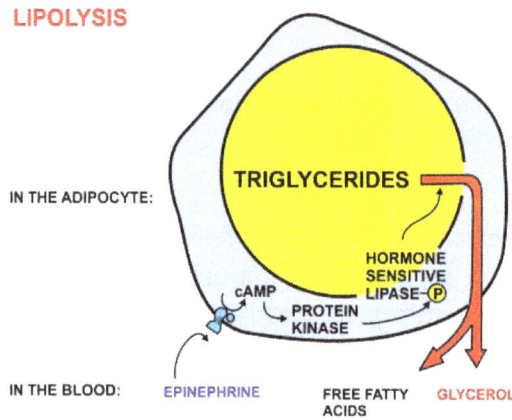

A diagrammatic illustration of the process of lipolysis (in a fat cell) induced by high epinephrine and low insulin levels in the blood. Epinephrine binds to a beta-adrenergic receptor in the cell wall of the adipocyte, which causes cAMP to be generated inside the cell. The cAMP activates a protein kinase, which phosphorylates and thus, in turn, activates a hormone-sensitive lipase in the fat cell. This lipase cleaves free fatty acids from their attachment to glycerol in the fat stored in the fat droplet of the adipocyte. The free fatty acids and glycerol are then released into the blood. However more recent studies have shown that adipose triglyceride lipase has to first convert triacylglycerides to diacylglycerides, and that hormone-sensitive lipase converts the diacylglycerides to monoglycerides and free fatty acids. Monoglycerides are hydrolyzed by monoglyceride lipase. The activity of hormone sensitive lipase is regulated by the circulation hormones insulin, glucagon, norepinephrine, and epinephrine, as shown in the diagram.

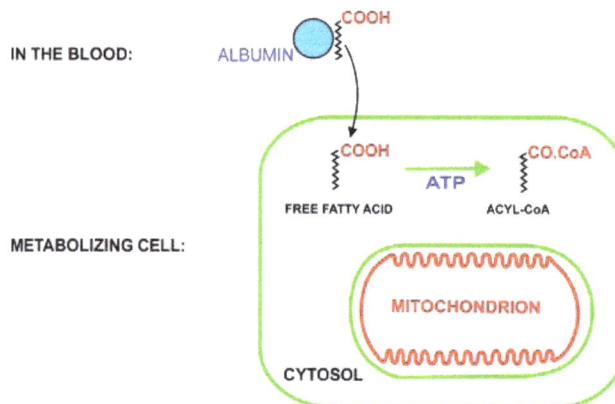

A diagrammatic illustration of the transport of free fatty acids in the blood attached to plasma albumin, its diffusion across the cell membrane using a protein transporter, and its activation, using ATP, to form acyl-CoA in the cytosol. The illustration is, for diagrammatic purposes, of a 12 carbon fatty acid. Most fatty acids in human plasma are 16 or 18 carbon atoms long.

**TRANSFER
INTO THE
MITOCHONDRION**

CAT IS INHIBITED BY **MALONYL- CoA**

ACYL- CoA
IN CYTOSOL   CO.CoA

CARNITINE   CAT

CO.CoA

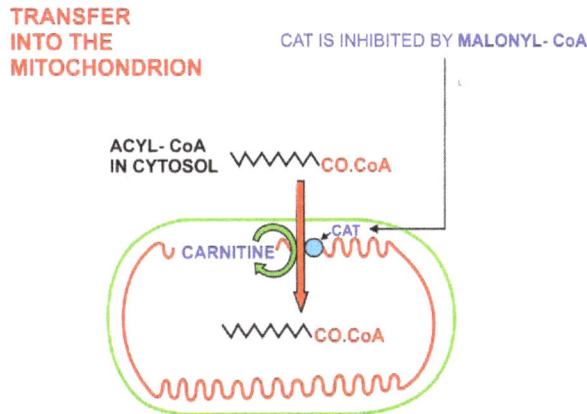

A diagrammatic illustration of the transfer of an acyl-CoA molecule across the inner membrane of the mitochondrion by carnitine-acyl-CoA transferase (CAT). The illustrated acyl chain is, for diagrammatic purposes, only 12 carbon atoms long. Most fatty acids in human plasma are 16 or 18 carbon atoms long. CAT is inhibited by high concentrations of malonyl-CoA (the first committed step in fatty acid synthesis) in the cytoplasm. This means that fatty acid synthesis and fatty acid catabolism cannot occur simultaneously in any given cell.

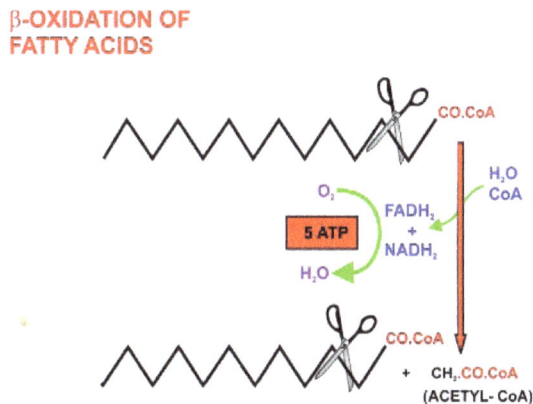

**β-OXIDATION OF
FATTY ACIDS**

CO.CoA

O_2

H_2O
CoA

5 ATP

$FADH_2$
+
$NADH_2$

H_2O

CO.CoA

+ CH_3.CO.CoA
(ACETYL- CoA)

A diagrammatic illustration of the process of the beta-oxidation of an acyl-CoA molecule in the mitochodrial matrix. During this process an acyl-CoA molecule which is 2 carbons shorter than it was at the beginning of the process is formed. Acetyl-CoA, water and 5 ATP molecules are the other products of each beta-oxidative event, until the entire acyl-CoA molecule has been reduced to a set of acetyl-CoA molecules.

Fatty acids are released, between meals, from the fat depots in adipose tissue, where they are stored as triglycerides, as follows:

- Lipolysis, the removal of the fatty acid chains from the glycerol to which they are bound in their storage form as triglycerides (or fats), is carried out by lipases. These lipases are activated by high epinephrine and glucagon levels in the blood (or norepinephrine secreted by sympathetic nerves in adipose tissue), caused by declining blood glucose levels after meals, which simultaneously lowers the insulin level in the blood.

- Once freed from glycerol, the free fatty acids enter the blood, which transports them, attached to plasma albumin, throughout the body.

- Long chain free fatty acids enter the metabolizing cells (i.e. most living cells in the body except red blood cells and neurons in the central nervous system) through specific transport proteins, such as the SLC27 family fatty acid transport protein. Red blood cells do not contain mitochondria and are therefore incapable of metabolizing fatty acids; the tissues of the central nervous system cannot use fatty acids, despite containing mitochondria, because fatty acids cannot cross the blood brain barrier into the interstitial fluids that bathe these cells.

- Once inside the cell long-chain-fatty-acid—CoA ligase catalyzes the reaction between a fatty acid molecule with ATP (which is broken down to AMP and inorganic pyrophosphate) to give a fatty acyl-adenylate, which then reacts with free coenzyme A to give a fatty acyl-CoA molecule.

- In order for the acyl-CoA to enter the mitochondrion the carnitine shuttle is used:

1. Acyl-CoA is transferred to the hydroxyl group of carnitine by carnitine palmitoyltransferase I, located on the cytosolic faces of the outer and inner mitochondrial membranes.

2. Acyl-carnitine is shuttled inside by a carnitine-acylcarnitine translocase, as a carnitine is shuttled outside.

3. Acyl-carnitine is converted back to acyl-CoA by carnitine palmitoyltransferase II, located on the interior face of the inner mitochondrial membrane. The liberated carnitine is shuttled back to the cytosol, as an acyl-CoA is shuttled into the matrix.

- Beta oxidation, in the mitochondrial matrix, then cuts the long carbon chains of the fatty acids (in the form of acyl-CoA molecules) into a series of two-carbon (acetate) units, which, combined with co-enzyme A, form molecules of acetyl CoA, which condense with oxaloacetate to form citrate at the "beginning" of the citric acid cycle. It is convenient to think of this reaction as marking the "starting point" of the cycle, as this is when fuel - acetyl-CoA - is added to the cycle, which will be dissipated as CO_2 and H_2O with the release of a substantial quantity of energy captured in the form of ATP, during the course of each turn of the cycle.

  Briefly, the steps in β-oxidation (the initial breakdown of free fatty acids into acetyl-CoA) are as follows:

1. Dehydrogenation by acyl-CoA dehydrogenase, yielding 1 $FADH_2$

2. Hydration by enoyl-CoA hydratase

3. Dehydrogenation by 3-hydroxyacyl-CoA dehydrogenase, yielding 1 $NADH + H^+$

4. Cleavage by thiolase, yielding 1 acetyl-CoA and a fatty acid that has now been shortened by 2 carbons (forming a new, shortened acyl-CoA)

This β-oxidation reaction is repeated until the fatty acid has been completely reduced to acetyl-CoA or, in, the case of fatty acids with odd numbers of carbon atoms, acetyl-CoA and 1 molecule of propionyl-CoA per molecule of fatty acid. Each β-oxidative cut of the acyl-CoA molecule yields 5 ATP molecules.

- The acetyl-CoA produced by β-oxidation enters the citric acid cycle in the mitochondrion by combining with oxaloacetate to form citrate. This results in the complete combustion of the acetyl-CoA to CO_2 and water. The energy released in this process is captured in the form of 1 GTP and 11 ATP molecules per acetyl-CoA molecule oxidized. This is the fate of acetyl-CoA wherever β-oxidation of fatty acids occurs, except under certain circumstances in the liver. In the liver oxaloacetate can be wholly or partially diverted into the gluconeogenic pathway during fasting, starvation, a low carbohydrate diet, prolonged strenuous exercise, and in uncontrolled type 1 diabetes mellitus. Under these circumstances oxaloacetate is hydrogenated to malate which is then removed from the mitochondrion to be converted into glucose in the cytoplasm of the liver cells, from where it is released into the blood. In the liver, therefore, oxaloacetate is unavailable for condensation with acetyl-CoA when significant gluconeogenesis has been stimulated by low (or absent) insulin and high glucagon concentrations in the blood. Under these circumstances acetyl-CoA is diverted to the formation of acetoacetate and beta-hydroxybutyrate. Acetoacetate, beta-hydroxybutyrate, and their spontaneous breakdown product, acetone, are frequently, but confusingly, known as ketone bodies (as they are not "bodies" at all, but water-soluble chemical substances). The ketone bodies are released by the liver into the blood. All cells with mitochondria can take ketone bodies up from the blood and reconvert them into acetyl-CoA, which can then be used as fuel in their citric acid cycles, as no other tissue can divert its oxaloacetate into the gluconeogenic pathway in the way that this can occur in the liver. Unlike free fatty acids, ketone bodies can cross the blood-brain barrier and are therefore available as fuel for the cells of the central nervous system, acting as a substitute for glucose, on which these cells normally survive. The occurrence of high levels of ketone bodies in the blood during starvation, a low carbohydrate diet, prolonged heavy exercise and uncontrolled type 1 diabetes mellitus is known as ketosis, and, in its extreme form, in out-of-control type 1 diabetes mellitus, as ketoacidosis.

The glycerol released by lipase action is phosphorylated by glycerol kinase in the liver (the only tissue in which this reaction can occur), and the resulting glycerol 3-phosphate is oxidized to dihydroxyacetone phosphate. The glycolytic enzyme triose phosphate isomerase converts this compound to glyceraldehyde 3-phosphate, which is oxidized via glycolysis, or converted to glucose via gluconeogenesis.

Fatty Acids as an Energy Source

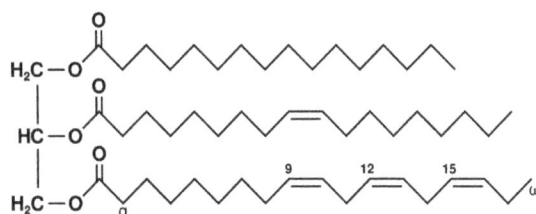

Example of an unsaturated fat triglyceride. Left part: glycerol, right part from top to bottom: palmitic acid, oleic acid, alpha-linolenic acid. Chemical formula: $C_{55}H_{98}O_6$

Fatty acids, stored as triglycerides in an organism, are an important source of energy because they are both reduced and anhydrous. The energy yield from a gram of fatty acids is approximately 9 kcal (37 kJ), compared to 4 kcal (17 kJ) for carbohydrates. Since the hydrocarbon portion of fatty acids is hydrophobic, these molecules can be stored in a relatively anhydrous (water-free) environment. Carbohydrates, on the other hand, are more highly hydrated. For example, 1 g of glycogen can bind approximately 2 g of water, which translates to 1.33 kcal/g (4 kcal/3 g). This means that fatty acids can hold more than six times the amount of energy per unit of storage mass. Put another way, if the human body relied on carbohydrates to store energy, then a person would need to carry 31 kg (67.5 lb) of hydrated glycogen to have the energy equivalent to 4.6 kg (10 lb) of fat.

Hibernating animals provide a good example for utilizing fat reserves as fuel. For example, bears hibernate for about 7 months, and, during this entire period, the energy is derived from degradation of fat stores. Migrating birds similarly build up large fat reserves before embarking on their intercontinental journeys.

Thus the young adult human's fat stores average between about 10–20 kg, but varies greatly depending on age, gender, and individual disposition. By contrast the human body stores only about 400 g of glycogen, of which 300 g is locked inside the skeletal muscles and is unavailable to the body as a whole. The 100 g or so of glycogen stored in the liver is depleted within one day of starvation. Thereafter the glucose that is released into the blood by the liver for general use by the body tissues, has to be synthesized from the glucogenic amino acids and a few other gluconeogenic substrates, which do not include fatty acids.

Animals Can Synthesize Carbohydrates From the Glycerol Portion of Triglycerides but not From the Fatty Acid Portion

Fatty acids are broken down to acetyl-CoA by means of beta oxidation inside the mitochondria, whereas fatty acids are synthesized from acetyl-CoA outside the mitochondria, in the cytosol. The two pathways are distinct, not only in where they occur, but also in the reactions that occur, and the substrates that are used. The two pathways are mutually inhibitory, preventing the acetyl-CoA produced by beta-oxidation from entering the synthetic pathway via the acetyl-CoA carboxylase reaction. It can also not be converted to pyruvate as the pyruvate decarboxylase reaction is irreversible. Instead the acetyl-CoA produced by the beta-oxidation of fatty acids condenses with oxaloacetate, to enter the citric acid cycle. During each turn of the cycle, two carbon atoms leave the cycle as CO_2 in the decarboxylation reactions catalyzed by isocitrate dehydrogenase and alpha-ketoglutarate dehydrogenase. Thus each turn of the citric acid cycle oxidizes an acetyl-CoA unit while regenerating the oxaloacetate molecule with which the acetyl-CoA had originally combined to form citric acid. The decarboxylation reactions occur before malate is formed in the cycle. This is the only substance that can be removed from the mitochondrion to enter the gluconeogenic pathway to form glucose or glycogen in the liver or any other tissue. There can therefore be no net conversion of fatty acids into glucose.

The energy in the fat stores is therefore extracted directly via the beta-oxidation of their fatty acids, and their combustion in the citric acid cycle, and never via their conversion to carbohydrates.

The glycerol released into the blood during the lipolysis of triglycerides in adipose tissue can only be taken up by the liver. Here it is converted into glycerol 3-phosphate by the action of glycerol kinase which hydrolyzes one molecule of ATP per glycerol molecule which is phosphorylated. Glycerol 3-phosphate is then oxidized to dihydroxyacetone phosphate, which is, in turn, converted into glyceraldehyde 3-phosphate by the enzyme triose phosphate isomerase. From here the three carbon atoms of the original glycerol can be oxidized via glycolysis, or converted to glucose via gluconeogenesis.

Only plants possess the enzymes to convert acetyl-CoA into oxaloacetate from which malate can be formed to ultimately be converted to glucose.

Other Functions and uses of Fatty Acids

Intracellular Signaling

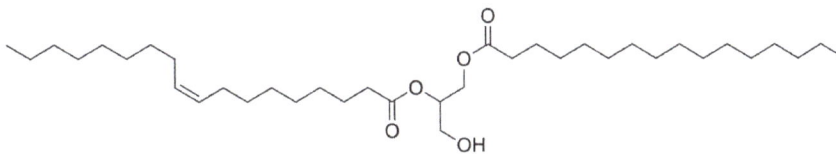

Chemical structure of the diglyceride 1-palmitoyl-2-oleoyl-glycerol

Fatty acids are an integral part of the phospholipids that make up the bulk of the plasma membranes, or cell membranes, of cells. These phospholipids can be cleaved into diacylglycerol (DAG) and inositol trisphosphate (IP_3) through hydrolysis of the phospholipid, phosphatidylinositol 4,5-bisphosphate (PIP_2), by the cell membrane bound enzyme phospholipase C (PLC).

An example of a diacyl-glycerol shown on the right. This DAG is 1-palmitoyl-2-oleoyl-glycerol, which contains side-chains derived from palmitic acid and oleic acid. Diacylglycerols can also have many other combinations of fatty acids attached at either the C-1 and C-2 positions or the C-1 and C-3 positions of the glycerol molecule. 1,2 disubstituted glycerols are always chiral, 1,3 disubstituted glycerols are chiral if the substituents are different from each other.

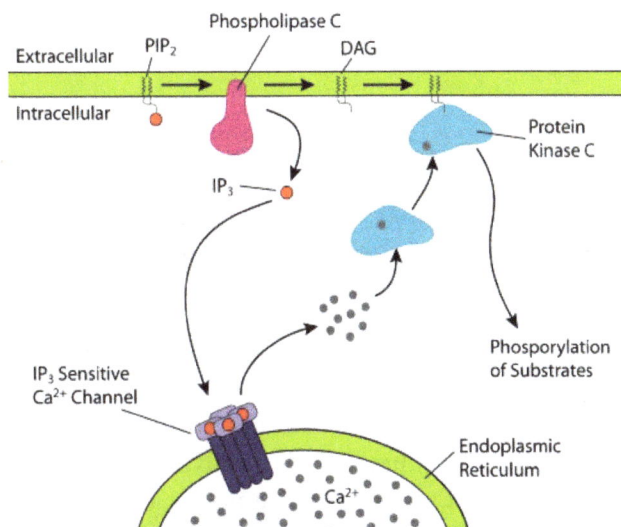

PIP_2 cleavage to IP_3 and DAG. IP_3 initiates intracellular calcium release, while DAG activates PKC (protein kinase C). Note: PLC (phospholipase C) is not an intermediate, as possibly suggested by the diagram, but is the enzyme that catalyzes the IP3/DAG separation.

Inositol trisphosphate (IP$_3$) functions as an intracellular second messenger, which initiates the intracellular release of calcium ions (which activates intracellular enzymes, causes the release of hormones and neurotransmitters from the cells in which they are stored, and causes smooth muscle contraction when released by IP$_3$), and the activation of protein kinase C (PKC), which is then translocated from the cell cytoplasm to the cell membrane. Although inositol trisphosphate, (IP$_3$), diffuses into the cytosol, diacylglycerol (DAG) remains within the plasma membrane, due to its hydrophobic properties. IP$_3$ stimulates the release of calcium ions from the smooth endoplasmic reticulum, whereas DAG is a physiological activator of protein kinase C (PKC), promoting its translocation from the cytosol to the plasma membrane. PKC is a multifunctional protein kinase which phosphorylates serine and threonine residues in many target proteins. However PKC is only active in the presence of calcium ions, and it is DAG that increases the affinity of PKC for Ca^{2+} and thereby renders it active at the physiological intracellular levels of this ion.

Diacylglycerol and IP$_3$ act transiently because both are rapidly metabolized. This is important as their message function should not linger after the message has been" received" by their target molecules. DAG can be phosphorylated to phosphatidate or it can be it can be hydrolysed to glycerol and its constituent fatty acids. IP$_3$ is rapidly converted to into derivatives that that do not open calcium ion channels.

Eicosanoid Paracrine Hormones

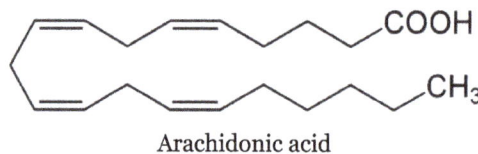

Arachidonic acid

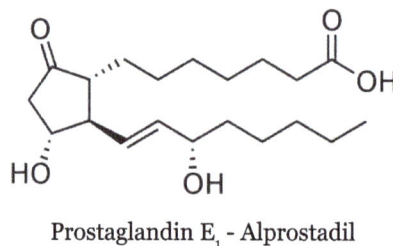

Prostaglandin E$_1$ - Alprostadil

The prostaglandins are a group of physiologically active lipid compounds having diverse hormone-like effects in animals. Prostaglandins have been found in almost every tissue in humans and other animals. They are enzymatically derived from arachidonic acid a 20-carbon polyunsaturated fatty acid. Every prostaglandin therefore contains 20 carbon atoms, including a 5-carbon ring. They are a subclass of eicosanoids and form the prostanoid class of fatty acid derivatives.

The prostaglandins are synthesized in the cell membrane by the cleavage of arachidonate from the phospholipids that make up the membrane. This is catalyzed either by phospholipase A$_2$ acting directly on a membrane phospholipid, or by a lipase acting on DAG (diacyl-glycerol). The arachidonate is then acted upon by the cyclooxygenase component of prostaglandin synthase. This forms a cyclopentane ring in roughly the middle of the fatty acid chain. The reaction also adds 4 oxygen atoms derived from two molecules of O$_2$. The resulting molecule is prostaglandin G$_2$ which is converted by the hydroperoxidase component of the enzyme complex into prostaglandin

H_2. This highly unstable compound is rapidly transformed into other prostaglandins, prostacyclin and thromboxanes. These are then released into the interstitial fluids surrounding the cells that have manufactured the eicosanoid hormone.

If arachidonate is acted upon by a lipoxygenase instead of cyclooxygenase, Hydroxyeicosatetraenoic acids and leukotrienes are formed. They also act as local hormones.

Prostaglandins were originally believed to leave the cells via passive diffusion because of their high lipophilicity. The discovery of the prostaglandin transporter (PGT, SLCO2A1), which mediates the cellular uptake of prostaglandin, demonstrated that diffusion alone cannot explain the penetration of prostaglandin through the cellular membrane. The release of prostaglandin has now also been shown to be mediated by a specific transporter, namely the multidrug resistance protein 4 (MRP4, ABCC4), a member of the ATP-binding cassette transporter superfamily. Whether MRP4 is the only transporter releasing prostaglandins from the cells is still unclear.

The structural differences between prostaglandins account for their different biological activities. A given prostaglandin may have different and even opposite effects in different tissues. The ability of the same prostaglandin to stimulate a reaction in one tissue and inhibit the same reaction in another tissue is determined by the type of receptor to which the prostaglandin binds. They act as autocrine or paracrine factors with their target cells present in the immediate vicinity of the site of their secretion. Prostaglandins differ from endocrine hormones in that they are not produced at a specific site but in many places throughout the human body.

Prostaglandins have two derivatives: prostacyclins and thromboxanes. Prostacyclins are powerful locally acting vasodilators and inhibit the aggregation of blood platelets. Through their role in vasodilation, prostacyclins are also involved in inflammation. They are synthesized in the walls of blood vessels and serve the physiological function of preventing needless clot formation, as well as regulating the contraction of smooth muscle tissue. Conversely, thromboxanes (produced by platelet cells) are vasoconstrictors and facilitate platelet aggregation. Their name comes from their role in clot formation (thrombosis).

Dietary Sources of Fatty Acids, their Digestion, Absorption, Transport in the Blood and Storage

A significant proportion of the fatty acids in the body are obtained from the diet, in the form of triglycerides of either animal or plant origin. The fatty acids in the fats obtained from land animals tend to be saturated, whereas the fatty acids in the triglycerides of fish and plants are often polyunsaturated and therefore present as oils.

These triglycerides, cannot be absorbed by the intestine. They are broken down into mono- and di-glycerides plus free fatty acids (but no free glycerol) by pancreatic lipase, which forms a 1:1 complex with a protein called colipase (also a constituent of pancreatic juice), which is necessary for its activity. The activated complex can work only at a water-fat interface. Therefore, it is essential that fats are first emulsified by bile salts for optimal activity of these enzymes. The digestion products consisting of a mixture of tri-, di- and monoglycerides and free fatty acids, which, together with the other fat soluble contents of the diet (e.g. the fat soluble vitamins and cholesterol) and bile salts form mixed micelles, in the watery duodenal contents (see diagrams below).

SOAPY LAYER
SOAP = BILE SALTS AND
PHOSPHATIDYL CHOLINE ("LECITHIN")

FAT DROPLET

FAT DROPLET

EMULSION DROPLETS
OF FAT STABILIZED BY
BILE SALTS,
IN THE PROCESS
OF BEING DIGESTED
BY PANCREATIC LIPASE

COLIPASE   LIPASE

MICELLE FORMATION

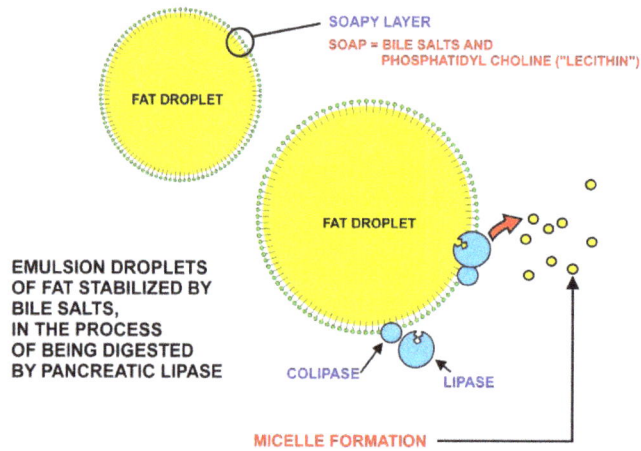

Dietary fats are emulsified in the duodenum by soaps in the form of bile salts and phospholipids, such as phosphatidylcholine. The fat droplets thus formed can be attacked by pancreatic lipase.

CHOLIC ACID

COOH
OH
HO   OH

COOH
OH
OH
OH

HYDROPHOBIC BACK   HYDROPHILIC FRONT

STANDARD
STRUCTURAL FORMULA

SEMI-REALISTIC
3D REPRESENTATION
OF MOLECULAR
STRUCTURE

HIGHLY DIAGRAMMATIC
3D STRUCTURE

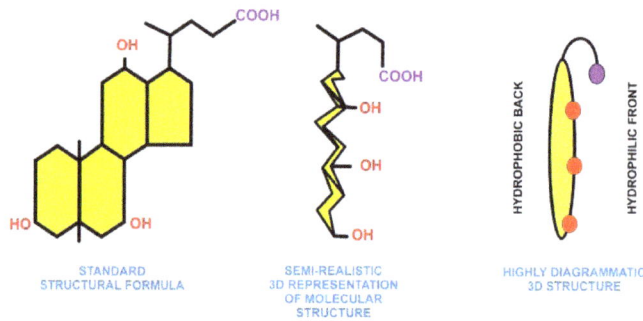

Structure of a bile acid (cholic acid), represented in the standard form, a semi-realistic 3D form, and a diagrammatic 3D form

MICELLES

3-4 nm

CHOLIC
ACID
MICELLE

MIXED MICELLE:
CHOLIC ACID
AND FATTY ACID

MIXED MICELLE WITH
FATTY ACIDS,
MONO- AND DI-GLYCERIDES
FATTY VITAMINS AND
CHOLESTEROL

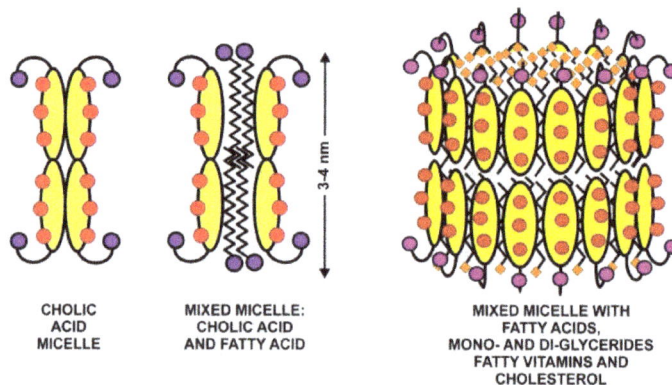

Diagrammatic illustration of mixed micelles formed in the duodenum in the presence of bile acids (e.g. cholic acid) and the digestion products of fats, the fat soluble vitamins and cholesterol.

The contents of these micelles (but not the bile salts) enter the enterocytes (epithelial cells lining the small intestine) where they are resynthesized into triglycerides, and packaged into chylomicrons which are released into the lacteals (the capillaries of the lymph system of the intestines). These lacteals drain into the thoracic duct which empties into the venous blood at the junction of the left jugular and left subclavian veins on the lower left hand side of the neck. This means that the fat soluble products of digestion are discharged directly into the general circulation, without first passing through the liver, as all other digestion products do. The reason for this peculiarity is unknown.

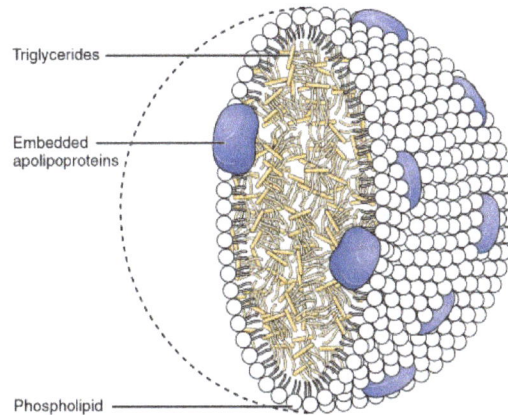

Triglycerides

Embedded
apolipoproteins

Phospholipid

A shematic diagram of a chylomicron.

The chylomicrons circulate throughout the body, giving the blood plasma a milky, or creamy appearance after a fatty meal. Lipoprotein lipase on the endothelial surfaces of the capillaries, especially in adipose tissue, but to a lesser extent also in other tissues, partially digests the chylomicrons into free fatty acids, glycerol and chylomicron remnants. The fatty acids are absorbed by the adipocytes, but the glycerol and chylomicron remnants remain in the blood plasma, ultimately to be removed from the circulation by the liver. The free fatty acids released by the digestion of the chylomicrons are absorbed by the adipocytes, where they are resynthesized into triglycerides using glycerol derived from glucose in the glycolytic pathway. These triglycerides are stored, until needed for the fuel requirements of other tissues, in the fat droplet of the adipocyte.

The liver absorbs a proportion of the glucose from the blood in the portal vein coming from the intestines. After the liver has replenished its glycogen stores (which amount to only about 100 g of glycogen when full) much of the rest of the glucose is converted into fatty acids as described below. These fatty acids are combined with glycerol to form triglycerides which are packaged into droplets very similar to chylomicrons, but known as very low-density lipoproteins (VLDL). These VLDL droplets are handled in exactly the same manner as chylomicrons, except that the VLDL remnant is known as an intermediate-density lipoprotein, (IDL), which is capable of scavenging cholesterol from the blood. This converts IDL into low-density lipoprotein, (LDL), which is taken up by cells that require cholesterol for incorporation into their cell membranes or for synthetic purposes (e.g. the formation of the steroid hormones). The remainder of the LDLs is removed by the liver.

Adipose tissue and lactating mammary glands also take up glucose from the blood for conversion into triglycerides. This occurs in the same way as it does in the liver, except that these tissues do not release the triglycerides thus produced as VLDL into the blood. Adipose tissue cells store the triglycerides in their fat droplets, ultimately to release them again as free fatty acids and glycerol into the blood (as described above), when the plasma concentration of insulin is low, and that of glucagon and/or epinephrine is high. Mammary glands discharge the fat (as cream fat droplets) into the milk that they produce under the influence of the anterior pituitary hormone prolactin.

All cells in the body need to manufacture and maintain their cell walls and the membranes of their organelles. Whether they rely for this entirely on free fatty acids absorbed from the blood, or are able to synthesize their own fatty acids from the blood glucose, is not known. The cells of the central nervous system will almost certainly have the capability of manufacturing their own fatty acids, as these molecules cannot reach them through the blood brain barrier, while, on the other hand, no cell in the body can manufacture the required essential fatty acids which have to be obtained from the diet and delivered to each cell via the blood.

Fatty Acid Synthesis

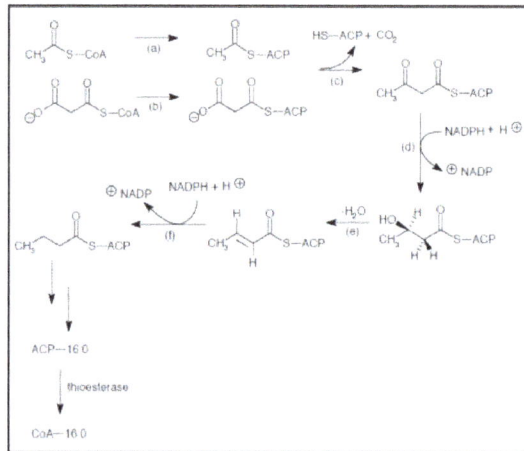

Synthesis of saturated fatty acids via Fatty Acid Synthase II in E. coli

Much like β-oxidation, straight-chain fatty acid synthesis occurs via the six recurring reactions shown below, until the 16-carbon palmitic acid is produced.

The diagrams presented show how fatty acids are synthesized in microorganisms and list the enzymes found in Escherichia coli. These reactions are performed by fatty acid synthase II (FASII), which in general contain multiple enzymes that act as one complex. FASII is present in prokaryotes, plants, fungi, and parasites, as well as in mitochondria.

In animals, as well as some fungi such as yeast, these same reactions occur on fatty acid synthase I (FASI), a large dimeric protein that has all of the enzymatic activities required to create a fatty acid. FASI is less efficient than FASII; however, it allows for the formation of more molecules, including "medium-chain" fatty acids via early chain termination.

Once a 16:0 carbon fatty acid has been formed, it can undergo a number of modifications, resulting in desaturation and/or elongation. Elongation, starting with stearate (18:0), is performed mainly in the ER by several membrane-bound enzymes. The enzymatic steps involved in the elongation process are principally the same as those carried out by FAS, but the four principal successive steps of the elongation are performed by individual proteins, which may be physically associated.

Step	Enzyme	Reaction	Description
(a)	Acetyl CoA:ACP trans-acylase		Activates acetyl CoA for reaction with malonyl-ACP
(b)	Malonyl CoA:ACP trans-acylase		Activates malonyl CoA for reaction with acetyl-ACP
(c)	3-ketoacyl-ACP synthase		Reacts priming acetyl-ACP with chain-extending malonyl-ACP.
(d)	3-ketoacyl-ACP reductase		Reduces the carbon 3 ketone to a hydroxyl group
(e)	3-Hydroxyacyl ACP dehydrase		Removes water
(f)	Enoyl-ACP reductase		Reduces the C2-C3 double bond.

Abbreviations: ACP – Acyl carrier protein, CoA – Coenzyme A, NADP – Nicotinamide adenine dinucleotide phosphate.

Note that during fatty synthesis the reducing agent is NADPH, whereas NAD is the oxidizing agent in beta-oxidation (the breakdown of fatty acids to acetyl-CoA). This difference exemplifies a general principle that NADPH is consumed during biosynthetic reactions, whereas NADH is generated in energy-yielding reactions. (Thus NADPH is also required for the synthesis of cholesterol from acetyl-CoA; while NADH is generated during glycolysis.) The source of the NADPH is two-fold. When malate is oxidatively decarboxylated by "NADP$^+$-linked malic enzyme" pyruvate, CO_2 and NADPH are formed. NADPH is also formed by the pentose phosphate pathway which converts glucose into ribose, which can be used in synthesis of nucleotides and nucleic acids, or it can be catabolized to pyruvate.

Glycolytic end Products are used in the Conversion of Carbohydrates into Fatty Acids

In humans, fatty acids are formed from carbohydrates predominantly in the liver and adipose tissue, as well as in the mammary glands during lactation. The cells of the central nervous system probably also make most of the fatty acids needed for the phospholipids of their extensive membranes from glucose, as blood-born fatty acids cannot cross the blood brain barrier to reach these cells. However, how the essential fatty acids, which mammals cannot synthesize themselves, but are nevertheless important components of cell membranes (and other functions described above) reach them is unknown.

The pyruvate produced by glycolysis is an important intermediary in the conversion of carbohydrates into fatty acids and cholesterol. This occurs via the conversion of pyruvate into acetyl-CoA in the mitochondrion. However, this acetyl CoA needs to be transported into cytosol where the synthesis of fatty acids and cholesterol occurs. This cannot occur directly. To obtain cytosolic acetyl-CoA, citrate (produced by the condensation of acetyl CoA with oxaloacetate) is removed from the citric acid cycle and carried across the inner mitochondrial membrane into the cytosol. There it is cleaved by ATP citrate lyase into acetyl-CoA and oxaloacetate. The oxaloacetate is returned to mitochondrion as malate (and then converted back into oxaloacetate to transfer more acetyl-CoA out of the mitochondrion). The cytosolic acetyl-CoA is carboxylated by acetyl CoA carboxylase into malonyl CoA, the first committed step in the synthesis of fatty acids.

Regulation of Fatty Acid Synthesis

Acetyl-CoA is formed into malonyl-CoA by acetyl-CoA carboxylase, at which point malonyl-CoA is destined to feed into the fatty acid synthesis pathway. Acetyl-CoA carboxylase is the point of regulation in saturated straight-chain fatty acid synthesis, and is subject to both phosphorylation and allosteric regulation. Regulation by phosphorylation occurs mostly in mammals, while allosteric regulation occurs in most organisms. Allosteric control occurs as feedback inhibition by palmitoyl-CoA and activation by citrate. When there are high levels of palmitoyl-CoA, the final product of saturated fatty acid synthesis, it allosterically inactivates acetyl-CoA carboxylase to prevent a build-up of fatty acids in cells. Citrate acts to activate acetyl-CoA carboxylase under high levels, because high levels indicate that there is enough acetyl-CoA to feed into the Krebs cycle and produce energy.

High plasma levels of insulin in the blood plasma (e.g. after meals) cause the dephosphorylation of acetyl-CoA carboxylase, thus promoting the formation of malonyl-CoA from acetyl-CoA, and consequently the conversion of carbohydrates into fatty acids, while epinephrine and glucagon (released into the blood during starvation and exercise) cause the phosphorylation of this enzyme, inhibiting lipogenesis in favor of fatty acid oxidation via beta-oxidation.

Disorders

Disorders of fatty acid metabolism can be described in terms of, for example, hypertriglyceridemia (too high level of triglycerides), or other types of hyperlipidemia. These may be familial or acquired.

Familial types of disorders of fatty acid metabolism are generally classified as inborn errors of lipid metabolism. These disorders may be described as fatty oxidation disorders or as a *lipid storage disorders*, and are any one of several inborn errors of metabolism that result from enzyme defects affecting the ability of the body to oxidize fatty acids in order to produce energy within muscles, liver, and other cell types.

Beta Oxidation

In biochemistry and metabolism, beta-oxidation is the catabolic process by which fatty acid molecules are broken down in the cytosol in prokaryotes and in the mitochondria in eukaryotes to generate acetyl-CoA, which enters the citric acid cycle, and NADH and $FADH_2$, which are co-enzymes used in the electron transport chain. It is named as such because the beta carbon of the fatty acid undergoes oxidation to a carbonyl group. Various mechanisms have evolved to handle the large variety of fatty acids.

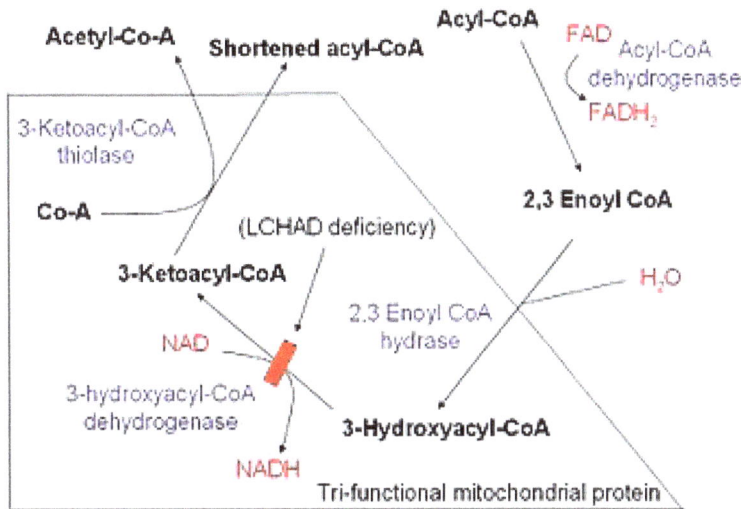

Schematic demonstrating mitochondrial fatty acid beta-oxidation and effects of long-chain 3-hydroxyacyl-coenzyme A dehydrogenase deficiency, LCHAD deficiency

Overview

Fatty acid catabolism consists of:

1. Activation and membrane transport of free fatty acids by binding to coenzyme A.

2. Oxidation of the beta carbon to a carbonyl group.

3. Cleavage of two-carbon segments resulting in acetyl-CoA.

4. Oxidation of acetyl-CoA to carbon dioxide in the citric acid cycle.

5. Electron transfer from electron carriers to the electron transfer chain in oxidative phosphorylation.

General Mechanism

Once the fatty acid is inside the mitochondrial matrix, beta-oxidation occurs by cleaving two carbons every cycle to form acetyl-CoA. The process consists of 4 steps.

1. A long-chain fatty acid is dehydrogenated to create a trans double bond between C2 and C3. This is catalyzed by acyl CoA dehydrogenase to produce trans-delta 2-enoyl CoA. It uses FAD as an electron acceptor and it is reduced to $FADH_2$.

2. Trans-delta2-enoyl CoA is hydrated at the double bond to produce L-3-hydroxyacyl CoA by enoyl-CoA hydratase.

3. L-3-hydroxyacyl CoA is dehydrogenated again to create 3-ketoacyl CoA by 3-hydroxyacyl CoA dehydrogenase. This enzyme uses NAD as an electron acceptor.

4. Thiolysis occurs between C2 and C3 (alpha and beta carbons) of 3-ketoacyl CoA. Thiolase enzyme catalyzes the reaction when a new molecule of coenzyme A breaks the bond by nucleophilic attack on C3. This releases the first two carbon units, as acetyl CoA, and a fatty acyl CoA minus two carbons. The process continues until all of the carbons in the fatty acid are turned into acetyl CoA.

Fatty acids are oxidized by most of the tissues in the body. However, some tissues such as the red blood cells (which do not contain mitochondria), and cells of the central nervous system (because fatty acids cannot cross the blood-brain barrier into the interstitial fluids that bathe these cells) do not use fatty acids for their energy requirements, but instead use carbohydrates.

Because many fatty acids are not fully saturated or do not have an even number of carbons, several different mechanisms have evolved, described below.

Even-numbered Saturated Fatty Acids

Once inside the mitochondria, each cycle of β-oxidation, liberating a two carbon unit (acetyl-CoA), occurs in a sequence of four reactions:

Description	Diagram	Enzyme	End product
Dehydrogenation by FAD: The first step is the oxidation of the fatty acid by Acyl-CoA-Dehydrogenase. The enzyme catalyzes the formation of a double bond between the C-2 and C-3.		acyl CoA dehydrogenase	trans-Δ^2-enoyl-CoA
Hydration: The next step is the hydration of the bond between C-2 and C-3. The reaction is stereospecific, forming only the L isomer.		enoyl CoA hydratase	L-β-hydroxyacyl CoA
Oxidation by NAD⁺: The third step is the oxidation of L-β-hydroxyacyl CoA by NAD⁺. This converts the hydroxyl group into a keto group.		3-hydroxyacyl-CoA dehydrogenase	β-ketoacyl CoA
Thiolysis: The final step is the cleavage of β-ketoacyl CoA by the thiol group of another molecule of Coenzyme A. The thiol is inserted between C-2 and C-3.		β-ketothiolase	An acetyl-CoA molecule, and an acyl-CoA molecule that is two carbons shorter

This process continues until the entire chain is cleaved into acetyl CoA units. The final cycle produces two separate acetyl CoAs, instead of one acyl CoA and one acetyl CoA. For every cycle, the Acyl CoA unit is shortened by two carbon atoms. Concomitantly, one molecule of $FADH_2$, NADH and acetyl CoA are formed.

Odd-numbered Saturated Fatty Acids

In general, fatty acids with an odd number of carbons are found in the lipids of plants and some marine organisms. Many ruminant animals form a large amount of 3-carbon propionate during the fermentation of carbohydrates in the rumen.

Chains with an odd-number of carbons are oxidized in the same manner as even-numbered chains, but the final products are propionyl-CoA and succinyl-CoA.

Propionyl-CoA is first carboxylated using a bicarbonate ion into D-stereoisomer of methylmalonyl-CoA, in a reaction that involves a biotin co-factor, ATP, and the enzyme propionyl-CoA carboxylase. The bicarbonate ion's carbon is added to the middle carbon of propionyl-CoA, forming a D-methylmalonyl-CoA. However, the D conformation is enzymatically converted into the L conformation by methylmalonyl-CoA epimerase, then it undergoes intramolecular rearrangement, which is catalyzed by methylmalonyl-CoA mutase (requiring B_{12} as a coenzyme) to form succinyl-CoA. The succinyl-CoA formed can then enter the citric acid cycle.

However, whereas acetyl-CoA enters the citric acid cycle by condensing with an existing molecule of oxaloacetate, succinyl-CoA enters the cycle as a principal in its own right. Thus the succinate just adds to the population of circulating molecules in the cycle and undergoes no net metabolization while in it. When this infusion of citric acid cycle intermediates exceeds cataplerotic demand (such as for aspartate or glutamate synthesis), some of them can be extracted to the gluconeogenesis pathway, in the liver and kidneys, through phosphoenolpyruvate carboxykinase, and converted to free glucose.

Unsaturated Fatty Acids

β-Oxidation of unsaturated fatty acids poses a problem since the location of a cis bond can prevent the formation of a trans-Δ^2 bond. These situations are handled by an additional two enzymes, Enoyl CoA isomerase or 2,4 Dienoyl CoA reductase.

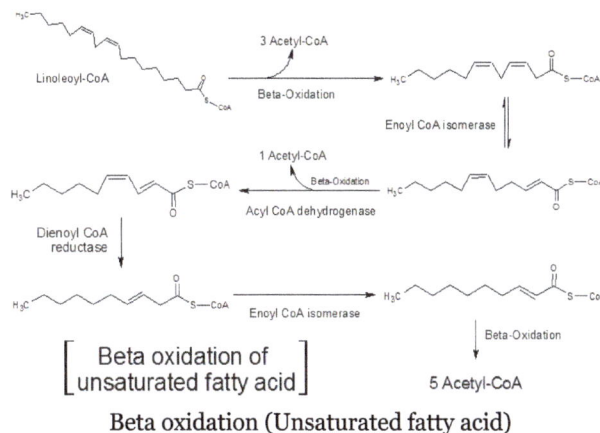

Beta oxidation (Unsaturated fatty acid)

Whatever the conformation of the hydrocarbon chain, β-oxidation occurs normally until the acyl CoA (because of the presence of a double bond) is not an appropriate substrate for acyl CoA dehydrogenase, or enoyl CoA hydratase:

- If the acyl CoA contains a *cis-Δ³ bond*, then *cis-Δ³*-Enoyl CoA isomerase will convert the bond to a *trans-Δ²* bond, which is a regular substrate.

- If the acyl CoA contains a *cis-Δ⁴ double bond*, then its dehydrogenation yields a 2,4-dienoyl intermediate, which is not a substrate for enoyl CoA hydratase. However, the enzyme 2,4 Dienoyl CoA reductase reduces the intermediate, using NADPH, into *trans-Δ³*-enoyl CoA. As in the above case, this compound is converted into a suitable intermediate by 3,2-Enoyl CoA isomerase.

To summarize:

- *Odd-numbered* double bonds are handled by the isomerase.

- *Even-numbered* double bonds by the reductase (which creates an odd-numbered double bond)

Peroxisomal Beta-oxidation

Fatty acid oxidation also occurs in peroxisomes when the fatty acid chains are too long to be handled by the mitochondria. The same enzymes are used in peroxisomes as in the mitochondrial matrix, and acetyl-CoA is generated. It is believed that very long chain (greater than C-22) fatty acids, branched fatty acids, some prostaglandins and leukotrienes undergo initial oxidation in peroxisomes until octanoyl-CoA is formed, at which point it undergoes mitochondrial oxidation.

One significant difference is that oxidation in peroxisomes is not coupled to ATP synthesis. Instead, the high-potential electrons are transferred to O_2, which yields H_2O_2. It does generate heat however. The enzyme catalase, found exclusively in peroxisomes, converts the hydrogen peroxide into water and oxygen.

Peroxisomal β-oxidation also requires enzymes specific to the peroxisome and to very long fatty acids. There are three key differences between the enzymes used for mitochondrial and peroxisomal β-oxidation:

1. The NADH formed in the third oxidative step cannot be reoxidized in the peroxisome, so reducing equivalents are exported to the cytosol.

2. β-oxidation in the peroxisome requires the use of a peroxisomal carnitine acyltransferase (instead of carnitine acyltransferase I and II used by the mitochondria) for transport of the activated acyl group into the mitochondria for further breakdown.

3. The first oxidation step in the peroxisome is catalyzed by the enzyme acyl-CoA oxidase.

4. The β-ketothiolase used in peroxisomal β-oxidation has an altered substrate specificity, different from the mitochondrial β-ketothiolase.

Peroxisomal oxidation is induced by a high-fat diet and administration of hypolipidemic drugs like clofibrate.

Energy Yield

The ATP yield for every oxidation cycle is theoretically at maximum yield 17, as NADH produces 3 ATP, $FADH_2$ produces 2 and a full rotation of the citric acid cycle produces 12. In practice it's closer to 14 ATP for a full oxidation cycle as in practice the theoretical yield isn't attained - it's generally closer to 2.5 ATP per NADH molecule produced, 1.5 for each $FADH_2$ Molecule produced and this equates to 10 per cycle of the TCA(according to the P/O ratio), broken down as follows:

Source	ATP	Total
1 $FADH_2$	x 1.5 ATP	= 1.5 ATP (Theoretically 2 ATP)
1 NADH	x 2.5 ATP	= 2.5 ATP (Theoretically 3 ATP)
1 acetyl CoA	x 10 ATP	= 10 ATP (Theoretically 12 ATP)
TOTAL		= 14 ATP

For an even-numbered saturated fat (C_{2n}), n - 1 oxidations are necessary, and the final process yields an additional acetyl CoA. In addition, two equivalents of ATP are lost during the activation of the fatty acid. Therefore, the total ATP yield can be stated as:

$$(n - 1) * 14 + 10 - 2 = \text{total ATP}$$

or

$$14n-6 \text{ (alternatively)}$$

For instance, the ATP yield of palmitate (C_{16}, $n = 8$) is:

$$(8 - 1) * 14 + 10 - 2 = 106 \text{ ATP}$$

Represented in table form:

Source	ATP	Total
7 $FADH_2$	x 1.5 ATP	= 10.5 ATP
7 NADH	x 2.5 ATP	= 17.5 ATP
8 acetyl CoA	x 10 ATP	= 80 ATP
Activation		= -2 ATP
NET		= 106 ATP

For sources that use the larger ATP production numbers described above, the total would be 129 ATP ={(8-1)*17+12-2} equivalents per palmitate.

Beta-oxidation of unsaturated fatty acids changes the ATP yield due to the requirement of two possible additional enzymes.

History and Discovery

In 1904, the German chemist Franz Knoop elucidated the steps in beta-oxidation by feeding dogs odd- and even-chain ω-phenyl fatty acids, such as ω-phenylvaleric acid and ω-phenylbutyric acid, respectively. The mechanism of beta-oxidation, i.e. successive removal of two carbons, was realized when it was discovered that the odd-chain ω-phenylvaleric acid was metabolized to hippuric acid, and that the even-chain ω-phenylbutyric acid was metabolized to phenaceturic acid. At this time, any reaction mechanism involving oxidation at the beta carbon was as yet unknown in organic chemistry.

Clinical Significance

There are at least 25 enzymes and specific transport proteins in the β-oxidation pathway. Of these, 18 have been associated with human disease as inborn errors of metabolism.

Amino Acid Synthesis

Amino acid synthesis is the set of biochemical processes (metabolic pathways) by which the various amino acids are produced from other compounds. The substrates for these processes are various compounds in the organism's diet or growth media. Not all organisms are able to synthesise all amino acids. Humans are excellent example of this, since humans can only synthesise 11 of the 20 standard amino acids (aka non-essential amino acid), and in time of accelerated growth, histidine, can be considered an essential amino acid.

A fundamental problem for biological systems is to obtain nitrogen in an easily usable form. This problem is solved by certain microorganisms capable of reducing the inert N≡N molecule (nitrogen gas) to two molecules of ammonia in one of the most remarkable reactions in biochemistry. Ammonia is the source of nitrogen for all the amino acids. The carbon backbones come from the glycolytic pathway, the pentose phosphate pathway, or the citric acid cycle.

In amino acid production, one encounters an important problem in biosynthesis, namely stereochemical control. Because all amino acids except glycine are chiral, biosynthetic pathways must generate the correct isomer with high fidelity. In each of the 19 pathways for the generation of chiral amino acids, the stereochemistry at the α-carbon atom is established by a transamination reaction that involves pyridoxal phosphate. Almost all the transaminases that catalyze these reactions descend from a common ancestor, illustrating once again that effective solutions to biochemical problems are retained throughout evolution.

Biosynthetic pathways are often highly regulated such that building-blocks are synthesized only when supplies are low. Very often, a high concentration of the final product of a pathway inhibits the activity of enzymes that function early in the pathway. Often present are allosteric enzymes capable of sensing and responding to concentrations of regulatory species. These enzymes are similar in functional properties to aspartate transcarbamoylase and its regulators. Feedback and allosteric mechanisms ensure that all twenty amino acids are maintained in sufficient amounts for protein synthesis and other processes.

Nitrogen Fixation

Microorganisms use ATP and reduced ferredoxin, a powerful reductant, to reduce atmospheric nitrogen (N_2) to ammonia (NH_3). An iron-molybdenum cluster in nitrogenase deftly catalyzes the fixation of N_2, a very inert molecule. Higher organisms consume the fixed nitrogen to synthesize amino acids, nucleotides, and other nitrogen-containing biomolecules. The major points of entry of ammonia into metabolism are glutamine or glutamate.

Transamination

Most amino acids are synthesized from α-ketoacids, and later transaminated from another amino acid, usually glutamate. The enzyme involved in this reaction is an aminotransferase.

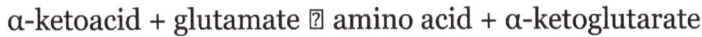

α-ketoacid + glutamate ⮂ amino acid + α-ketoglutarate

Glutamate itself is formed by amination of α-ketoglutarate:

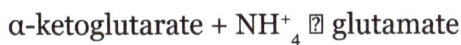

α-ketoglutarate + NH^+_4 ⮂ glutamate

From Intermediates of the Citric Acid Cycle and Other Pathways

Of the basic set of twenty amino acids (not counting selenocysteine), there are eight that human beings cannot synthesize. In addition, the amino acids arginine, cysteine, glycine, glutamine, histidine, proline, serine, and tyrosine are considered conditionally essential, meaning they are not normally required in the diet, but must be supplied exogenously to specific populations that do not synthesize it in adequate amounts. For example, enough arginine is synthesized by the urea cycle to meet the needs of an adult but perhaps not those of a growing child. Amino acids that must be obtained from the diet are called essential amino acids. Nonessential amino acids are produced in the body. The pathways for the synthesis of nonessential amino acids are quite simple. Glutamate dehydrogenase catalyzes the reductive amination of α-ketoglutarate to glutamate. A transamination reaction takes place in the synthesis of most amino acids. At this step, the chirality of the amino acid is established. Alanine and aspartate are synthesized by the transamination of pyruvate and oxaloacetate, respectively. Glutamine is synthesized from NH4+ and glutamate, and asparagine is synthesized similarly. Proline and arginine are derived from glutamate. Serine, formed from 3-phosphoglycerate, is the precursor of glycine and cysteine. Tyrosine is synthesized by the hydroxylation of phenylalanine, an essential amino acid. The pathways for the biosynthesis of essential amino acids are much more complex than those for the nonessential ones. Activated Tetrahydrofolate, a carrier of one-carbon units, plays an important role in the metabolism of amino acids and nucleotides. This coenzyme carries one-carbon units at three oxidation states, which are interconvertible: most reduced—methyl; intermediate—methylene; and most oxidized—formyl, formimino, and methenyl. The major donor of activated methyl groups is S-adenosylmethionine, which is synthesized by the transfer of an adenosyl group from ATP to the sulfur atom of methionine. S-Adenosylhomocysteine is formed when the activated methyl group is transferred to an acceptor. It is hydrolyzed to adenosine and homocysteine, the latter of which is then methylated to methionine to complete the activated methyl cycle.

Cortisol inhibits protein synthesis.

Regulation by Feedback Inhibition

Most of the pathways of amino acid biosynthesis are regulated by feedback inhibition, in which the committed step is allosterically inhibited by the final product. Branched pathways require extensive interaction among the branches that includes both negative and positive regulation. The regulation of glutamine synthetase from *E. coli* is a striking demonstration of cumulative feedback inhibition and of control by a cascade of reversible covalent modifications.

α-Ketoglutarates

The α-ketoglutarate family of amino acid synthesis (synthesis of glutamate, glutamine, proline and arginine) begins with α-ketoglutarate, an intermediate in the Citric Acid Cycle. The concentration of α-ketoglutarate is dependent on the activity and metabolism within the cell along with the regulation of enzymatic activity. In *E. coli* citrate synthase, the enzyme involved in the condensation reaction initiating the Citric Acid Cycle is strongly inhibited by α-ketoglutarate feedback inhibition and can be inhibited by DPNH as well high concentrations of ATP. This is one of the initial regulations of the α-ketoglutarate family of amino acid synthesis.

The regulation of the synthesis of glutamate from α-ketoglutarate is subject to regulatory control of the Citric Acid Cycle as well as mass action dependent on the concentrations of reactants involved due to the reversible nature of the transamination and glutamate dehydrogenase reactions.

The conversion of glutamate to glutamine is regulated by glutamine synthetase (GS) and is a highly significant step in nitrogen metabolism. This enzyme is regulated by at least four different mechanisms: 1. Repression and depression due to nitrogen levels; 2. Activation and inactivation due to enzymatic forms (taut and relaxed); 3. Cumulative feedback inhibition through end product metabolites; and 4. Alterations of the enzyme due to adenylation and deadenylation. In rich nitrogenous media or growth conditions containing high quantities of ammonia there is a low level of GS, whereas in limiting quantities of ammonia the specific activity of the enzyme is 20-fold higher. The confirmation of the enzyme plays a role in regulation depending on if GS is in the taut or relaxed form. The taut form of GS is fully active but, the removal of manganese converts the enzyme to the relaxed state. The specific conformational state occurs based on the binding of specific divalent cations and is also related to adenylation. The feedback inhibition of GS is due to a cumulative feedback due to several metabolites including L-tryptophan, L-histidine, AMP, CTP, glucosamine-6-phosphate and carbamyl phosphate, alanine, and glycine. An excess of any one product does not individually inhibit the enzyme but a combination or accumulation of all the end products have a strong inhibitory effect on the synthesis of glutamine. Glutamine synthase activity is also inhibited via adenylation. The adenylation activity is catalyzed by the bifunctional adenylyltransferase/adenylyl removal (AT/AR) enzyme. Glutamine and a regulatory protein called PII act together to stimulate adenylation.

The regulation of proline biosynthesis can be dependent on the initial controlling step through negative feedback inhibition. In *E. coli*, proline allosterically inhibits Glutamate 5-kinase which catalyzes the reaction from L-glutamate to an unstable intermediate L-γ-Glutamyl phosphate.

Arginine synthesis also utilizes negative feedback as well as repression through a repressor encoded by the gene *argR*. The gene product of *argR*, ArgR an aporepressor, and arginine as a corepressor affect the operon of arginine biosynthesis. The degree of repression is determined by the concentrations of the repressor protein and corepressor level.

Erythrose 4-phosphate and Phosphoenolpyruvate

Phenylalanine, tyrosine, and tryptophan are known as the aromatic amino acids. The synthesis of all three share a common beginning to their pathways; the formation of chorismate from phosphoenolpyruvate (PEP) and erythrose 4- phosphate (E4P). The first step, condensation of 3-deoxy-D-arabino-heptulosonic acid 7-phosphate (DAHP) from PEP/E4P, uses three isoenzymes AroF, AroG, and AroH. Each one of these has its synthesis regulated from tyrosine, phenylalanine, and tryptophan, respectively. These isoenzymes all have the ability to help regulate synthesis of DAHP by the method of feedback inhibition. This acts in the cell by monitoring the concentrations of each of the three aromatic amino acids. When there is too much of any one of them, that one will allosterically control the DAHP synthetase by "turning it off". With the first step of the common pathway shut off, synthesis of the three amino acids can not proceed. The rest of the enzymes in the common pathway (conversion of DAHP to chorismate) appear to be synthesized constitutively, except for shikimate kinase which can be inhibited by shikimate through linear mixed-type inhibition. If too much shikimate has been produced then it can bind to shikimate kinase to stop further production.

Besides the regulations described above, each amino acids terminal pathway can be regulated. These terminal pathways progress from chorismate to the final end product, either tyrosine, phenylalanine, or tryptophan. Each one of these pathways is regulated in a similar fashion to the common pathway; with feedback inhibition on the first committed step of the pathway.

Tyrosine and phenylalanine share the same initial step in their terminal pathways, chorismate converted to prephenate which is converted to an amino acid-specific intermediate. This process is mediated by a phenylalanine (PheA) or tyrosine (TyrA) specific chorismate mutase-prephenate dehydrogenase. The reason for the amino acid-specific enzymes is because PheA uses a simple dehydrogenase to convert prephenate to phenylpyruvate, while TyrA uses a NAD-dependent dehydrogenase to make 4-hydroxylphenylpyruvate. Both PheA and TyrA are feedback inhibited by their respective amino acids. Tyrosine can also be inhibited at the transcriptional level by the TyrR repressor. TyrR binds to the TyrR boxes on the operon near the promoter of the gene that it wants to repress.

In the terminal-tryptophan synthesis pathway, the initial step converts chorismate to anthranilate using anthranilate synthase. This enzyme requires either ammonia or glutamine as the amino group donor. Anthranilate synthase is regulated by the gene products of trpE and trpD. trpE encodes the first subunit, which binds to chorismate and moves the amino group from the donor to chorismate. trpD encodes the second subunit, which is simply used to bind glutamine and use it as the amino group donor so that the amine group can transfer to the chorismate. Anthranilate synthase is also regulated by feedback inhibition. The finished product of tryptophan, once produced in great enough quantities, is able to act as the co-repressor to the TrpR repressor which represses expression of the trp operon.

Oxaloacetate/Aspartate

The oxaloacetate/aspartate family of amino acids is composed of lysine, asparagine, methionine, threonine, and isoleucine. Aspartate can be converted into lysine, asparagine, methionine and threonine. Threonine also gives rise to isoleucine. All of these amino acids contain different mechanisms for their regulation, some being more complex than others. All the enzymes in this biosynthetic pathway are subject to regulation via feedback inhibition and/or repression at the genetic level. As is typical in highly branched metabolic pathways, there is additional regulation at each branch point of the pathway. This type of regulatory scheme allows control over the total flux of the aspartate pathway in addition to the total flux of individual amino acids. The aspartate pathway uses L-aspartic acid as the precursor for the biosynthesis of one fourth of the building block amino acids. Without this pathway, protein synthesis would not be possible.

Aspartate

The enzyme aspartokinase, which catalyzes the phosphorylation of aspartate and initiates its conversion into other amino acids, can be broken up into 3 isozymes, AK-I, II and III. AK-I is feedback inhibited by threonine, while AK-II and III are inhibited by lysine. As a sidenote, AK-III catalyzes the phosphorylation of aspartic acid that is the commitment step in this biosynthetic pathway. The higher the concentration of threonine or lysine, the more aspartate kinase becomes downregulated.

Lysine

Lysine is synthesized from aspartate via the diaminopimelate (DAP) pathway. The initial two stages of the DAP pathway are catalyzed by aspartokinase and aspartate semialdehyde dehydrogenase and play a key role in the biosynthesis of lysine, threonine and methionine. There are two bifunctional aspartokinase/homoserine dehydrogenases, ThrA and MetL, in addition to a monofunctional aspartokinase, LysC. Transcription of aspartokinase genes is regulated by concentrations of the subsequently produced amino acids, lysine, threonine and methionine. The higher these amino acids concentrations, the less the gene is transcribed. ThrA and LysC are also feed-back inhibited by threonine and lysine. Finally, DAP decarboxylase LysA mediates the last step of the lysine synthesis and is common for all studied bacterial species. The formation of aspartate kinase (AK), which catalyzes the phosphorylation of aspartate and initiates its conversion into other amino acids, is also inhibited by both lysine and threonine, which prevents the formation of the amino acids derived from aspartate. Additionally, high lysine concentrations inhibit the activity of dihydrodipicolinate synthase (DHPS). So, in addition to inhibiting the first enzyme of the aspartate families biosynthetic pathway, lysine also inhibits the activity of the first enzyme after the branch point, i.e. the enzyme that is specific for lysine's own synthesis.

Asparagine

There are two different asparagine synthetases found in bacterial species. These two synthetases, which are both referred to as the AsnC protein, are coded for by two genes: AsnA and AsnB. AsnC is autogenously regulated, which is where the product of a structural gene regulates the expression of the operon in which the genes reside. The stimulating effect of AsnC on AsnA transcription is downregulated by asparagine. However, the autoregulation of AsnC is not affected by asparagine.

Methionine

Methionine synthesis is under tight regulation. The repressor protein MetJ, in cooperation with the corepressor protein S-adenosyl-methionine, mediates the repression of methionine's biosynthetic pathway. Recently, a new regulator focus, MetR has been identified. The MetR protein is required for MetE and MetH gene expression and functions as a transactivator of transcription for these genes. MetR transcriptional activity is regulated by homocystein, which is the metabolic precursor of methionine. It is also known that vitamin B12 can repress MetE gene expression, which is mediated by the MetH holoenzyme.

Threonine

The biosynthesis of threonine is regulated via allosteric regulation of its precursor, homoserine, by structurally altering the enzyme homoserine dehydrogenase. This reaction occurs at a key branch point in the pathway, with the substrate homoserine serving as the precursor for the biosynthesis of lysine, methionine, threonin and isoleucine. High levels of threonine result in low levels of homoserine synthesis. The synthesis of aspartate kinase (AK), which catalyzes the phosphorylation of aspartate and initiates its conversion into other amino acids, is feed-back inhibited by lysine, isoleucine, and threonine, which prevents the synthesis of the amino acids derived from aspartate. So, in addition to inhibiting the first enzyme of the aspartate families biosynthetic pathway, threonine also inhibits the activity of the first enzyme after the branch point, i.e. the enzyme that is specific for threonine's own synthesis.

Isoleucine

The enzymes threonine deaminase, dihydroxy acid dehydrase and transaminase are controlled by end-product regulation. I.e. the presence of isoleucine will downregulate the formation of all three enzymes, resulting in the downregulation of threonine biosynthesis. High concentrations of isoleucine also result in the downregulation of aspartate's conversion into the aspartyl-phosphate intermediate, hence halting further biosynthesis of lysine, methionine, threonine, and isoleucine.

Ribose 5-phosphates

The synthesis of histidine in "E. coli" is a complex pathway involving 10 reactions and 10 enzymes. Synthesis begins with 5-phosphoribosyl-pyrophosphate (PRPP) and finishes with histidine and occurs through the reactions of the following enzymes:

HisG-> HisE/HisI-> HisA-> HisH-> HisF-> HisB-> HisC-> HisB-> HisD (HisE/I and HisB are both bifunctional enzymes)

All of the enzymes are coded for on the his operon. This operon has a distinct block of the leader sequence, called block 1:

Met-Thr-Arg-Val-Gln-Phe-Lys-His-His-His-His-His-His-His-Pro-Asp

This leader sequence is very important for the regulation of histidine in "E. coli". The *his* operon operates under a system of coordinated regulation where all the gene products will be repressed or depressed equally. The main factor in the repression or derepression of histidine synthesis is the concentration of histidine charged tRNAs. The regulation of histidine is actually quite simple considering the complexity of its biosynthesis pathway and, it closely resembles regulation of tryptophan. In this system the full leader sequence has 4 blocks of complementary strands that can form hairpin loops structures. Block one, shown above, is the key to regulation. When histidine charged tRNA levels are low in the cell the ribosome will stall at the string of His residues in block 1. This stalling of the ribosome will allow complementary strands 2 and 3 to form a hairpin loop. The loop formed by strands 2 and 3 forms an anti-terminator and translation of the *his* genes will continue and histidine will be produced. However when histidine charged tRNA levels are high the ribosome will not stall at block 1, this will not allow strands 2 and 3 to form a hairpin. Instead strands 3 and 4 will form a hairpin loop further downstream of the ribosome. The hairpin loop formed by strands 3 and 4 is a terminating loop, when the ribosome comes into contact with the loop, it will be "knocked off" the transcript. When the ribosome is removed the *his* genes will not be translated and histidine will not be produced by the cell.

3-Phosphoglycerates

Serine

Serine is the first amino acid in this family to be produced; it is then modified to produce both glycine and cysteine (and many other biologically important molecules). Serine is formed from 3-phosphoglycerate in the following pathway:

3-phosphoglycerate-> phosphohydroxyl-pyruvate-> phosphoserine-> serine

The conversion from 3-phosphoglycerate to phosphohydroxyl-pyruvate is achieved by the enzyme phosphoglycerate dehydrogenase. This enzyme is the key regulatory step in this pathway. Phosphoglycerate dehydrogenase is regulated by the concentration of serine in the cell. At high concentrations this enzyme will be inactive and serine will not be produced. At low concentrations of serine the enzyme will be fully active and serine will be produced by the bacterium. Since serine is the first amino acid produced in this family both glycine and cysteine will be regulated by the available concentration of serine in the cell.

Glycine

Glycine is synthesized from serine using the enzyme serine hydromethyltransferase (SHMT), which is coded by the gene *glyA*. The enzyme effectively removes a hydroxyl group from serine and replaces it with a methyl group to yield glycine. This reaction is the only way *E. coli* can produce glycine. The regulation of *glyA* is very complex and is known to incorporate serine, glycine, methionine, purines, thymine, and folates however, the full mechanism has yet to be elucidated. The methionine gene product MetR and the methionine intermediate homocysteine are known to positively regulate glyA. Homocysteine is a coactivator of *glyA* and must act in concert with MetR. On the other hand, PurR, a protein which plays a role in purine synthesis and S-adeno-sylmethionine are known to down regulate *glyA*. PurR binds directly to the control region of *glyA* and effectively turns the gene off so that glycine will not be produced by the bacterium.

Cysteine

Cysteine is a very important molecule for a bacterium's survival. This amino acid harbors a sulfur atom and can actively participate in disulfide bond formation. The genes required for the synthesis of cysteine are coded for on the *cys* regulon. The integration of sulfur into the molecule is positively regulated by CysB. CysB is the main focus of cysteine regulation. Effective inducers of this regulon are N-acetyl-serine (NAS) and very small amounts of reduced sulfur. CysB functions by binding to

DNA half sites on the *cys* regulon. These half sites differ in quantity and arrangement depending on the promoter of interest. There is however one half site that is conserved. It lies just upstream of the -35 site of the promoter. There are also multiple accessory sites depending on the promoter. In the absence of the inducer, NAS, CysB will bind the DNA and cover many of the accessory half sites. Without the accessory half sites the regulon cannot be transcribed and cysteine will not be produced. It is believed that the presence of NAS causes CysB to undergo a conformational change. This conformational change allows CysB to bind properly to all the half sites and causes the recruitment of the RNA polymerase. The RNA polymerase will then transcribe the *cys* regulon and cysteine will be produced.

Further regulation is required for this pathway, however. CysB can actually down regulate its own transcription by binding to its own DNA sequence and blocking the RNA polymerase. In this case NAS will act to disallow the binding of CysB to its own DNA sequence. OAS is a precursor of NAS, cysteine itself can inhibit CysE which functions to create OAS. Without the necessary OAS, NAS will not be produced and cysteine will not be produced. There are two other negative regulators of cysteine. These are the molecules sulfide and thiosulfate, they act to bind to CysB and they compete with NAS for the binding of CysB.

Pyruvates

Pyruvate is the end result of glycolysis and can feed into both the TCA cycle and fermentation processes. Reactions beginning with either one or two molecules of pyruvate cause the synthesis of alanine, valine, and leucine. Feedback inhibition of final products is the main method of inhibition, and, in *E. coli*, the *ilvEDA* operon also plays a part in this regulation.

Alanine

Alanine is produced by the transamination of one molecule of pyruvate using two alternate steps: 1) conversion of glutamate to α-ketoglutarate using a glutamate-alanine transaminase, and 2) conversion of valine to α-ketoisovalerate via Transaminase C.

Not much is known about the regulation of alanine synthesis. The only definite method is the bacterium's ability to repress Transaminase C activity by either valine or leucine. Other than that, alanine biosynthesis does not seem to be regulated.

Valine

Valine is produced by a four-enzyme pathway. It begins with the reaction of two pyruvate molecules catalyzed by Acetohydroxy acid synthase yielding α-acetolactate. Step two is the NADPH+ + H+ - dependent reduction of α-acetolactate and migration of the methane groups to produce α, β-dihydroxyisovalerate. This is catalyzed by Acetohydroxy isomeroreductase. The third reaction is the dehydration reaction of α, β-dihydroxyisovalerate catalyzed by Dihydroxy acid dehydrase resulting in α-ketoisovalerate. Finally, a transamination catalyzed either by an alanine-valine transaminase or a glutamate-valine transaminase results in valine.

Valine performs feedback inhibition to inhibit the Acetohydroxy acid synthase used to combine the first two pyruvate molecules.

Leucine

The leucine synthesis pathway diverges from the valine pathway beginning with α-ketoisovalerate. α-Isopropylmalate synthase reacts with this substrate and Acetyl CoA to produce α-isopropylmalate. An isomerase then isomerizes α-isopropylmalate to β-isopropylmalate. The third step is the NAD+-dependent oxidation of β-isopropylmalate via the action of a dehydrogenase to yield α-ketoisocaproate. Finally is the transamination via the action of a glutamate-leucine transaminase to result in leucine.

Leucine, like valine, regulates the first step of its pathway by inhibiting the action of the α-Isopropylmalate synthase. Because leucine is synthesized by a diversion from the valine synthetic pathway, the feedback inhibition of valine on its pathway also can inhibit the synthesis of leucine.

ilvEDA operon

The genes that encode both the Dihydroxy acid dehydrase used in the creation of α-ketoisovalerate and Transaminase E, as well as other enzymes are encoded on the ilvEDA operon. This operon is bound and inactivated by valine, leucine, and isoleucine. (Isoleucine is not a direct derivative of pyruvate, but is produced by the use of many of the same enzymes used to produce valine and, indirectly, leucine.) When one of these amino acids is limited, the gene furthest from the amino-acid binding site of this operon can be transcribed. When a second of these amino acids is limited, the next-closest gene to the binding site can be transcribed, and so forth.

Amino Acids as Precursors to Other Biomolecules

Amino acids are precursors of a variety of biomolecules. Glutathione (γ-Glu-Cys-Gly) serves as a sulfhydryl buffer and detoxifying agent. Glutathione peroxidase, a selenoenzyme, catalyzes the reduction of hydrogen peroxide and organic peroxides by glutathione. Nitric oxide, a short-lived messenger, is formed from arginine. Porphyrins are synthesized from glycine and succinyl CoA, which condense to give δ-aminolevulinate. Two molecules of this intermediate become linked to form porphobilinogen. Four molecules of porphobilinogen combine to form a linear tetrapyrrole, which cyclizes to uroporphyrinogen III. Oxidation and side-chain modifications lead to the synthesis of protoporphyrin IX, which acquires an iron atom to form heme.

Fermentation

Fermentation is a metabolic process that converts sugar to acids, gases, or alcohol. It occurs in yeast and bacteria, and also in oxygen-starved muscle cells, as in the case of lactic acid fermentation. Fermentation is also used more broadly to refer to the bulk growth of microorganisms on a growth medium, often with the goal of producing a specific chemical product. French microbiologist Louis Pasteur is often remembered for his insights into fermentation and its microbial causes. The science of fermentation is known as zymology.

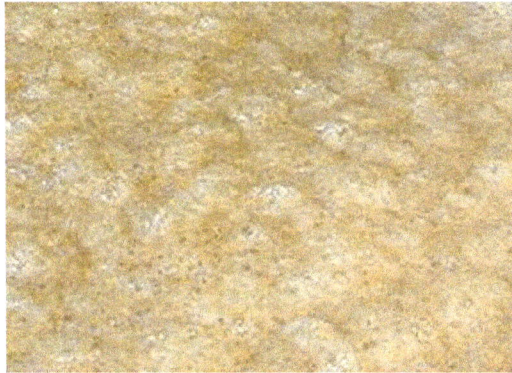

Fermentation in progress: Bubbles of CO_2 form a froth on top of the fermentation mixture.

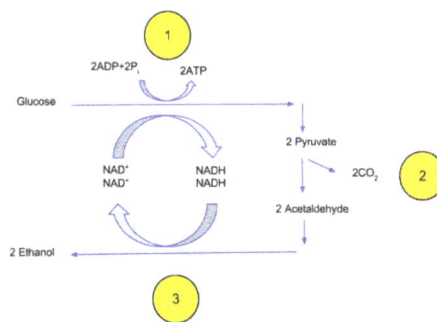

Overview of ethanol fermentation. One glucose molecule breaks down into two pyruvate molecules (1). The energy from this exothermic reaction is used to bind inorganic phosphates to ATP and convert NAD+ to NADH. The two pyruvates are then broken down into two acetaldehyde molecules and give off two CO2 molecules as a waste product (2). The acetaldehyde is then reduced into ethanol using the energy and hydrogen from NADH; in this process the NADH is oxidized into NAD+ so that the cycle may repeat (3).

Fermentation takes place when the electron transport chain is unusable (often due to lack of a final electron receptor, such as oxygen), and becomes the cell's primary means of ATP (energy) production. It turns NADH and pyruvate produced in glycolysis into NAD^+ and an organic molecule (which varies depending on the type of fermentation; see examples below). In the presence of O_2, NADH and pyruvate are used to generate ATP in respiration. This is called oxidative phosphorylation, and it generates much more ATP than glycolysis alone. For that reason, cells generally benefit from avoiding fermentation when oxygen is available, the exception being obligate anaerobes which cannot tolerate oxygen.

The first step, glycolysis, is common to all fermentation pathways:

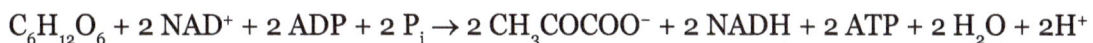

$$C_6H_{12}O_6 + 2\ NAD^+ + 2\ ADP + 2\ P_i \rightarrow 2\ CH_3COCOO^- + 2\ NADH + 2\ ATP + 2\ H_2O + 2H^+$$

Pyruvate is CH_3COCOO^-. P_i is inorganic phosphate. Two ADP molecules and two P_i are converted to two ATP and two water molecules via substrate-level phosphorylation. Two molecules of NAD^+ are also reduced to NADH.

In oxidative phosphorylation the energy for ATP formation is derived from an electrochemical proton gradient generated across the inner mitochondrial membrane (or, in the case of bacteria, the plasma membrane) via the electron transport chain. Glycolysis has substrate-level phosphorylation (ATP generated directly at the point of reaction).

Humans have used fermentation to produce food and beverages since the Neolithic age. For example, fermentation is used for preservation in a process that produces lactic acid as found in such sour foods as pickled cucumbers, kimchi and yogurt, as well as for producing alcoholic beverages such as wine and beer. Fermentation can even occur within the stomachs of animals, such as humans.

Definitions

To many people, fermentation simply means the production of alcohol: grains and fruits are fermented to produce beer and wine. If a food soured, one might say it was 'off' or fermented. Here are some definitions of fermentation. They range from informal, general usage to more scientific definitions.

1. Preservation methods for food via microorganisms (general use).

2. Any process that produces alcoholic beverages or acidic dairy products (general use).

3. Any large-scale microbial process occurring with or without air (common definition used in industry).

4. Any energy-releasing metabolic process that takes place only under anaerobic conditions (becoming more scientific).

5. Any metabolic process that releases energy from a sugar or other organic molecules, does not require oxygen or an electron transport system, and uses an organic molecule as the final electron acceptor (most scientific).

Examples

Fermentation does not necessarily have to be carried out in an anaerobic environment. For example, even in the presence of abundant oxygen, yeast cells greatly prefer fermentation to aerobic respiration, as long as sugars are readily available for consumption (a phenomenon known as the Crabtree effect). The antibiotic activity of hops also inhibits aerobic metabolism in yeast.

Fermentation reacts NADH with an endogenous, organic electron acceptor. Usually this is pyruvate formed from the sugar during the glycolysis step. During fermentation, pyruvate is metabolized to various compounds through several processes:

-   ethanol fermentation, aka alcoholic fermentation, is the production of ethanol and carbon dioxide

-   lactic acid fermentation refers to two means of producing lactic acid:

1. homolactic fermentation is the production of lactic acid exclusively

2. heterolactic fermentation is the production of lactic acid as well as other acids and alcohols.

Sugars are the most common substrate of fermentation, and typical examples of fermentation products are ethanol, lactic acid, carbon dioxide, and hydrogen gas (H_2). However, more exotic compounds can be produced by fermentation, such as butyric acid and acetone. Yeast carries out fermentation in the production of ethanol in beers, wines, and other alcoholic drinks, along with the production of large quantities of carbon dioxide. Fermentation occurs in mammalian muscle during periods of intense exercise where oxygen supply becomes limited, resulting in the creation of lactic acid.

Chemistry

Comparison of aerobic respiration and most known fermentation types in eucaryotic cell.
Numbers in circles indicate counts of carbon atoms in molecules, C6 is glucose $C_6H_{12}O_6$, C1 carbon dioxide CO_2. Mitochondrial outer membrane is omitted.

Fermentation products contain chemical energy (they are not fully oxidized), but are considered waste products, since they cannot be metabolized further without the use of oxygen.

Ethanol Fermentation

The chemical equation below shows the alcoholic fermentation of glucose, whose chemical formula is $C_6H_{12}O_6$. One glucose molecule is converted into two ethanol molecules and two carbon dioxide molecules:

$$C_6H_{12}O_6 \rightarrow 2\,C_2H_5OH + 2\,CO_2$$

C_2H_5OH is the chemical formula for ethanol.

Before fermentation takes place, one glucose molecule is broken down into two pyruvate molecules. This is known as glycolysis.

Lactic Acid Fermentation

Homolactic fermentation (producing only lactic acid) is the simplest type of fermentation. The pyruvate from glycolysis undergoes a simple redox reaction, forming lactic acid. It is unique because it is one of the only respiration processes to not produce a gas as a byproduct. Overall, one molecule of glucose (or any six-carbon sugar) is converted to two molecules of lactic acid: $C_6H_{12}O_6 \rightarrow 2\,CH_3CHOHCOOH$ It occurs in the muscles of animals when they need energy faster than the blood can supply oxygen. It also occurs in some kinds of bacteria (such as lactobacilli) and some fungi. It is this type of bacteria that converts lactose into lactic acid in yogurt, giving it its sour taste. These lactic acid bacteria can carry out either homolactic fermentation, where the end-product is mostly lactic acid, or

Heterolactic fermentation, where some lactate is further metabolized and results in ethanol and carbon dioxide (via the phosphoketolase pathway), acetate, or other metabolic products, e.g.: $C_6H_{12}O_6 \rightarrow CH_3CHOHCOOH + C_2H_5OH + CO_2$ If lactose is fermented (as in yogurts and cheeses), it is first converted into glucose and galactose (both six-carbon sugars with the same atomic formula): $C_{12}H_{22}O_{11} + H_2O \rightarrow 2\ C_6H_{12}O_6$

Heterolactic fermentation is in a sense intermediate between lactic acid fermentation, and other types, e.g. alcoholic fermentation. The reasons to go further and convert lactic acid into anything else are:

- The acidity of lactic acid impedes biological processes; this can be beneficial to the fermenting organism as it drives out competitors who are unadapted to the acidity; as a result the food will have a longer shelf-life (part of the reason foods are purposely fermented in the first place); however, beyond a certain point, the acidity starts affecting the organism that produces it.

- The high concentration of lactic acid (the final product of fermentation) drives the equilibrium backwards (Le Chatelier's principle), decreasing the rate at which fermentation can occur, and slowing down growth

- Ethanol, that lactic acid can be easily converted to, is volatile and will readily escape, allowing the reaction to proceed easily. CO_2 is also produced, however it's only weakly acidic, and even more volatile than ethanol.

- Acetic acid (another conversion product) is acidic, and not as volatile as ethanol; however, in the presence of limited oxygen, its creation from lactic acid releases a lot of additional energy. It is a lighter molecule than lactic acid, that forms fewer hydrogen bonds with its surroundings (due to having fewer groups that can form such bonds), and thus more volatile and will also allow the reaction to move forward more quickly.

- If propionic acid, butyric acid and longer monocarboxylic acids are produced, the amount of acidity produced per glucose consumed will decrease, as with ethanol, allowing faster growth.

Aerobic Respiration

In aerobic respiration, the pyruvate produced by glycolysis is oxidized completely, generating additional ATP and NADH in the citric acid cycle and by oxidative phosphorylation. However, this can occur only in the presence of oxygen. Oxygen is toxic to organisms that are obligate anaerobes, and is not required by facultative anaerobic organisms. In the absence of oxygen, one of the fermentation pathways occurs in order to regenerate NAD^+; lactic acid fermentation is one of these pathways.

Hydrogen Gas Production in Fermentation

Hydrogen gas is produced in many types of fermentation (mixed acid fermentation, butyric acid fermentation, caproate fermentation, butanol fermentation, glyoxylate fermentation), as a way to regenerate NAD^+ from NADH. Electrons are transferred to ferredoxin, which in turn is oxidized by hydrogenase, producing H_2. Hydrogen gas is a substrate for methanogens and sulfate reducers, which keep the concentration of hydrogen low and favor the production of such an energy-rich compound, but hydrogen gas at a fairly high concentration can nevertheless be formed, as in flatus.

As an example of mixed acid fermentation, bacteria such as *Clostridium pasteurianum* ferment glucose producing butyrate, acetate, carbon dioxide and hydrogen gas: The reaction leading to acetate is:

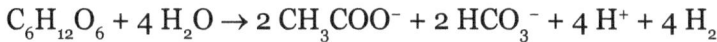

$$C_6H_{12}O_6 + 4\ H_2O \rightarrow 2\ CH_3COO^- + 2\ HCO_3^- + 4\ H^+ + 4\ H_2$$

Glucose could theoretically be converted into just CO_2 and H_2, but the global reaction releases little energy.

Methane Gas Production in Fermentation

Acetic acid can also undergo a dismutation reaction to produce methane and carbon dioxide:

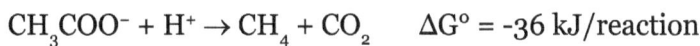

$$CH_3COO^- + H^+ \rightarrow CH_4 + CO_2 \qquad \Delta G° = \text{-36 kJ/reaction}$$

This disproportionation reaction is catalysed by methanogen archaea in their fermentative metabolism. One electron is transferred from the carbonyl function (e^- donor) of the carboxylic group to the methyl group (e^- acceptor) of acetic acid to respectively produce CO_2 and methane gas.

History of Human Use

The use of fermentation, particularly for beverages, has existed since the Neolithic and has been documented dating from 7000–6600 BCE in Jiahu, China, 5000 BCE in India, Ayurveda mentions many Medicated Wines, 6000 BCE in Georgia, 3150 BCE in ancient Egypt, 3000 BCE in Babylon, 2000 BCE in pre-Hispanic Mexico, and 1500 BC in Sudan. Fermented foods have a religious significance in Judaism and Christianity. The Baltic god Rugutis was worshiped as the agent of fermentation.

The first solid evidence of the living nature of yeast appeared between 1837 and 1838 when three publications appeared by C. Cagniard de la Tour, T. Swann, and F. Kuetzing, each of whom independently concluded as a result of microscopic investigations that yeast is a living organism that reproduces by budding. It is perhaps because wine, beer, and bread were each basic foods in Europe that most of the early studies on fermentation were done on yeasts, with which they were made. Soon, bacteria were also discovered; the term was first used in English in the late 1840s, but it did not come into general use until the 1870s, and then largely in connection with the new germ theory of disease.

Louis Pasteur (1822–1895), during the 1850s and 1860s, showed that fermentation is initiated by living organisms in a series of investigations. In 1857, Pasteur showed that lactic acid fermentation is caused by living organisms. In 1860, he demonstrated that bacteria cause souring in milk, a process formerly thought to be merely a chemical change, and his work in identifying the role of microorganisms in food spoilage led to the process of pasteurization. In 1877, working to improve the French brewing industry, Pasteur published his famous paper on fermentation, "*Etudes sur la Bière*", which was translated into English in 1879 as "Studies on fermentation". He defined fermentation (incorrectly) as "Life without air", but correctly showed that specific types of microorganisms cause specific types of fermentations and specific end-products.

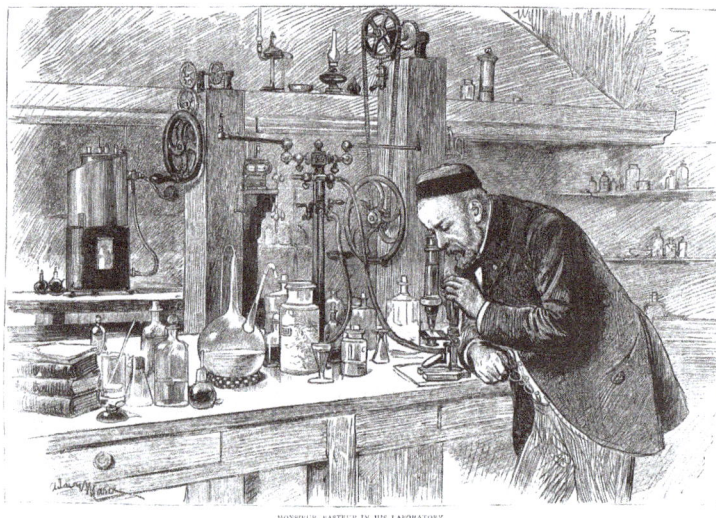

Louis Pasteur in his laboratory

Although showing fermentation to be the result of the action of living microorganisms was a breakthrough, it did not explain the basic nature of the fermentation process, or prove that it is caused by the microorganisms that appear to be always present. Many scientists, including Pasteur, had unsuccessfully attempted to extract the fermentation enzyme from yeast. Success came in 1897 when the German chemist Eduard Buechner ground up yeast, extracted a juice from them, then found to his amazement that this "dead" liquid would ferment a sugar solution, forming carbon dioxide and alcohol much like living yeasts. Buechner's results are considered to mark the birth of biochemistry. The "unorganized ferments" behaved just like the organized ones. From that time on, the term enzyme came to be applied to all ferments. It was then understood that fermentation is caused by enzymes that are produced by microorganisms. In 1907, Buechner won the Nobel Prize in chemistry for his work.

Advances in microbiology and fermentation technology have continued steadily up until the present. For example, in the late 1970s, it was discovered that microorganisms could be mutated with physical and chemical treatments to be higher-yielding, faster-growing, tolerant of less oxygen, and able to use a more concentrated medium. Strain selection and hybridization developed as well, affecting most modern food fermentations. Other approaches to advancing the fermentation industry has been done by companies such as BioTork, a biotechnology company that naturally evolves microorganisms to improve fermentation processes. This approach differs from the more popular genetic modification, which has become the current industry standard.

Etymology

The word *ferment* is derived from the Latin verb *fervere*, which means 'to boil'. It is thought to have been first used in the late fourteenth century in alchemy, but only in a broad sense. It was not used in the modern scientific sense until around 1600.

Oxidative Phosphorylation

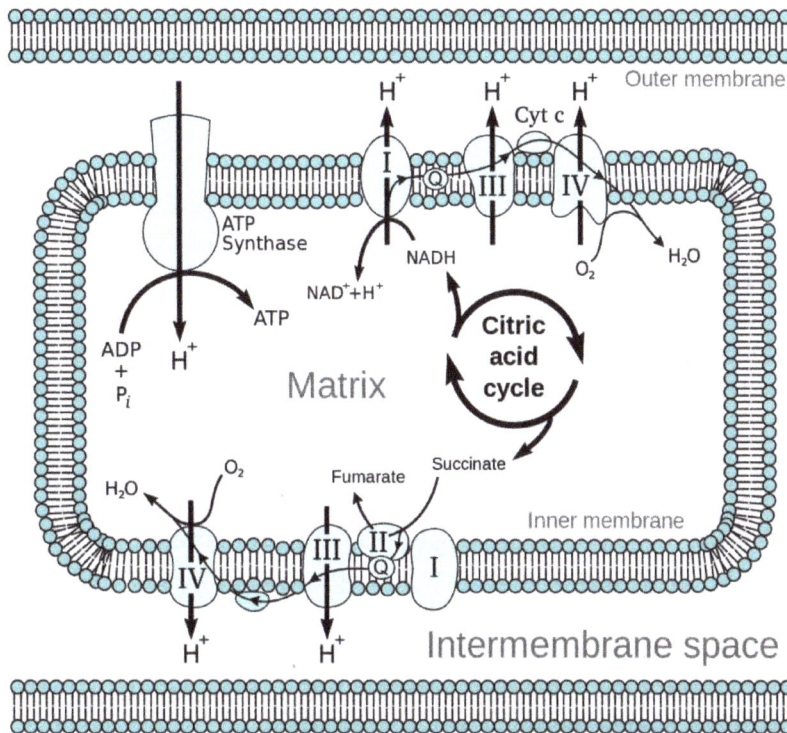

The electron transport chain in the cell is the site of oxidative phosphorylation in prokaryotes. The NADH and succinate generated in the citric acid cycle are oxidized, releasing energy to power the ATP synthase.

Oxidative phosphorylation (or OXPHOS in short) is the metabolic pathway in which cells use enzymes to oxidize nutrients, thereby releasing energy which is used to reform ATP. In most eukaryotes, this takes place inside mitochondria. Almost all aerobic organisms carry out oxidative phosphorylation. This pathway is probably so pervasive because it is a highly efficient way of releasing energy, compared to alternative fermentation processes such as anaerobic glycolysis.

During oxidative phosphorylation, electrons are transferred from electron donors to electron acceptors such as oxygen, in redox reactions. These redox reactions release energy, which is used to form ATP. In eukaryotes, these redox reactions are carried out by a series of protein complexes within the inner membrane of the cell's mitochondria, whereas, in prokaryotes, these proteins are located in the cells' intermembrane space. These linked sets of proteins are called electron transport chains. In eukaryotes, five main protein complexes are involved, whereas in prokaryotes many different enzymes are present, using a variety of electron donors and acceptors.

The energy released by electrons flowing through this electron transport chain is used to transport protons across the inner mitochondrial membrane, in a process called *electron transport*. This generates potential energy in the form of a pH gradient and an electrical potential across this membrane. This store of energy is tapped by allowing protons to flow back across the membrane and down this gradient, through a large enzyme called ATP synthase; this process is known as chemiosmosis. This enzyme uses this energy to generate ATP from adenosine diphosphate (ADP), in a phosphorylation reaction. This reaction is driven by the proton flow, which forces the rotation of a part of the enzyme; the ATP synthase is a rotary mechanical motor.

Although oxidative phosphorylation is a vital part of metabolism, it produces reactive oxygen species such as superoxide and hydrogen peroxide, which lead to propagation of free radicals, damaging cells and contributing to disease and, possibly, aging (senescence). The enzymes carrying out this metabolic pathway are also the target of many drugs and poisons that inhibit their activities.

Overview of Energy Transfer by Chemiosmosis

Oxidative phosphorylation works by using energy-releasing chemical reactions to drive energy-requiring reactions: The two sets of reactions are said to be *coupled*. This means one cannot occur without the other. The flow of electrons through the electron transport chain, from electron donors such as NADH to electron acceptors such as oxygen, is an exergonic process – it releases energy, whereas the synthesis of ATP is an endergonic process, which requires an input of energy. Both the electron transport chain and the ATP synthase are embedded in a membrane, and energy is transferred from electron transport chain to the ATP synthase by movements of protons across this membrane, in a process called *chemiosmosis*. In practice, this is like a simple electric circuit, with a current of protons being driven from the negative N-side of the membrane to the positive P-side by the proton-pumping enzymes of the electron transport chain. These enzymes are like a battery, as they perform work to drive current through the circuit. The movement of protons creates an electrochemical gradient across the membrane, which is often called the *proton-motive force*. It has two components: a difference in proton concentration (a H^+ gradient, ΔpH) and a difference in electric potential, with the N-side having a negative charge.

ATP synthase releases this stored energy by completing the circuit and allowing protons to flow down the electrochemical gradient, back to the N-side of the membrane. This kinetic energy drives the rotation of part of the enzymes structure and couples this motion to the synthesis of ATP.

The two components of the proton-motive force are thermodynamically equivalent: In mitochondria, the largest part of energy is provided by the potential; in alkaliphile bacteria the electrical energy even has to compensate for a counteracting inverse pH difference. Inversely, chloroplasts operate mainly on ΔpH. However, they also require a small membrane potential for the kinetics of ATP synthesis. At least in the case of the fusobacterium *P. modestum* it drives the counter-rotation of subunits a and c of the F_O motor of ATP synthase.

The amount of energy released by oxidative phosphorylation is high, compared with the amount produced by anaerobic fermentation. Glycolysis produces only 2 ATP molecules, but somewhere between 30 and 36 ATPs are produced by the oxidative phosphorylation of the 10 NADH and 2 succinate molecules made by converting one molecule of glucose to carbon dioxide and water, while each cycle of beta oxidation of a fatty acid yields about 14 ATPs. These ATP yields are theoretical maximum values; in practice, some protons leak across the membrane, lowering the yield of ATP.

Electron and Proton Transfer Molecules

The electron transport chain carries both protons and electrons, passing electrons from donors to acceptors, and transporting protons across a membrane. These processes use both soluble and protein-bound transfer molecules. In mitochondria, electrons are transferred within the inter-membrane space by the water-soluble electron transfer protein cytochrome c. This carries only electrons, and these are transferred by the reduction and oxidation of an iron atom that the protein holds within a heme group in its structure. Cytochrome c is also found in some bacteria, where it is located within the periplasmic space.

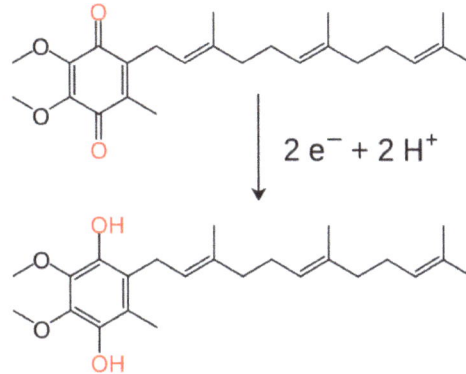

Reduction of coenzyme Q from its ubiquinone form (Q) to the reduced ubiquinol form (QH$_2$).

Within the inner mitochondrial membrane, the lipid-soluble electron carrier coenzyme Q10 (Q) carries both electrons and protons by a redox cycle. This small benzoquinone molecule is very hydrophobic, so it diffuses freely within the membrane. When Q accepts two electrons and two protons, it becomes reduced to the *ubiquinol* form (QH$_2$); when QH$_2$ releases two electrons and two protons, it becomes oxidized back to the *ubiquinone* (Q) form. As a result, if two enzymes are arranged so that Q is reduced on one side of the membrane and QH$_2$ oxidized on the other, ubiquinone will couple these reactions and shuttle protons across the membrane. Some bacterial electron transport chains use different quinones, such as menaquinone, in addition to ubiquinone.

Within proteins, electrons are transferred between flavin cofactors, iron–sulfur clusters, and cytochromes. There are several types of iron–sulfur cluster. The simplest kind found in the electron transfer chain consists of two iron atoms joined by two atoms of inorganic sulfur; these are called [2Fe–2S] clusters. The second kind, called [4Fe–4S], contains a cube of four iron atoms and four sulfur atoms. Each iron atom in these clusters is coordinated by an additional amino acid, usually by the sulfur atom of cysteine. Metal ion cofactors undergo redox reactions without binding or releasing protons, so in the electron transport chain they serve solely to transport electrons through proteins. Electrons move quite long distances through proteins by hopping along chains of these cofactors. This occurs by quantum tunnelling, which is rapid over distances of less than 1.4×10^{-9} m.

Eukaryotic Electron Transport Chains

Many catabolic biochemical processes, such as glycolysis, the citric acid cycle, and beta oxidation, produce the reduced coenzyme NADH. This coenzyme contains electrons that have a high transfer potential; in other words, they will release a large amount of energy upon oxidation. However, the cell does not release this energy all at once, as this would be an uncontrollable reaction. Instead, the electrons are removed from NADH and passed to oxygen through a series of enzymes that each release a small amount of the energy. This set of enzymes, consisting of complexes I through IV, is called the electron transport chain and is found in the inner membrane of the mitochondrion. Succinate is also oxidized by the electron transport chain, but feeds into the pathway at a different point.

In eukaryotes, the enzymes in this electron transport system use the energy released from the oxidation of NADH to pump protons across the inner membrane of the mitochondrion. This causes protons to build up in the intermembrane space, and generates an electrochemical gradient across the membrane. The energy stored in this potential is then used by ATP synthase to produce ATP. Oxidative phosphorylation in the eukaryotic mitochondrion is the best-understood example of this process. The mitochondrion is present in almost all eukaryotes, with the exception of anaerobic protozoa such as *Trichomonas vaginalis* that instead reduce protons to hydrogen in a remnant mitochondrion called a hydrogenosome.

Typical respiratory enzymes and substrates in eukaryotes.		
Respiratory enzyme	**Redox pair**	**Midpoint potential (Volts)**
NADH dehydrogenase	NAD^+ / NADH	-0.32
Succinate dehydrogenase	FMN or FAD / $FMNH_2$ or $FADH_2$	-0.20
Cytochrome bc_1 complex	Coenzyme $Q10_{ox}$ / Coenzyme $Q10_{red}$	$+0.06$
Cytochrome bc_1 complex	Cytochrome b_{ox} / Cytochrome b_{red}	$+0.12$
Complex IV	Cytochrome c_{ox} / Cytochrome c_{red}	$+0.22$
Complex IV	Cytochrome a_{ox} / Cytochrome a_{red}	$+0.29$
Complex IV	O_2 / HO^-	$+0.82$
Conditions: pH = 7		

NADH-coenzyme Q Oxidoreductase (Complex I)

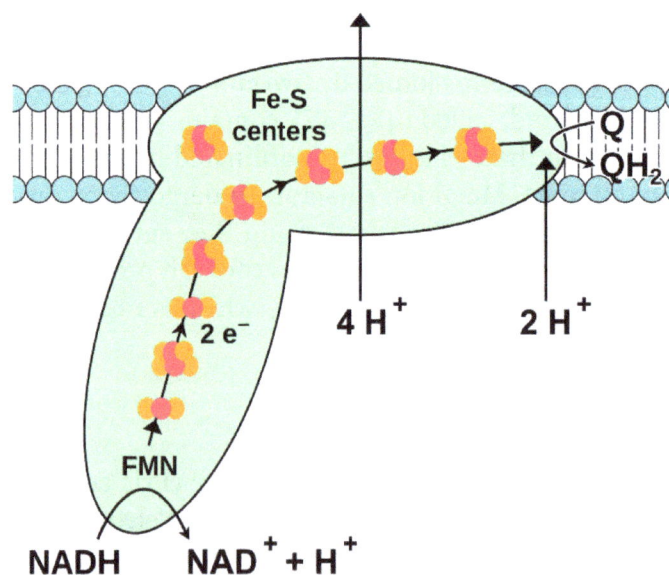

Complex I or NADH-Q oxidoreductase. The abbreviations are discussed in the text. In all diagrams of respiratory complexes in this article, the matrix is at the bottom, with the intermembrane space above.

NADH-coenzyme Q oxidoreductase, also known as *NADH dehydrogenase* or *complex I*, is the first protein in the electron transport chain. Complex I is a giant enzyme with the mammalian complex I having 46 subunits and a molecular mass of about 1,000 kilodaltons (kDa). The structure is known in detail only from a bacterium; in most organisms the complex resembles a boot with a large "ball" poking out from the membrane into the mitochondrion. The genes that encode the individual proteins are contained in both the cell nucleus and the mitochondrial genome, as is the case for many enzymes present in the mitochondrion.

The reaction that is catalyzed by this enzyme is the two electron oxidation of NADH by coenzyme Q10 or *ubiquinone* (represented as Q in the equation below), a lipid-soluble quinone that is found in the mitochondrion membrane:

The start of the reaction, and indeed of the entire electron chain, is the binding of a NADH molecule to complex I and the donation of two electrons. The electrons enter complex I via a prosthetic group attached to the complex, flavin mononucleotide (FMN). The addition of electrons to FMN converts it to its reduced form, $FMNH_2$. The electrons are then transferred through a series of iron–sulfur clusters: the second kind of prosthetic group present in the complex. There are both [2Fe–2S] and [4Fe–4S] iron–sulfur clusters in complex I.

As the electrons pass through this complex, four protons are pumped from the matrix into the intermembrane space. Exactly how this occurs is unclear, but it seems to involve conformational changes in complex I that cause the protein to bind protons on the N-side of the membrane and release them on the P-side of the membrane. Finally, the electrons are transferred from the chain of iron–sulfur clusters to a ubiquinone molecule in the membrane. Reduction of ubiquinone also contributes to the generation of a proton gradient, as two protons are taken up from the matrix as it is reduced to ubiquinol (QH_2).

Succinate-Q Oxidoreductase (Complex II)

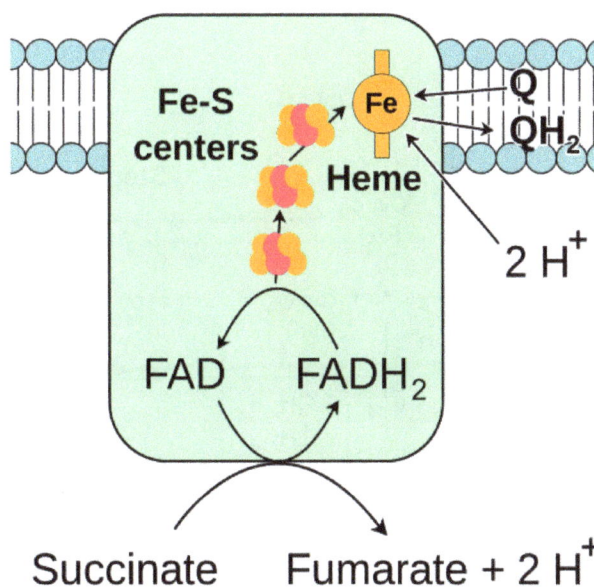

Complex II: Succinate-Q oxidoreductase.

Succinate-Q oxidoreductase, also known as *complex II* or *succinate dehydrogenase*, is a second entry point to the electron transport chain. It is unusual because it is the only enzyme that is part of both the citric acid cycle and the electron transport chain. Complex II consists of four protein subunits and contains a bound flavin adenine dinucleotide (FAD) cofactor, iron–sulfur clusters, and a heme group that does not participate in electron transfer to coenzyme Q, but is believed to be important in decreasing production of reactive oxygen species. It oxidizes succinate to fumarate and reduces ubiquinone. As this reaction releases less energy than the oxidation of NADH, complex II does not transport protons across the membrane and does not contribute to the proton gradient.

In some eukaryotes, such as the parasitic worm *Ascaris suum*, an enzyme similar to complex II, fumarate reductase (menaquinol:fumarate oxidoreductase, or QFR), operates in reverse to oxidize ubiquinol and reduce fumarate. This allows the worm to survive in the anaerobic environment of the large intestine, carrying out anaerobic oxidative phosphorylation with fumarate as the electron acceptor. Another unconventional function of complex II is seen in the malaria parasite *Plasmodium falciparum*. Here, the reversed action of complex II as an oxidase is important in regenerating ubiquinol, which the parasite uses in an unusual form of pyrimidine biosynthesis.

Electron Transfer Flavoprotein-Q Oxidoreductase

Electron transfer flavoprotein-ubiquinone oxidoreductase (ETF-Q oxidoreductase), also known as *electron transferring-flavoprotein dehydrogenase*, is a third entry point to the electron transport chain. It is an enzyme that accepts electrons from electron-transferring flavoprotein in the mitochondrial matrix, and uses these electrons to reduce ubiquinone. This enzyme contains a flavin and a [4Fe–4S] cluster, but, unlike the other respiratory complexes, it attaches to the surface of the membrane and does not cross the lipid bilayer.

In mammals, this metabolic pathway is important in beta oxidation of fatty acids and catabolism of amino acids and choline, as it accepts electrons from multiple acetyl-CoA dehydrogenases. In plants, ETF-Q oxidoreductase is also important in the metabolic responses that allow survival in extended periods of darkness.

Q-cytochrome C Oxidoreductase (Complex III)

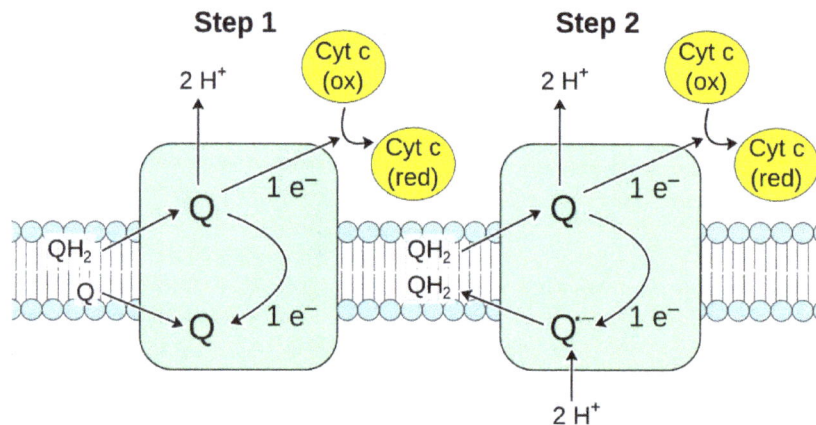

The two electron transfer steps in complex III: Q-cytochrome c oxidoreductase. After each step, Q (in the upper part of the figure) leaves the enzyme.

Q-cytochrome c oxidoreductase is also known as *cytochrome c reductase, cytochrome bc₁ complex,* or simply *complex III*. In mammals, this enzyme is a dimer, with each subunit complex containing 11 protein subunits, an [2Fe-2S] iron–sulfur cluster and three cytochromes: one cytochrome c_1 and two b cytochromes. A cytochrome is a kind of electron-transferring protein that contains at least one heme group. The iron atoms inside complex III's heme groups alternate between a reduced ferrous (+2) and oxidized ferric (+3) state as the electrons are transferred through the protein.

The reaction catalyzed by complex III is the oxidation of one molecule of ubiquinol and the reduction of two molecules of cytochrome c, a heme protein loosely associated with the mitochondrion. Unlike coenzyme Q, which carries two electrons, cytochrome c carries only one electron.

As only one of the electrons can be transferred from the QH_2 donor to a cytochrome c acceptor at a time, the reaction mechanism of complex III is more elaborate than those of the other respiratory complexes, and occurs in two steps called the Q cycle. In the first step, the enzyme binds three substrates, first, QH_2, which is then oxidized, with one electron being passed to the second substrate, cytochrome c. The two protons released from QH_2 pass into the intermembrane space. The third substrate is Q, which accepts the second electron from the QH_2 and is reduced to Q^-, which is the ubisemiquinone free radical. The first two substrates are released, but this ubisemiquinone intermediate remains bound. In the second step, a second molecule of QH_2 is bound and again passes its first electron to a cytochrome c acceptor. The second electron is passed to the bound ubisemiquinone, reducing it to QH_2 as it gains two protons from the mitochondrial matrix. This QH_2 is then released from the enzyme.

As coenzyme Q is reduced to ubiquinol on the inner side of the membrane and oxidized to ubiquinone on the other, a net transfer of protons across the membrane occurs, adding to the proton gradient. The rather complex two-step mechanism by which this occurs is important, as it increases the efficiency of proton transfer. If, instead of the Q cycle, one molecule of QH_2 were used to directly reduce two molecules of cytochrome c, the efficiency would be halved, with only one proton transferred per cytochrome c reduced.

Cytochrome C Oxidase (Complex IV)

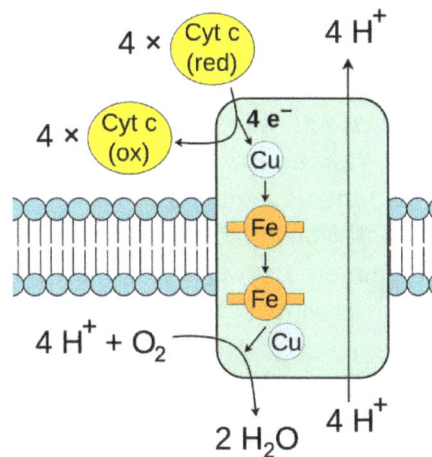

Complex IV: cytochrome c oxidase.

Cytochrome c oxidase, also known as *complex IV*, is the final protein complex in the electron transport chain. The mammalian enzyme has an extremely complicated structure and contains 13 subunits, two heme groups, as well as multiple metal ion cofactors – in all, three atoms of copper, one of magnesium and one of zinc.

This enzyme mediates the final reaction in the electron transport chain and transfers electrons to oxygen, while pumping protons across the membrane. The final electron acceptor oxygen, which is also called the *terminal electron acceptor*, is reduced to water in this step. Both the direct pumping of protons and the consumption of matrix protons in the reduction of oxygen contribute to the proton gradient. The reaction catalyzed is the oxidation of cytochrome c and the reduction of oxygen:

Alternative Reductases and Oxidases

Many eukaryotic organisms have electron transport chains that differ from the much-studied mammalian enzymes described above. For example, plants have alternative NADH oxidases, which oxidize NADH in the cytosol rather than in the mitochondrial matrix, and pass these electrons to the ubiquinone pool. These enzymes do not transport protons, and, therefore, reduce ubiquinone without altering the electrochemical gradient across the inner membrane.

Another example of a divergent electron transport chain is the *alternative oxidase*, which is found in plants, as well as some fungi, protists, and possibly some animals. This enzyme transfers electrons directly from ubiquinol to oxygen.

The electron transport pathways produced by these alternative NADH and ubiquinone oxidases have lower ATP yields than the full pathway. The advantages produced by a shortened pathway are not entirely clear. However, the alternative oxidase is produced in response to stresses such as cold, reactive oxygen species, and infection by pathogens, as well as other factors that inhibit the full electron transport chain. Alternative pathways might, therefore, enhance an organisms' resistance to injury, by reducing oxidative stress.

Organization of Complexes

The original model for how the respiratory chain complexes are organized was that they diffuse freely and independently in the mitochondrial membrane. However, recent data suggest that the complexes might form higher-order structures called supercomplexes or "respirasomes." In this model, the various complexes exist as organized sets of interacting enzymes. These associations might allow channeling of substrates between the various enzyme complexes, increasing the rate and efficiency of electron transfer. Within such mammalian supercomplexes, some components would be present in higher amounts than others, with some data suggesting a ratio between complexes I/II/III/IV and the ATP synthase of approximately 1:1:3:7:4. However, the debate over this supercomplex hypothesis is not completely resolved, as some data do not appear to fit with this model.

Prokaryotic Electron Transport Chains

In contrast to the general similarity in structure and function of the electron transport chains in eukaryotes, bacteria and archaea possess a large variety of electron-transfer enzymes. These use an equally wide set of chemicals as substrates. In common with eukaryotes, prokaryotic electron transport uses the energy released from the oxidation of a substrate to pump ions across a membrane and generate an electrochemical gradient. In the bacteria, oxidative phosphorylation in *Escherichia coli* is understood in most detail, while archaeal systems are at present poorly understood.

The main difference between eukaryotic and prokaryotic oxidative phosphorylation is that bacteria and archaea use many different substances to donate or accept electrons. This allows prokaryotes to grow under a wide variety of environmental conditions. In *E. coli*, for example, oxidative phosphorylation can be driven by a large number of pairs of reducing agents and oxidizing agents, which are listed below. The midpoint potential of a chemical measures how much energy is released when it is oxidized or reduced, with reducing agents having negative potentials and oxidizing agents positive potentials.

Respiratory enzymes and substrates in *E. coli*.		
Respiratory enzyme	**Redox pair**	**Midpoint potential (Volts)**
Formate dehydrogenase	Bicarbonate / Formate	−0.43
Hydrogenase	Proton / Hydrogen	−0.42
NADH dehydrogenase	NAD^+ / NADH	−0.32
Glycerol-3-phosphate dehydrogenase	DHAP / Gly-3-P	−0.19
Pyruvate oxidase	Acetate + Carbon dioxide / Pyruvate	?
Lactate dehydrogenase	Pyruvate / Lactate	−0.19
D-amino acid dehydrogenase	2-oxoacid + ammonia / D-amino acid	?
Glucose dehydrogenase	Gluconate / Glucose	−0.14
Succinate dehydrogenase	Fumarate / Succinate	+0.03
Ubiquinol oxidase	Oxygen / Water	+0.82
Nitrate reductase	Nitrate / Nitrite	+0.42
Nitrite reductase	Nitrite / Ammonia	+0.36
Dimethyl sulfoxide reductase	DMSO / DMS	+0.16
Trimethylamine *N*-oxide reductase	TMAO / TMA	+0.13
Fumarate reductase	Fumarate / Succinate	+0.03

As shown above, *E. coli* can grow with reducing agents such as formate, hydrogen, or lactate as electron donors, and nitrate, DMSO, or oxygen as acceptors. The larger the difference in midpoint potential between an oxidizing and reducing agent, the more energy is released when they react. Out of these compounds, the succinate/fumarate pair is unusual, as its midpoint potential is close to zero. Succinate can therefore be oxidized to fumarate if a strong oxidizing agent such as oxygen is available, or fumarate can be reduced to succinate using a strong reducing agent such as formate. These alternative reactions are catalyzed by succinate dehydrogenase and fumarate reductase, respectively.

Some prokaryotes use redox pairs that have only a small difference in midpoint potential. For example, nitrifying bacteria such as *Nitrobacter* oxidize nitrite to nitrate, donating the electrons to oxygen. The small amount of energy released in this reaction is enough to pump protons and generate ATP, but not enough to produce NADH or NADPH directly for use in anabolism. This problem is solved by using a nitrite oxidoreductase to produce enough proton-motive force to run part of the electron transport chain in reverse, causing complex I to generate NADH.

Prokaryotes control their use of these electron donors and acceptors by varying which enzymes are produced, in response to environmental conditions. This flexibility is possible because different oxidases and reductases use the same ubiquinone pool. This allows many combinations of enzymes to function together, linked by the common ubiquinol intermediate. These respiratory chains therefore have a modular design, with easily interchangeable sets of enzyme systems.

In addition to this metabolic diversity, prokaryotes also possess a range of isozymes – different enzymes that catalyze the same reaction. For example, in *E. coli*, there are two different types of ubiquinol oxidase using oxygen as an electron acceptor. Under highly aerobic conditions, the cell uses an oxidase with a low affinity for oxygen that can transport two protons per electron. However, if levels of oxygen fall, they switch to an oxidase that transfers only one proton per electron, but has a high affinity for oxygen.

ATP Synthase (complex V)

ATP synthase, also called *complex V*, is the final enzyme in the oxidative phosphorylation pathway. This enzyme is found in all forms of life and functions in the same way in both prokaryotes and eukaryotes. The enzyme uses the energy stored in a proton gradient across a membrane to drive the synthesis of ATP from ADP and phosphate (P_i). Estimates of the number of protons required to synthesize one ATP have ranged from three to four, with some suggesting cells can vary this ratio, to suit different conditions.

This phosphorylation reaction is an equilibrium, which can be shifted by altering the proton-motive force. In the absence of a proton-motive force, the ATP synthase reaction will run from right to left, hydrolyzing ATP and pumping protons out of the matrix across the membrane. However, when the proton-motive force is high, the reaction is forced to run in the opposite direction; it proceeds from left to right, allowing protons to flow down their concentration gradient and turning ADP into ATP. Indeed, in the closely related vacuolar type H+-ATPases, the hydrolysis reaction is used to acidify cellular compartments, by pumping protons and hydrolysing ATP.

ATP synthase is a massive protein complex with a mushroom-like shape. The mammalian enzyme complex contains 16 subunits and has a mass of approximately 600 kilodaltons. The portion embedded within the membrane is called F_O and contains a ring of c subunits and the proton channel. The stalk and the ball-shaped headpiece is called F_1 and is the site of ATP synthesis. The ball-shaped complex at the end of the F_1 portion contains six proteins of two different kinds (three α subunits and three β subunits), whereas the "stalk" consists of one protein: the γ subunit, with the tip of the stalk extending into the ball of α and β subunits. Both the α and β subunits bind nucleotides, but only the β subunits catalyze the ATP synthesis reaction. Reaching along the side of the F_1 portion and back into the membrane is a long rod-like subunit that anchors the α and β subunits into the base of the enzyme.

As protons cross the membrane through the channel in the base of ATP synthase, the F_O proton-driven motor rotates. Rotation might be caused by changes in the ionization of amino acids in the ring of c subunits causing electrostatic interactions that propel the ring of c subunits past the proton channel. This rotating ring in turn drives the rotation of the central axle (the γ subunit stalk) within the α and β subunits. The α and β subunits are prevented from rotating themselves by the side-arm, which acts as a stator. This movement of the tip of the γ subunit within the ball of α and β subunits provides the energy for the active sites in the β subunits to undergo a cycle of movements that produces and then releases ATP.

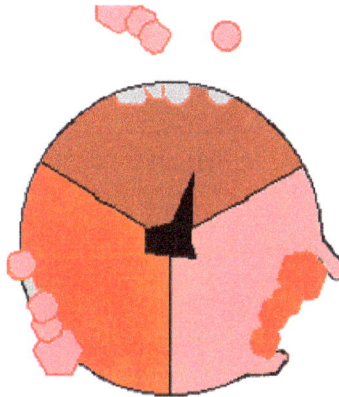

Mechanism of ATP synthase. ATP is shown in red, ADP and phosphate in pink and the rotating γ subunit in black.

This ATP synthesis reaction is called the *binding change mechanism* and involves the active site of a β subunit cycling between three states. In the "open" state, ADP and phosphate enter the active site (shown in brown in the diagram). The protein then closes up around the molecules and binds them loosely – the "loose" state (shown in red). The enzyme then changes shape again and forces these molecules together, with the active site in the resulting "tight" state (shown in pink) binding the newly produced ATP molecule with very high affinity. Finally, the active site cycles back to the open state, releasing ATP and binding more ADP and phosphate, ready for the next cycle.

In some bacteria and archaea, ATP synthesis is driven by the movement of sodium ions through the cell membrane, rather than the movement of protons. Archaea such as *Methanococcus* also contain the A_1A_O synthase, a form of the enzyme that contains additional proteins with little similarity in sequence to other bacterial and eukaryotic ATP synthase subunits. It is possible that, in some species, the A_1A_O form of the enzyme is a specialized sodium-driven ATP synthase, but this might not be true in all cases.

Reactive Oxygen Species

Molecular oxygen is an ideal terminal electron acceptor because it is a strong oxidizing agent. The reduction of oxygen does involve potentially harmful intermediates. Although the transfer of four electrons and four protons reduces oxygen to water, which is harmless, transfer of one or two electrons produces superoxide or peroxide anions, which are dangerously reactive.

These reactive oxygen species and their reaction products, such as the hydroxyl radical, are very harmful to cells, as they oxidize proteins and cause mutations in DNA. This cellular damage might contribute to disease and is proposed as one cause of aging.

The cytochrome c oxidase complex is highly efficient at reducing oxygen to water, and it releases very few partly reduced intermediates; however small amounts of superoxide anion and peroxide are produced by the electron transport chain. Particularly important is the reduction of coenzyme Q in complex III, as a highly reactive ubisemiquinone free radical is formed as an intermediate in the Q cycle. This unstable species can lead to electron "leakage" when electrons transfer directly to oxygen, forming superoxide. As the production of reactive oxygen species by these proton-pumping complexes is greatest at high membrane potentials, it has been proposed that mitochondria regulate their activity to maintain the membrane potential within a narrow range that balances ATP production against oxidant generation. For instance, oxidants can activate uncoupling proteins that reduce membrane potential.

To counteract these reactive oxygen species, cells contain numerous antioxidant systems, including antioxidant vitamins such as vitamin C and vitamin E, and antioxidant enzymes such as superoxide dismutase, catalase, and peroxidases, which detoxify the reactive species, limiting damage to the cell.

Inhibitors

There are several well-known drugs and toxins that inhibit oxidative phosphorylation. Although any one of these toxins inhibits only one enzyme in the electron transport chain, inhibition of any step in this process will halt the rest of the process. For example, if oligomycin inhibits ATP synthase, protons cannot pass back into the mitochondrion. As a result, the proton pumps are unable to operate, as the gradient becomes too strong for them to overcome. NADH is then no longer oxidized and the citric acid cycle ceases to operate because the concentration of NAD$^+$ falls below the concentration that these enzymes can use.

Compounds	Use	Site of action	Effect on oxidative phosphorylation
Cyanide Carbon monoxide Azide Hydrogen sulfide	Poisons	Complex IV	Inhibit the electron transport chain by binding more strongly than oxygen to the Fe–Cu center in cytochrome c oxidase, preventing the reduction of oxygen.
Oligomycin	Antibiotic	Complex V	Inhibits ATP synthase by blocking the flow of protons through the F_o subunit.
CCCP 2,4-Dinitrophenol	Poisons, weight-loss[N 1]	Inner membrane	Ionophores that disrupt the proton gradient by carrying protons across a membrane. This ionophore uncouples proton pumping from ATP synthesis because it carries protons across the inner mitochondrial membrane.
Rotenone	Pesticide	Complex I	Prevents the transfer of electrons from complex I to ubiquinone by blocking the ubiquinone-binding site.
Malonate and oxaloacetate	Poisons	Complex II	Competitive inhibitors of succinate dehydrogenase (complex II).
Antimycin A	Piscicide	Complex III	Binds to the Qi site of cytochrome c reductase, thereby inhibiting the oxidation of ubiquinol.

Not all inhibitors of oxidative phosphorylation are toxins. In brown adipose tissue, regulated proton channels called uncoupling proteins can uncouple respiration from ATP synthesis. This rapid respiration produces heat, and is particularly important as a way of maintaining body temperature for hibernating animals, although these proteins may also have a more general function in cells' responses to stress.

History

The field of oxidative phosphorylation began with the report in 1906 by Arthur Harden of a vital role for phosphate in cellular fermentation, but initially only sugar phosphates were known to be involved. However, in the early 1940s, the link between the oxidation of sugars and the generation of ATP was firmly established by Herman Kalckar, confirming the central role of ATP in energy transfer that had been proposed by Fritz Albert Lipmann in 1941. Later, in 1949, Morris Friedkin and Albert L. Lehninger proved that the coenzyme NADH linked metabolic pathways such as the citric acid cycle and the synthesis of ATP. The term *oxidative phosphorylation* was coined by Volodymyr Belitser (uk) in 1939.

For another twenty years, the mechanism by which ATP is generated remained mysterious, with scientists searching for an elusive "high-energy intermediate" that would link oxidation and phosphorylation reactions. This puzzle was solved by Peter D. Mitchell with the publication of the chemiosmotic theory in 1961. At first, this proposal was highly controversial, but it was slowly accepted and Mitchell was awarded a Nobel prize in 1978. Subsequent research concentrated on purifying and characterizing the enzymes involved, with major contributions being made by David E. Green on the complexes of the electron-transport chain, as well as Efraim Racker on the ATP synthase. A critical step towards solving the mechanism of the ATP synthase was provided by Paul D. Boyer, by his development in 1973 of the "binding change" mechanism, followed by his radical proposal of rotational catalysis in 1982. More recent work has included structural studies on the enzymes involved in oxidative phosphorylation by John E. Walker, with Walker and Boyer being awarded a Nobel Prize in 1997.

References

- Cox, David L. Nelson, Michael M. (2008). Lehninger principles of biochemistry (5th ed.). New York: W.H. Freeman. p. 26. ISBN 978-0-7167-7108-1.

- Pratt, Donald Voet, Judith G. Voet, Charlotte W. (2013). Fundamentals of biochemistry : life at the molecular level (4th ed.). Hoboken, NJ: Wiley. pp. 441–442. ISBN 978-0470-54784-7.

- Reece, Jane B. (2011). Campbell biology / Jane B. Reece ... [et al.]. (9th ed.). Boston: Benjamin Cummings. p. 143. ISBN 978-0-321-55823-7.

- Berg, Jeremy M.; Tymoczko, John L.; Stryer, Lubert; Gatto, Gregory J. (2012). Biochemistry (7th ed.). New York: W.H. Freeman. p. 429. ISBN 1429229365.

- Clarke, Jeremy M. Berg; John L. Tymoczko; Lubert Stryer. Web content by Neil D. (2002). Biochemistry (5. ed., 4. print. ed.). New York, NY [u.a.]: W. H. Freeman. pp. 578–579. ISBN 0716730510.

- Eichhorn, Peter H. Raven ; Ray F. Evert ; Susan E. (2011). Biology of plants (8. ed.). New York, NY: Freeman. pp. 100–106. ISBN 978-1-4292-1961-7.

- Cox, David L. Nelson, Michael M. (2008). Lehninger principles of biochemistry (5th ed.). New York: W.H. Freeman. pp. 25–27. ISBN 978-0-7167-7108-1.

- Choffnes, Eileen R.; Relman,, David A.; Academies, Leslie Pray, rapporteurs, Forum on Microbial Threat, Board on Global Health, Institute of Medicine of the National (2011). The science and applications of synthetic and systems biology workshop summary. Washington, D.C.: National Academies Press. p. 135. ISBN 978-0-309-21939-6.

- White, David (1995). The physiology and biochemistry of prokaryotes. New York [u.a.]: Oxford Univ. Press. p. 133. ISBN 0-19-508439-X.

- Weckwerth, edited by Wolfram (2006). Metabolomics methods and protocols. Totowa, N.J.: Humana Press. p. 177. ISBN 1597452440.

- Kohlmeier M (2015). "Leucine". Nutrient Metabolism: Structures, Functions, and Genes (2nd ed.). Academic Press. pp. 385–388. ISBN 9780123877840. Retrieved 6 June 2016. Figure 8.57: Metabolism of L-LEUCINE

- Stryer, Lubert (1995). "Fatty acid metabolism.". In: Biochemistry. (Fourth ed.). New York: W.H. Freeman and Company. pp. 603–628. ISBN 0 7167 2009 4.

- Nelson, Randy F. (2005). An introduction to behavioral endocrinology (3rd ed.). Sunderland, Mass: Sinauer Associates. p. 100. ISBN 0-87893-617-3.

- Smith, Sareen S. Gropper, Jack L.; Smith, Jack S (2013). Advanced nutrition and human metabolism (6th ed.). Belmont, CA: Wadsworth/Cengage Learning. ISBN 1133104053.

- Williams, Peter L.; Warwick, Roger; Dyson, Mary; Bannister, Lawrence H. (1989). "Angiology.". In: Gray's Anatomy (Thirty-seventh ed.). Edinburgh: Churcill Livingstone. pp. 841–843. ISBN 0443 041776.

- Voet, Donald; Judith G. Voet; Charlotte W. Pratt (2006). Fundamentals of Biochemistry, 2nd Edition. John Wiley and Sons, Inc. pp. 547, 556. ISBN 0-471-21495-7.

Nutritional Deficiencies

This chapter serves as a source to understand nutritional deficiencies. Nutritional deficiencies are the result of your body not getting enough of the nutrients it needs. The major categories of nutritional deficiencies are discussed in this chapter; those include mineral deficiency, vitamin deficiency, protein-energy malnutrition, kwashiorkor and marasmus. Malnutrition has serious implications like marasmus and kwashiorkor; this chapter helps in the understanding of these deficiencies and is of great importance to broaden the existing knowledge of nutritional deficiencies.

Mineral Deficiency

Mineral deficiency is a lack of dietary minerals, the micronutrients that are needed for an organism's proper health. The cause may be a poor diet, impaired uptake of the minerals that are consumed or a dysfunction in the organism's use of the mineral after it is absorbed. These deficiencies can result in many disorders including anemia and goitre. Examples of mineral deficiency include, zinc deficiency, iron deficiency, and magnesium deficiency.

Vitamin Deficiency

A vitamin deficiency can cause a disease or syndrome known as an avitaminosis or hypovitaminosis. This usually refers to a long-term deficiency of a vitamin. When caused by inadequate nutrition it can be classed as a *primary deficiency*, and when due to an underlying disorder such as malabsorption it can be classed as a *secondary deficiency*. An underlying disorder may be metabolic as in a defect converting tryptophan to niacin. It can also be the result of lifestyle choices including smoking and alcohol consumption.

Examples are vitamin A deficiency, folate deficiency, (scurvy), vitamin D deficiency, vitamin E deficiency, and vitamin K deficiency. In the medical literature, any of these may also be called by names on the pattern of *hypovitaminosis* or *avitaminosis + [letter of vitamin]*, for example, hypovitaminosis A, hypovitaminosis C, hypovitaminosis D.

Conversely hypervitaminosis is the syndrome of symptoms caused by over-retention of fat-soluble vitamins in the body.

Types

- Vitamin A is important in growth and development, in the immune system and in eyesight. Its deficiency can cause problems in these areas, particularly in vision, notably night blindness and xerophthalmia.

- Thiamine (vitamin B1) deficiency can cause beriberi and Wernicke–Korsakoff syndrome.

- Riboflavin deficiency (vitamin B2) causes ariboflavinosis.

- Niacin (vitamin B3) deficiency causes pellagra.

- Pantothenic acid (vitamin B5) deficiency causes chronic paresthesia.

- Biotin (vitamin B7) deficiency negatively affects fertility and hair/skin growth. Deficiency can be caused by poor diet or genetic factors (such as mutations in the BTD gene.

- Folate (vitamin B9) deficiency is associated with numerous health problems. Fortification of certain foods with folate has drastically reduced the incidence of neural tube defects in countries where such fortification takes place. Deficiency can result from poor diet or genetic factors (such as mutations in the MTHFR gene that lead to compromised folate metabolism).

- Vitamin B12 (cobalamin) deficiency can lead to pernicious anemia, megaloblastic anemia, subacute combined degeneration of spinal cord,and methylmalonic acidemia among other conditions.

- Vitamin C (ascorbic acid) short-term deficiency can lead to weakness, weight loss and general aches and pains. Longer-term depletion may affect the connective tissue. Persistent vitamin C deficiency leads to scurvy.

- Vitamin D (cholecalciferol) deficiency is a known cause of rickets, and has been linked to numerous health problems.

- Vitamin E deficiency causes nerve problems due to poor conduction of electrical impulses along nerves due to changes in nerve membrane structure and function.

- Vitamin K (phylloquinone or menaquinone) deficiency causes impaired coagulation and has also been implicated in osteoporosis.

Protein–Energy Malnutrition

Protein–energy malnutrition (PEM) or protein–calorie malnutrition refers to a form of malnutrition where there is inadequate calorie or protein intake.

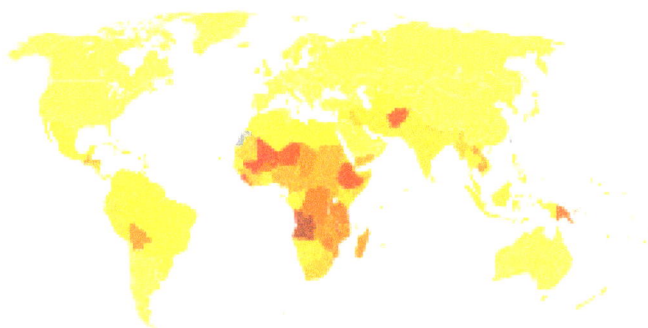

Disability-adjusted life year for protein–energy malnutrition per 100,000 inhabitants in 2004.

no data

less than 10

10–100

100–200

200–300

300–400

400–500

500–600

600–700

700–800

800–1000

1000–1350

more than 1350

Types include:

- Kwashiorkor (protein malnutrition predominant)

- Marasmus (deficiency in calorie intake)

- Marasmic Kwashiorkor (marked protein deficiency and marked calorie insufficiency signs present, sometimes referred to as the most severe form of malnutrition)

PEM is fairly common worldwide in both children and adults and accounts for 6 million deaths annually. In the industrialized world, PEM is predominantly seen in hospitals, is associated with disease, or is often found in the elderly.

Note that PEM may be secondary to other conditions such as chronic renal disease or cancer cachexia in which protein energy wasting may occur.

Protein–energy malnutrition affects children the most because they have less protein intake. The few rare cases found in the developed world are almost entirely found in small children as a result of fad diets, or ignorance of the nutritional needs of children, particularly in cases of milk allergy.

Prenatal Protein Malnutrition

Protein malnutrition is detrimental at any point in life, but protein malnutrition prenatally has been shown to have significant lifelong effects. During pregnancy, one should aim for a diet that consists of at least 20% protein for the health of the fetus. Diets that consist of less than 6% protein *in utero* have been linked with many deficits, including decreased brain weight, increased obesity, and impaired communication within the brain in some animals. Even diets of mild protein malnutrition (7.2%) have been shown to have lasting and significant effects in rats. The following are some studies in which prenatal protein deficiency has been shown to have unfavorable consequences.

- Decreased brain size: Protein deficiency has been shown to affect the size and composition of brains in rhesus monkeys. Monkeys whose mother had eaten a diet with an adequate amount of protein were shown to have no deficit in brain size or composition, even when their body weight amounted to less than one-half of that of the controls, whereas monkeys whose mothers had eaten low-protein diets were shown to have smaller brains regardless of the diet given after birth.

- Impaired neocortical long-term potentiation: Mild protein deficiency (in which 7.2% of the diet consists of protein) in rats has been shown to impair entorhinal cortex plasticity (visuospatial memory), noradrenergic function in the neocortex, and neocortical long-term potentiation.

- Altered fat distribution: Protein undernutrition can have varying effects depending on the period of fetal life during which the malnutrition occurred. Although there were not significant differences in the food intake, there were increased amounts of perirenal fat in rats that were protein-deprived during early (gestation days 0–7) and mid (gestation days 8–14) pregnancy, and throughout pregnancy, whereas rats that were protein-deprived only late in gestation (gestation days 15–22) were shown to have increased gonadal fat.

- Increased obesity: Mice exposed to a low-protein diet prenatally weighed 40% less than the control group at birth (intrauterine growth retardation). When fed a high-fat diet after birth, the prenatally undernourished mice were shown to have increased body weight and adiposity (body fat), while those who were adequately nourished prenatally did not show an increase in body weight or adiposity when fed the same high-fat diet after birth.

- Decreased birth weight, and gestation duration: Supplementation of protein and energy can lead to increased duration of gestation and higher birth weight. When fed a supplement containing protein, energy, and micronutrients, pregnant women showed more successful results during birth, including high birth weights, longer gestations, and fewer preterm births, than women who had consumed a supplement with micronutrients and low energy but no protein (although this finding may be due to the increase of energy in the supplements, not the increase of protein).

- Increased stress sensitivity: Male offspring of pregnant rats fed low-protein diets have been shown to exhibit blood pressure that is hyperresponsive to stress and salt.

- Decreased sperm quality: A low-protein diet during gestation in rats has been shown to affect the sperm quality of the male offspring in adulthood. The protein deficiency appeared to reduce sertoli cell number, sperm motility, and sperm count.

- Altered cardiac energy metabolism: Prenatal nutrition, specifically protein nutrition, may affect the regulation of cardiac energy metabolism through changes in specific genes.

- Increased passive stiffness: Intrauterine undernutrition was shown to increase passive stiffness in skeletal muscles in rats.

From these studies it is possible to conclude that prenatal protein nutrition is vital to the development of the fetus, especially the brain, the susceptibility to diseases in adulthood, and even gene expression. When pregnant females of various species were given low-protein diets, the offspring were shown to have many deficits. These findings highlight the great significance of adequate protein in the prenatal diet.

Epidemiology

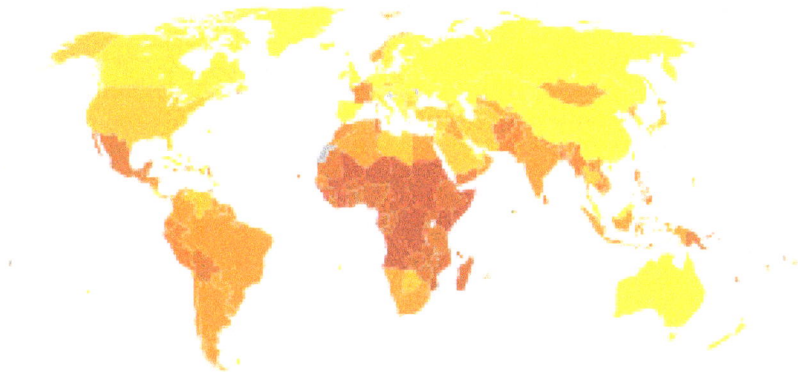

Deaths from protein-energy malnutrition per million persons in 2012

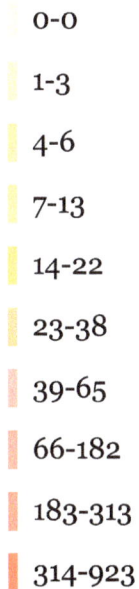

0-0

1-3

4-6

7-13

14-22

23-38

39-65

66-182

183-313

314-923

Although protein energy malnutrition is more common in low-income countries, children from higher-income countries are also affected, including children from large urban areas in low socio-economic neighborhoods. This may also occur in children with chronic diseases, and children who are institutionalized or hospitalized for a different diagnosis. Risk factors include a primary diagnosis of intellectual disability, cystic fibrosis, malignancy, cardiovascular disease, end stage renal disease, oncologic disease, genetic disease, neurological disease, multiple diagnoses, or prolonged hospitalization. In these conditions, the challenging nutritional management may get overlooked and underestimated, resulting in an impairment of the chances for recovery and the worsening of the situation.

PEM is fairly common worldwide in both children and adults and accounts for 6 million deaths annually. In the industrialized world, PEM is predominantly seen in hospitals, is associated with disease, or is often found in the elderly.

Co-morbidity

A large percentage of children that suffer from PEM also have other co-morbid conditions. The most common co-morbidities are diarrhea (72.2% of a sample of 66 subjects) and malaria (43.3%). However, a variety of other conditions have been observed with PEM, including sepsis, severe anaemia, bronchopneumonia, HIV, tuberculosis, scabies, chronic suppurative otitis media, rickets, and keratomalacia. These co-morbidities tax already malnourished children and may prolong hospital stays initially for PEM and may increase the likelihood of death.

Kashin–Beck Disease

Kashin–Beck disease (KBD) is a chronic, endemic osteochondropathy (disease of the bone), which is mainly distributed from northeastern to southwestern China involving 15 provinces. Tibet currently has the highest incidence rate of KBD in China. Southeast Siberia and North Korea are other affected areas KBD usually involves children ages 5–15 and to date more than a million individuals have suffered from KBD. The symptoms of KBD include joint pain, morning stiffness in the joints, disturbances of flexion and extension in the elbows, enlarged inter-phalangeal joints and limited motion in many joints of the body. Death of cartilage cells in the growth plate and articular surface is the basic pathologic feature; this can result in growth retardation and secondary osteoarthrosis. Histological diagnosis of KBD is particularly difficult; clinical and radiological examinations have proved to be the best means for identifying KBD. Little is known about the early stages of KBD before the visible appearance of the disease becomes evident in the destruction of the joints.

This disease has been recognized for over 150 years but its etiology has not yet been completely defined. Currently the accepted potential causes of KBD include mycotoxins present in grain, trace mineral deficiency in nutrition and high levels of fulvic acid in drinking water. Selenium and iodine have been considered the most important deficiencies associated with KBD. Mycotoxins produced by fungi can contaminate grain which may cause KBD because mycotoxins cause the production of free radicals. T-2 is the mycotoxin implicated with KBD, produced by members of several fungal genera. T-2 toxin can cause lesions in hematopoietic, lymphoid, gastrointestinal, and cartilage tissues, especially in physeal cartilage. Fulvic acid present in drinking water damages cartilage cells. Selenium supplementation in selenium deficient areas has been shown to prevent this disease. However, selenium supplementation in some areas showed no significant effect, proving that deficiency of selenium may not be the dominant cause in KBD. Recently a significant association between SNP rs6910140 of COL9A1 and Kashin–Beck disease was discovered genetically, suggesting a role of COL9A1 in the development of Kashin–Beck disease.

Distribution

Kashin–Beck disease occurrence is limited to 13 provinces and two autonomous regions of China. It has also been reported in Siberia and North Korea, but incidence in these regions is reported to have decreased with socio-economic development. In China, KBD is estimated to affect some 2 million to 3 million people across China, and 30 million are living in endemic areas. Life expectancy in KBD regions has been reported to be significantly decreased in relation to selenium deficiency and Keshan disease (endemic juvenile dilative cardiomyopathia).

The prevalence of KBD in Tibet varies strongly according to valleys and villages.

Prevalence of clinical symptoms suggestive of KBD reaches 100% in 5- to 15-year-old children in at least one village. Prevalence rates of over 50% are not uncommon. A clinical prevalence survey carried out in Lhasa prefecture yielded a figure of 11.4% for a study population of approximately 50,000 inhabitants. As in other regions of China, farmers are by far the most affected population group.

Etiology and Risk Factors

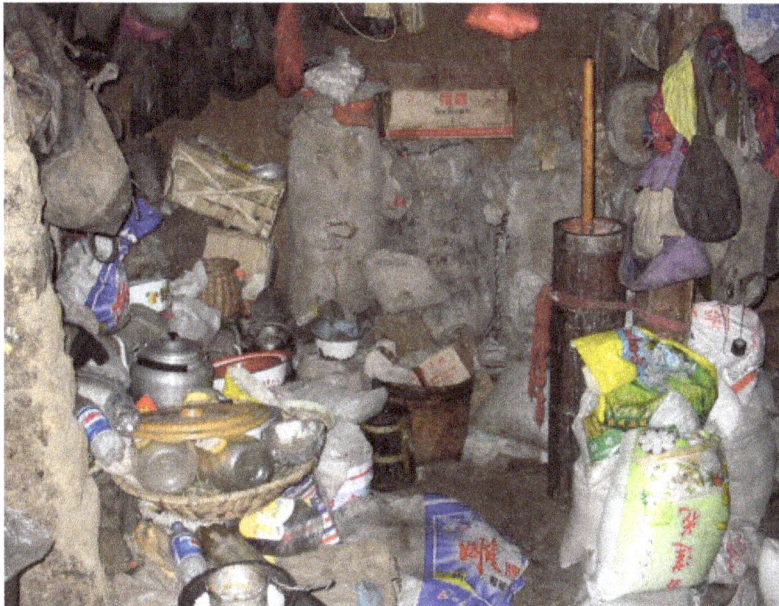

A dirty storage room

The etiology of KBD remains controversial. Studies of the pathogenesis and risk factors of KBD have proposed selenium deficiency, inorganic (manganese, phosphate...) and organic matter (humic and fulvic acids) in drinking water, fungi on self-produced storage grain (Alternaria sp., Fusarium sp.), producing trichotecene (T2) mycotoxins.

Nowadays, most authors accept that the aetiology of KBD is multifactorial, selenium deficiency being the underlying factor that predisposes the target cells (chondrocytes) to oxidative stress from free-radical carriers such as mycotoxins in storage grain and fulvic acid in drinking water.

In Tibet, epidemiological studies carried out in 1995–1996 by MSF and coll. showed that KBD was associated with iodine deficiency and with fungal contamination of barley grains by Alternaria sp., Trichotecium sp., Cladosporium sp. and Drechslera sp. Indications existed as well with respect to the role of organic matters in drinking water.

A severe selenium deficiency was documented as well, but selenium status was not associated with the disease, suggesting that selenium deficiency alone could not explain the occurrence of KBD in the villages under study.

An association with the gene Peroxisome Proliferator-Activated Receptor Gamma Coactivator 1 Beta (PPARGC1B) has been reported. This gene is a transcription factor and mutations in this gene would be expected to affect several other genes.

Treatment

Treatment of KBD is palliative. Surgical corrections have been made with success by Chinese and Russian orthopedists. By the end of 1992, Médecins Sans Frontières—Belgium started a physical therapy programme aiming at alleviating the symptoms of KBD patients with advanced joint impairment and pain (mainly adults), in Nyemo county, Lhasa prefecture. Physical therapy had significant effects on joint mobility and joint pain in KBD patients. Later on (1994–1996), the programme has been extended to several other counties and prefectures in Tibet.

Prevention

Prevention of Kashin–Beck Disease has a long history. Intervention strategies were mostly based on one of the three major etiologic theories.

Selenium supplementation, with or without additional antioxidant therapy (Vitamin E and Vitamin C) has been reported to be successful, but in other studies no significant decrease could be shown compared to a control group. Major drawbacks of selenium supplementation are logistic difficulties (daily or weekly intake, drug supply), potential toxicity (in case of less controlled supplementation strategies), associated iodine deficiency (that should be corrected before selenium supplementation to prevent further deterioration of thyroid status) and low compliance. The latter was certainly the case in Tibet, where a selenium supplementation has been implemented from 1987 to 1994 in areas of high endemicity.

With the mycotoxin theory in mind, backing of grains before storage was proposed in Guanxi province, but results are not reported in international literature. Changing from grain source has been reported to be effective in Heilongjiang province and North Korea.

With respect to the role of drinking water, changing of water sources to deep well water has been reported to decrease the X-ray metaphyseal detection rate in different settings.

In general, the effect of preventive measures however remains controversial, due to methodological problems (no randomised controlled trials), lack of documentation or, as discussed above, due to inconsistency of results.

Eponymy

The condition as named after Russian military physicians Evgeny Vladimirovich Bek (1865–1915) and Nicolai Ivanowich Kashin (1825–1872).

Kwashiorkor

Kwashiorkor is a form of severe protein–energy malnutrition characterized by edema, irritability, ulcerating dermatoses, and an enlarged liver with fatty infiltrates. Sufficient calorie intake, but with insufficient protein consumption, distinguishes it from marasmus. Kwashiorkor cases occur in areas of famine or poor food supply. Cases in the developed world are rare.

Jamaican pediatrician Cicely Williams introduced the name into the medical community in a 1935 *Lancet* article, two years after she published the disease's first formal description in the Western medical literature. The name is derived from the Ga language of coastal Ghana, translated as "the sickness the baby gets when the new baby comes" or "the disease of the deposed child", and reflecting the development of the condition in an older child who has been weaned from the breast when a younger sibling comes. Breast milk contains proteins and amino acids vital to a child's growth. In at-risk populations, kwashiorkor may develop after a mother weans her child from breast milk, replacing it with a diet high in carbohydrates, especially sugar.

Signs and Symptoms

The defining sign of kwashiorkor in a malnourished child is pitting edema (swelling of the ankles and feet). Other signs include a distended abdomen, an enlarged liver with fatty infiltrates, thinning hair, loss of teeth, skin depigmentation and dermatitis. Children with kwashiorkor often develop irritability and anorexia. Generally, the disease can be treated by adding protein to the diet; however, it can have a long-term impact on a child's physical and mental development, and in severe cases may lead to death.

In dry climates, marasmus is the more frequent disease associated with malnutrition. Another malnutrition syndrome includes cachexia, although it is often caused by underlying illnesses. These are important considerations in the treatment of the patients.

Causes

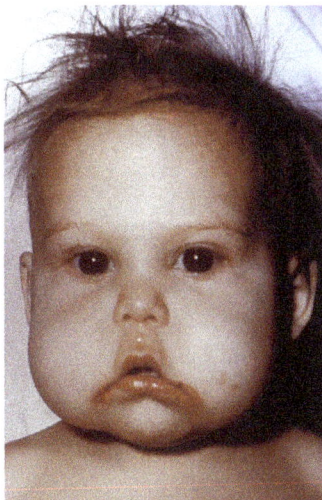

Child in the United States with symptoms of Kwashiorkor.

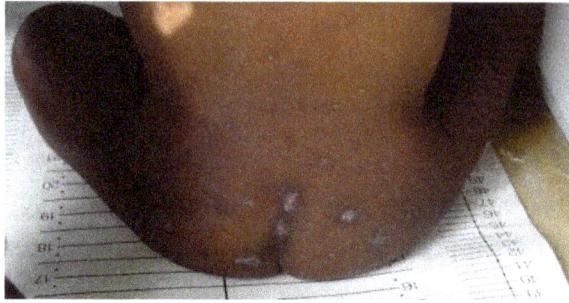

Typical ulcerating dermatosis seen on a Malawian child with kwashiorkor

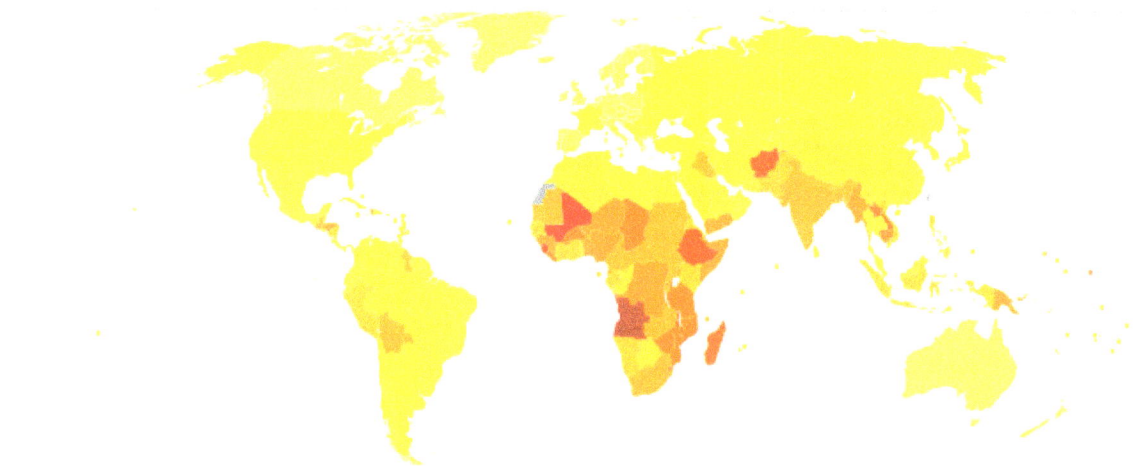

Disability-adjusted life year for protein–energy malnutrition per 100,000 inhabitants in 2002.

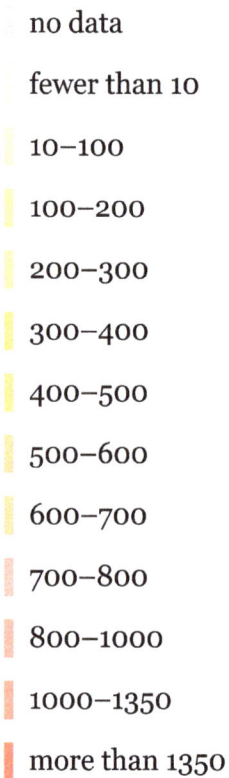

no data

fewer than 10

10–100

100–200

200–300

300–400

400–500

500–600

600–700

700–800

800–1000

1000–1350

more than 1350

Kwashiorkor is a severe form of malnutrition, caused by a deficiency in dietary protein. The extreme lack of protein causes an osmotic imbalance in the gastro-intestinal system causing swelling of the gut diagnosed as an edema or retention of water.

Extreme fluid retention observed in individuals suffering from kwashiorkor is a direct result of irregularities in the lymphatic system and an indication of capillary exchange. The lymphatic system serves three major purposes: fluid recovery, immunity, and lipid absorption. Victims of kwashiorkor commonly exhibit reduced ability to recover fluids, immune system failure, and low lipid absorption, all of which result from a state of severe undernourishment. Fluid recovery in the lymphatic system is accomplished by re-absorption of water and proteins which are then returned to the blood. Compromised fluid recovery results in the characteristic belly distension observed in highly malnourished children.

Capillary exchange between the lymphatic system and the bloodstream is stunted due to the inability of the body to effectively overcome the hydrostatic pressure gradient. Proteins, mainly albumin, are responsible for creating the colloid osmotic pressure (COP) observed in the blood and tissue fluids. The difference in the COP of the blood and tissue is called the oncotic pressure. The oncotic pressure is in direct opposition with the hydrostatic pressure and tends to draw water back into the capillary by osmosis. However, due to the lack of proteins, no substantial pressure gradient can be established to draw fluids from the tissue back into the blood stream. This results in the pooling of fluids, causing the swelling and distention of the abdomen.

The low protein intake leads to some specific signs: edema of the hands and feet, irritability, anorexia, a desquamative rash, hair discolouration, and a large fatty liver. The typical swollen abdomen is due to two causes: ascites because of hypoalbuminemia (low oncotic pressure), and enlarged fatty liver.

Ignorance of nutrition can be a cause. Latham, director of the Program in International Nutrition at Cornell University, along with Keith Rosenberg cited a case where parents who fed their child cassava failed to recognize malnutrition because of the edema caused by the syndrome and insisted the child was well-nourished despite the lack of dietary protein.

Protein should be supplied only for anabolic purposes. The catabolic needs should be satisfied with carbohydrate and fat. Protein catabolism involves the urea cycle, which is located in the liver and can easily overwhelm the capacity of an already damaged organ. The resulting liver failure can be fatal. This means in patients suffering from kwashiorkor, protein must be introduced back into the diet gradually. Clinical solutions include weaning the affected with milk products and increasing the intake of proteinaceous material to daily recommended amounts.

Marasmus

Marasmus is a form of severe malnutrition characterized by energy deficiency. A child with marasmus looks emaciated. Body weight is reduced to less than 60% of the normal (expected) body weight for the age. Marasmus occurrence increases prior to age 1, whereas kwashiorkor occurrence increases after 18 months. It can be distinguished from kwashiorkor in that kwashiorkor is protein deficiency with adequate energy intake whereas marasmus is inadequate energy intake in all forms, including protein. Protein wasting in kwashiorkor may lead to edema.

The prognosis is better than it is for kwashiorkor but half of severely malnourished children die due to unavailability of adequate treatment.

Signs and Symptoms

Marasmus is commonly represented by a shrunken, wasted appearance, loss of muscle mass and subcutaneous fat mass. Buttocks and upper limb muscle groups are usually more affected than others. Marasmus is not always linked to severe edema. Other symptoms of marasmus include unusual body temperature (hypothermia, pyrexia), anemia, edema, dehydration (as characterized with consistent thirst and shrunken eyes), hypovolemic shock (weak radial pulse, cold extremities, decreased consciousness), tachypnea (pneumonia, heart failure), abdominal manifestations (distension, decreased or metallic bowel sounds, large or small liver, blood or mucus in the stools), ocular manifestations (corneal lesions associated with vitamin A deficiency), dermal manifestations (evidence of infection, purpura, and ear, nose, and throat symptoms (otitis, rhinitis).

Causes

Marasmus is caused by a severe deficiency of nearly all nutrients, especially protein, carbohydrates, and lipids.

Treatment

It is necessary to treat not only the causes but also the complications of the disorder, including infections, dehydration, and circulation disorders, which are frequently lethal and lead to high mortality if ignored.

Ultimately, marasmus can progress to the point of no return when the body's ability for protein synthesis is lost. At this point, attempts to correct the disorder by giving food or protein are futile. Vitamin D will help to alleviate this problem.

Epidemiology

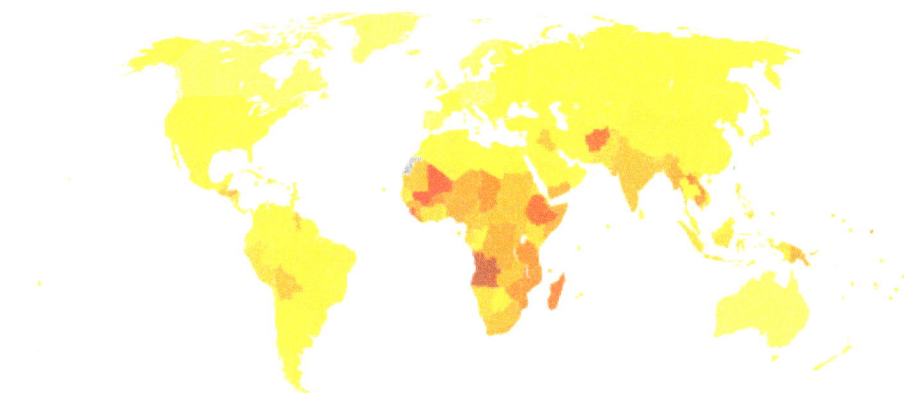

Disability-adjusted life year for protein-energy malnutrition per 100,000 inhabitants in 2002.

no data

less than 10

10–100

100–200

200–300

300–400

400–500

500–600

600–700

700–800

800–1000

1000–1350

more than 1350

References

- Saladin, Kenneth (2012). Anatomy and Physiology (6th ed.). New York: McGraw Hill. pp. 766–767, 809–811. ISBN 978-0-07-337825-1.

- Wen Y, Hao J, Xiao X, Wang W, Guo X, Lin W, Yang T, Liu X, Shen H, Tan L, Chen X, Tian Q, Deng HW, Zhang F (2016) PARGC1B gene is associated with Kashin-Beck disease in Han Chinese. Funct Integr Genomics

- Ubesie, Agozie C.; Ibeziako, Ngozi S.; Ndiokwelu, Chika I.; Uzoka, Chinyeaka M.; Nwafor, Chinelo A. (2012-01-01). "Under-five Protein Energy Malnutrition Admitted at the University of In Nigeria Teaching Hospital, Enugu: a 10 year retrospective review". Nutrition Journal. 11: 43. doi:10.1186/1475-2891-11-43. ISSN 1475-2891.

Permissions

All chapters in this book are published with permission under the Creative Commons Attribution Share Alike License or equivalent. Every chapter published in this book has been scrutinized by our experts. Their significance has been extensively debated. The topics covered herein carry significant information for a comprehensive understanding. They may even be implemented as practical applications or may be referred to as a beginning point for further studies.

We would like to thank the editorial team for lending their expertise to make the book truly unique. They have played a crucial role in the development of this book. Without their invaluable contributions this book wouldn't have been possible. They have made vital efforts to compile up to date information on the varied aspects of this subject to make this book a valuable addition to the collection of many professionals and students.

This book was conceptualized with the vision of imparting up-to-date and integrated information in this field. To ensure the same, a matchless editorial board was set up. Every individual on the board went through rigorous rounds of assessment to prove their worth. After which they invested a large part of their time researching and compiling the most relevant data for our readers.

The editorial board has been involved in producing this book since its inception. They have spent rigorous hours researching and exploring the diverse topics which have resulted in the successful publishing of this book. They have passed on their knowledge of decades through this book. To expedite this challenging task, the publisher supported the team at every step. A small team of assistant editors was also appointed to further simplify the editing procedure and attain best results for the readers.

Apart from the editorial board, the designing team has also invested a significant amount of their time in understanding the subject and creating the most relevant covers. They scrutinized every image to scout for the most suitable representation of the subject and create an appropriate cover for the book.

The publishing team has been an ardent support to the editorial, designing and production team. Their endless efforts to recruit the best for this project, has resulted in the accomplishment of this book. They are a veteran in the field of academics and their pool of knowledge is as vast as their experience in printing. Their expertise and guidance has proved useful at every step. Their uncompromising quality standards have made this book an exceptional effort. Their encouragement from time to time has been an inspiration for everyone.

The publisher and the editorial board hope that this book will prove to be a valuable piece of knowledge for students, practitioners and scholars across the globe.

Index

A

Aerobic Respiration, 88, 187, 220-222

Agricultural Productivity, 41, 151, 153

Amino Acid Synthesis, 69, 210, 212

Amino Acids, 7-8, 10-11, 13-14, 17, 25, 27-28, 30-32, 34, 49, 52, 59-60, 63-64, 66-69, 72, 83, 101-102, 108, 115, 118 119, 121-125, 148, 175, 189-190, 196, 210-211, 213-215, 218, 230, 235, 247

Amphibolic Pathway, 185, 188

Anabolic Pathway (anabolism), 187

Anammox, 94

Animal Nutrition, 17

Antinutrient, 25

Asparagine, 121-122, 211, 213-214

Aspartate, 69, 207, 210-211, 213-215

Atp Synthase (complex V), 234

B

Basal Metabolic Rate, 5, 58, 96, 99-100, 103-104

Beta Oxidation, 64, 191, 194, 196, 204, 207, 226-227, 230

Bodybuilding Supplements, 118-119

Breakdown Into Nutrients, 83

C

Cancer, 9, 14, 22-24, 30, 32-33, 35-36, 52-53, 108, 111 114, 126, 128-129, 178, 241

Carbohydrate Digestion, 83

Carbohydrates, 5, 8-10, 17, 24, 27-30, 35, 38, 41, 46-48, 50-52, 58-60, 62, 64, 67, 72, 81, 85, 94, 97, 100-102, 107, 112, 132, 146, 158, 186, 190-191, 196, 203-204, 206-207, 247, 250

Carbon Fixation, 65-67, 91

Cardiovascular Implications, 104

Catabolic Pathway (catabolism), 186

Celiac Disease, 171, 178

Cellular Respiration, 8, 58, 187

Child Malnutrition, 36, 157, 162

Cofactors, 62, 88-89, 185, 227, 232

Conjugation Machinery, 76

Cytochrome C Oxidase (complex Iv), 231

D

Diet (nutrition), 106

Dietary Mineral, 117

Dietary Supplement, 115-116, 118

Digestion, 16-17, 29, 58-59, 63, 74-75, 77-85, 100-101, 165, 199-201

E

Eating Disorder, 106-107, 134, 166-183

Electron Donors, 91, 225-226, 233-234

Energy For Reduction, 91

Energy From Light, 65-66, 87

Energy From Organic Compounds, 64

Energy Yield, 196, 209

Environmental Influences, 172

Environmental Nutrition, 18

Essential Amino Acid, 121, 124-125, 210-211

Essential Dietary Minerals, 31

Essential Fatty Acids, 10, 14, 29-30, 32, 108, 118, 202-203

Ethanol Fermentation, 219-221

Excessive, 8, 13, 21-22, 32-33, 54, 56, 107-108, 119, 126, 128, 130, 139, 166-167, 169, 174-175, 179, 190

F

Fat, 5, 7-9, 15, 22, 24-25, 27, 29, 33, 35, 47-49, 67, 81, 83, 85, 97-100, 102-103, 107, 112-116, 125-127, 129, 132, 134, 136-137, 139, 142, 144-145, 148, 152, 166, 174, 176, 182, 184, 191-193, 195-196, 199-202, 208-209, 239, 242, 249-250

Fatty Acid Metabolism, 185, 191, 204, 238

Fermentation, 17, 53, 65, 74, 81, 83, 88, 91, 185, 207, 217 226, 237

Ferrous Iron (fe2+) Oxidation, 93

Fiber, 8-9, 17, 26-27, 30, 35, 47, 112, 115, 126, 162

Folic Acid, 23, 35, 54-56, 155, 164-165

Food Sovereignty, 155

Fortified Foods, 44, 155

G

Gastrovascular Cavity, 77

Genetics, 17, 105, 130, 133-134, 170, 180

Glucose, 5, 8-9, 11, 28, 49, 51-52, 60, 64, 67, 70-71, 83-85, 101, 159, 186, 188-191, 193, 195-197, 201-203, 207, 219, 221-223, 226, 233

Glycans, 67

H

Healthy Diet, 1, 16, 31, 107-109, 111-114

Herbal Medicine, 117

Heterotrophic Microbial Metabolism, 87

Human Nutrition, 1, 26-27, 57, 61, 108, 123, 184

Hydrogen Oxidation, 93

Hypertension, 22, 33-34, 53, 108, 113, 129, 145, 166, 168

Hyponatremia, 22, 24, 33, 36, 168

I

Illnesses Caused By Improper Nutrient Consumption, 22

Inhibitors, 72, 236

Insufficient, 21, 31-33, 37, 41, 47, 98, 107, 130, 133, 146, 172, 190, 247

Intestinal Bacterial Flora, 16

Isoleucine, 121-122, 124, 213, 215, 218

K

Kashin-beck Disease, 244, 246, 251

Ketogenesis, 185, 189-191

Ketone Bodies, 67, 189-191, 195

Kwashiorkor, 2, 22, 33, 125, 146-148, 150, 239, 241, 247 250

L

Lactic Acid Fermentation, 53, 218, 220-223

Lipids, 8, 17, 27, 58-60, 62-63, 66-68, 83, 94, 114, 187, 207, 250

Longevity, 15, 103, 107, 112

Lysine, 121-124, 213-215

M

Macrominerals, 13-14, 22, 32

Macronutrients, 8, 22, 27-28, 38, 52, 100, 102, 113

Malnutrition, 2, 18, 20-21, 27, 32-33, 36-38, 40-43, 45, 47, 106, 125, 136, 145-157, 160-165, 184, 239-243, 247-251

Marasmus, 2, 22, 33, 125, 146, 148, 150, 239, 241, 247, 249-250

Mental Agility, 23, 34

Mental Disorders, 23, 34, 166-167

Metabolic Pathway, 70, 72, 185-186, 189, 225-226, 230

Metabolic Syndrome, 2, 24, 35, 129, 132

Metabolic Syndrome And Obesity, 35

Metabolism, 2, 4-6, 8, 10, 12-14, 16-18, 20, 22, 24, 26, 28, 30, 32, 34, 36, 38, 40, 42, 44, 46, 48, 50, 52, 54, 56-105, 108, 110, 112, 114, 116, 118, 120, 122, 124, 126, 128, 130, 132, 134, 136, 138, 140, 142, 144, 146, 148, 150, 152, 154, 156, 158, 160, 162, 164, 166, 168, 170, 172, 174, 176, 178, 180, 182, 184-238, 240, 242, 244, 246, 248, 250

Methionine, 121-124, 211, 213-216

Microbial Metabolism, 58, 85-87, 90-91

Mineral Deficiency, 239, 244

Minerals, 6, 8, 12-14, 20, 22, 24-25, 27, 31-32, 35, 37-38, 45, 49-52, 62, 75, 78, 81, 107-108, 110, 115-119, 121, 146 148, 157-158, 164, 185, 239

Morbidity, 39, 129, 244

Mortality, 36-37, 39, 42-43, 55, 120-121, 128-130, 139, 142, 161-163, 172, 183, 250

N

Nitrification, 65, 94

Nitrogen Fixation, 18, 95-96, 210

Nucleotides, 59-61, 66, 69, 72, 203, 211, 234

O

Obesity, 2-3, 7, 14, 19, 21-22, 24-26, 33, 35-38, 41, 43, 50, 106, 108, 113-114, 125-146, 148, 152, 166, 169, 173, 176, 181, 183-184, 241-242

Organization Of Complexes, 232

Oxidative Phosphorylation, 65-66, 69, 103, 185, 187, 191, 205, 219, 222, 225-226, 228, 230, 233-234, 236-237

P

Pathophysiology, 136, 176

Peroxisomal Beta-oxidation, 208

Personality Traits, 171, 177

Phagosome, 77

Phytochemicals, 8, 14, 16, 25, 32

Plant Nutrition, 17-18

Pregnancy, 7, 11, 47, 49, 53-57, 129-130, 139, 146, 164 165, 168, 241-242

Processed Foods, 24-26, 110

Prokaryotic Electron Transport Chains, 232

Protein, 5-8, 10-11, 15, 22, 24, 28, 30-31, 33, 35, 46, 48-53, 55, 61-62, 68-71, 74-76, 80-84, 95, 102, 108, 111-113, 118-119, 122-125, 146-150, 157, 160, 162, 164, 176, 186, 191-192, 194, 197-199, 202-203, 210-212, 214-216, 225, 227, 229-232, 234-235, 239-243, 247-251

Protein Digestion, 74-75, 83

Protein-energy Malnutrition, 125, 146-148, 160, 162, 240 241, 243, 247-248, 250

Proteins, 8, 10-11, 13-14, 17, 27, 30-32, 46, 49-50, 52, 57 60, 62-69, 71-73, 76, 78, 83, 85, 94, 97, 100-102, 105, 107, 118, 123-124, 186-187, 194, 198, 202, 210, 225, 227, 229, 234-236, 247, 249

Psychological, 14, 32, 115, 147, 157, 169-170, 172, 176, 178-179

R

Reactive Oxygen Species, 69, 226, 230, 232, 235-236

Redox Metabolism, 69

Ribose 5-phosphates, 215

S
Secretion Systems, 76
Sedentary Lifestyle, 129, 133
Social Determinants, 134
Sports Nutrition, 1, 46, 50, 52, 57
Sulfur Oxidation, 93-94
Survival Paradox, 130
Syntrophy, 90

T
Thermodynamics Of Living Organisms, 70
Threonine, 121-124, 198, 213-215
Trace Minerals, 13, 22, 32

U
Unbalanced, 21
Unsaturated Fatty Acids, 9, 29, 113, 207, 209

V
Vitamin Deficiency, 22, 36, 239
Vitamins, 6-8, 14, 17, 20, 24-27, 32-33, 35, 37-38, 45, 49
50, 52, 54-55, 61, 75, 81, 107-108, 110, 115-119, 121, 125,
146-149, 155, 157-158, 164, 185, 199-200, 236, 239

W
Water, 3-5, 7-9, 11-12, 15, 17-18, 24-25, 27, 29-31, 36, 44
45, 48-51, 56, 62-63, 66-67, 69, 74-75, 80-81, 83, 87, 95,
101, 112, 132, 149, 157-159, 163, 168, 186, 191, 193, 195
196, 199, 203, 208, 219, 226-227, 232-233, 235-236, 244-
246, 249

www.ingramcontent.com/pod-product-compliance
Lightning Source LLC
Chambersburg PA
CBHW061305190326
41458CB00011B/3766

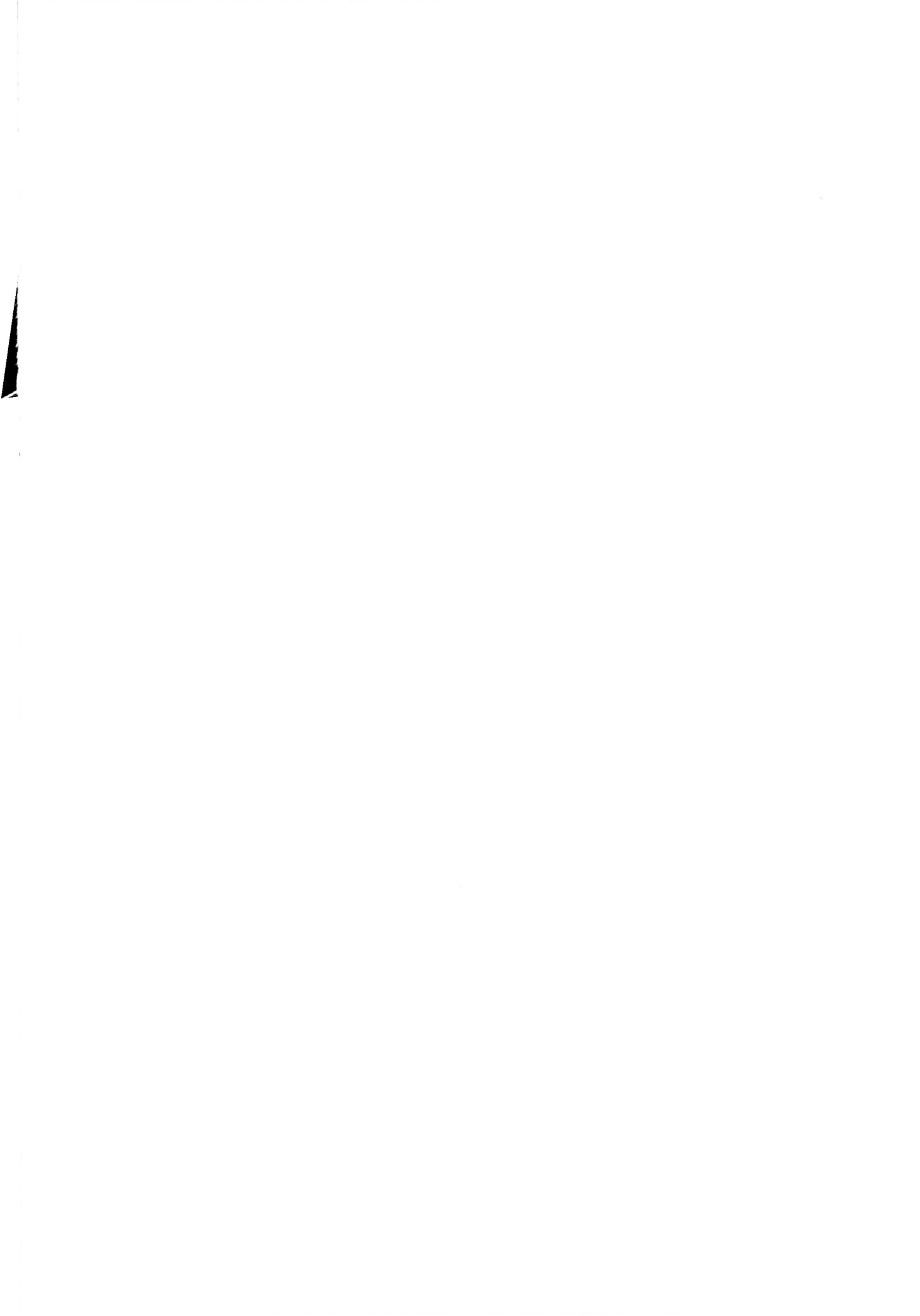